9/10 - 1
9/17 - 2,10
9/24 - 3,4
10/1
10/8 - 20
10/15 - 8,9
10/22 - 21 ?
10/29 -
11/5 - 11,12, App. B
11/12
11/19 - QUIZ
11/26 - 18, 16, 8,
          17, 14-13,
          19

A Clinical Guide to the Treatment of the Human Stress Response

Second Edition

The Plenum Series on Stress and Coping

Series Editor:
Donald Meichenbaum, *University of Waterloo, Waterloo, Ontario, Canada*

A Continuation Order Plan is available for this series. A continuation order will bring
delivery of each new volume immediately upon publication. Volumes are billed only upon
actual shipment. For further information please contact the publisher.

A Clinical Guide to the Treatment of the Human Stress Response
Second Edition

George S. Everly, Jr.
Loyola College in Maryland and
The Johns Hopkins University
Baltimore, Maryland

and

Jeffrey M. Lating
Loyola College in Maryland
Baltimore, Maryland

Kluwer Academic / Plenum Publishers
New York, Boston, Dordrecht, London, Moscow

ISBN: 0-306-46620-1

©2002 Kluwer Academic / Plenum Publishers
233 Spring Street, New York, New York 10013

http://www.wkap.nl/

10 9 8 7 6 5 4 3 2 1

A C.I.P. record for this book is available from the Library of Congress

To Marideth Rose Everly and to George S. Everly, Sr.,
both of whom have taught me some of the most important
lessons in life that I have ever learned

GSE

To Austin and Jenna, I am so grateful for the immense love,
joy, and balance you have brought to my life.

JML

Preface to the Second Edition

Over a decade has passed since the first edition of this critically acclaimed volume was published. Much is new, but much has remained the same. The reader will find that the primary efferent biological mechanisms of the stress response are largely the same as described in 1989. This underscores the brilliance of Selye, Cannon, Mason, Gellhorn, and Levi as they sought to elucidate the anatomical and physiological constituents of human stress. New information has been generated regarding the microanatomy, biochemistry, and genetic aspects of the human stress response. Furthermore, the anatomy and physiology of posttraumatic stress has been more thoroughly elucidated. The important role of cognitive processes in the determination of subsequent stress arousal remains underscored and has been empirically validated by subsequent research (Smith, Everly, & Johns, 1992, 1993). The "rediscovery" of the importance of positive psychology and optimism is consistent with our earlier etiological emphasis upon the cognitive–affective domain in the overall phenomenology of human stress.

But there have been even more dramatic changes in the field of human stress since our first edition was published. Since then, we have discovered that the stress response can affect virtually every cell in the human body, not only by virtue of direct neural, neuroendocrine, and endocrine mechanisms, but also by the more recent realization that psychological processes, through stress response mechanisms, can dramatically affect the human immune system, and as a result, one's vulnerability to autoimmune and communicable diseases. We have included a special chapter on the immune system to update and emphasize this important phenomenon.

Since the first edition was published, interest in posttraumatic stress has dramatically increased. School shootings, mass disasters, "airline rage," "road rage," violence in the workplace, and of course terrorism in the wake of September 11, have emerged as important stress-related issues. To respond to this interest, we have not only revised and expanded our chapter on posttraumatic stress, but we have also included a new chapter on crisis intervention as an empirically validated intervention for the mitigation of dysfunctional and disabling posttraumatic stress reactions.

Numerous clinical innovations have emerged since the first edition was published. Interventions such as Eye Movement Desensitization and Reprocessing (EMDR), Critical Incident Stress Debriefing (CISD), Crisis Management Briefings in response to mass disasters and terrorism, and Critical Incident Stress Management (CISM) have generated interest and programmatic utilization. Therefore, we have included a special section on innovations in clinical practice.

Since the first edition was published, a new interest in spirituality and religion as stress management tools has emerged. Spirituality, religion, and faith appear to exert generally positive effects upon health. In response, we have included a new chapter on these topics.

Dramatically new information has emerged in the area of dietary factors and stress. Dietary sympathomimetics, antioxidants, and cholesterol are all topics addressed in a new chapter on diet and stress.

Since the first edition was published, psychopharmacological intervention in the human stress response has significantly changed. The advent of selective serotonergic reuptake inhibitors (SSRIs) and increased utilization of anticonvulsant medications has expanded the basic pharmacopeia for the treatment of human stress.

Finally, new perspectives and research have emerged relevant to topics in our original edition, necessitating an updated presentation of those topics.

We believe that these additions, along with our efforts to update previously addressed topics, will make this textbook useful to students, practitioners, and faculty in the fields of psychology, psychiatry, medicine, nursing, social work, public health, business administration, and even public safety and emergency services. We hope that these updates will once again make this volume the standard textbook for the understanding and treatment of the human stress response.

GEORGE S. EVERLY, JR.
JEFFREY M. LATING

Acknowledgments

George S. Everly, Jr. wishes to thank the following individuals for their contributions, either direct or indirect, to the creation of this second edition: Theodore Millon, Ph.D., D.Sc., for his continued mentorship, Bertram Brown, M.D., M.P.H., for his support and guidance in international affairs, Jeffrey T. Mitchell, Ph.D., for his friendship and support over the last decade, but most of all, he thanks his family.

Jeffrey M. Lating wishes to thank Wayne Campbell, M.D., for his expertise and early review of the chapter on psychoneuroimmunology, and Stephen Bono, Ph.D. for his guidance, friendship, and support. Thanks also to Amos Zeichner, Ph.D., Don Wilmes, Ph.D., Lee McCabe, Ph.D. and Jennifer Haythornthwaite, Ph.D. for their continued mentorship. He would also like to thank his wife, Kathy Niager, Ph.D., whose patience and tolerance enables him to stay focused on his work.

Finally, both authors would like to thank Melvin Gravitz, Ph.D., Roger Page, Ph.D., Jason Noel, Pharm.D., Judy Curtis, Pharm.D. and Kristy Kelly, B.A. for their scholarly contributions. They are also indebted to Kristy Kelly, Jan Warrington, Psy.D., Thomas Winston Thorpe, Doris Manner, Nina Morrison, Phyllis Grupp, Kristy Burroughs, Mike D'Imperio, and Joanne Newbert for their editorial and production assistance in the development of the text, Dan Vaught and Steve Beck for their artistic contributions, and Eliot Werner, Sharon Panulla, Herman Makler, and Donald Meichenbaum, Ph.D., for their useful suggestions.

Contents

II: THE TREATMENT OF THE HUMAN STRESS RESPONSE

III. SPECIAL TOPICS IN THE TREATMENT OF THE HUMAN STRESS RESPONSE

APPENDIXES: SPECIAL CONSIDERATIONS IN
CLINICAL PRACTICE

I

The Nature of Human Stress

First study the science.
Then practice the art...
LEONARDO DA VINCI

Part I, the first of three parts that constitute this volume, is dedicated to an in-depth analysis of the nature of human stress. The six chapters of Part I explore stress phenomenology.

Chapter 1, entitled "The Concept of Stress," provides the reader with a working definition of the stress response derived from the Selyean tradition. This chapter also reviews other, related terms and concepts that provide a basic conceptual framework from which to study stress.

The purpose of Chapter 2, entitled "The Anatomy and Physiology of the Human Stress Response," is to examine the mechanisms that serve to "link" *stressor stimuli* with subsequent stress-related *target-organ arousal*. A systems model is constructed to assist the reader in understanding phenomenological processes. Also contained in this chapter is a comprehensive analysis of the physiological stress-response mechanisms originally studied by Walter Cannon and Hans Selye, and most recently updated with the latest published and unpublished research findings. A unique diagrammatic summary of the "multiaxial" nature of the physiological stress response is provided as a pedagogical tool.

Chapter 3, entitled "The Link from Stress Arousal to Disease," examines several major models of target-organ pathogenesis; that is, it is designed to explore the mechanisms that link stress arousal to subsequent target-organ disease and dysfunction. Thus, whereas Chapter 2 explored the link from stimulus to stress arousal, Chapter 3 explores the link from stress arousal to disease.

Chapter 4, entitled "Stress-Related Disease: A Review," is the logical extension of Chapters 2 and 3, and, as such, reviews common stress-related disorders that clinicians are likely to encounter during the course of clinical practice. Chapter 5, entitled "Psychoneuroimmunology," explores the burgeoning interest in how stress is related to neural and immune processes.

The final chapter in Part I, Chapter 6, entitled "Measurement of the Human Stress Response," employs the same systems model constructed in Chapter 2, details stress phenomenology, and uses it to superimpose technologies that may be considered for the measurement of human stress. By graphically depicting assessment technologies in relation to the systems model of the stress response, it facilitates greater phenomenological insight into the measurement process itself.

The fact that one-third of this volume, dedicated to the treatment of human stress, is a detailed discussion of phenomenology of the human stress responses bears witness to the wisdom of da Vinci when he proclaimed, "First study the science. Then practice the art which is born of that science."

1

The Concept of Stress

To study medicine without reading is like sailing an uncharted sea.

SIR WILLIAM OSLER, M.D.

STRESS, BEHAVIOR, AND HEALTH

Scientists investigating human health and disease are now reformulating the basic tenets upon which disease theory is based. For generations, the delivery of health care services was built upon the "one-germ, one-disease, one-treatment" formulations that arose from the work of Louis Pasteur. Although clearly one of the great advances in medicine, yielding massive gains against the infectious diseases that plagued humanity, the "germ theory" of disease also represents an intellectual quagmire that threatens to entrap us in a unidimensional quest to improve human health.

The germ theory of disease ignores the fact that by the year 1960, the primary causes of death in the United States were no longer microbial in nature. Rather, other pathogenic factors had emerged. Even three decades ago, it was noted, "New knowledge ... has increased the recognition that the etiology of poor health is multifactorial. The virulence of infection interacts with the particular susceptibility of the host" (American Psychological Association, 1976, p. 264). Thus, in addition to mere exposure to a pathogen, one's overall risk of ill health seems also to be greatly influenced by other factors. Recent evidence points toward health-related behavior patterns and overall lifestyle as important health determinants.

The significance of health-related behavior in the overall determination of health status is cogently discussed by Jonas Salk (1973) in his treatise *The Survival of the Wisest*. Salk argues that we are leaving the era in which the greatest threat to human health was microbial disease, only to

3

enter an era in which the greatest threat to human health resides in
humanity itself. He emphasizes that we must actively confront health-
eroding practices such as pollution, sedentary lifestyles, diets void of nutrients, and practices that disregard the fundamentals of personal and
interpersonal hygiene at the same time that we endeavor to treat disease.

Stress! While this word is relatively new in the English lexicon, few
words have had such far-reaching implications. Evidence of the adverse
effects of stress is well documented in innumerable sources. Homer's *Iliad*
describes the symptoms of posttraumatic stress as suffered by Achilles.
In *The New Testament*, Acts, Chapter 5, describes what may be the sudden
death syndrome as it befell Ananias and his wife Saphira, after being
confronted by Peter the Apostle, for withholding money intended for
missionary service.

Excessive stress has emerged as a significant challenge to public
health. More than 30 years ago, the Office of the U.S. Surgeon General
declared that when stress reaches excessive proportions, psychological
changes can be so dramatic as to have serious implications for both mental and physical health (U.S. Public Health Service, 1979). More recently,
the Global Burden of Disease Study (Murray & Lopez, 1996) revealed that
mental illnesses represent a significant contributor to the burden of global
disease. The disability-adjusted life year (DALY) represents the number of
years of life lost to premature death and disability; the disease burdens are
listed by selected illnesses:

Cardiovascular diseases	18.6 DALY
Mental illnesses (including stress and suicide)	15.4 DALY
Malignant diseases	15.0 DALY
Respiratory diseases	4.8 DALY
Alcohol use	4.7 DALY
Infectious diseases	2.8 DALY
Drug use	1.5 DALY

It should be noted that mental illnesses not only rank as the second most
burdensome disease process, but also, consistent with the observations of
Salk (1973) almost 30 years ago, infectious diseases represent significantly
less of a global burden upon health compared to mental disorders and
alcohol and drug use. According to the U.S. Surgeon General (U.S.
Department of Health and Human Services, 1999), for persons ages
18–54 years, anxiety and stress-related diseases are the major contributors
to the mental illness in the United States, with more than twice the prevalence (16.4%) of mood disorders (7.1%). Stress seems to have reached
almost epidemic proportions. Table 1.1 underscores the role that stress
may play as a public health challenge.

Table 1.1. Stress and Trauma as Public Health Challenges

- Recent evidence suggests that 90% of adults in the United States will be exposed to a traumatic event during their lifetime (Breslau et al., 1998).
- Suicide rates have been seen to increase in the first year after an earthquake, in the first 2 years after a hurricane, and 4 years after a flood (Krug et al., 1998).
- United States citizens ages 12 years or older experienced 37 million crimes in 1996 (Bureau of Justice Statistics, 1997).
- The lifetime prevalence of criminal victimization was assessed among female health management organization patients and found to be about 57%.
- Each year, approximately 1 million persons become victims of violent crime at work (Bachman, 1994).
- The prevalence of posttraumatic stress disorder (PTSD) was found to be 13% in a sample of suburban law enforcement officers (Robinson, Sigman, & Wilson, 1997).
- Law enforcement officers are 8.6 times more likely to die from suicide than from homicide and 3.1 times more likely to die from suicide than from accidental circumstances (Violanti, 1996).
- Of the clinical health care staff sampled, 62% reported being exposed to a traumatic stressor at work (Caldwell, 1992).
- In 2001, the terrorist attacks against the World Trade Center and the Pentagon focus terrorism in the United States.
- The prevalence of posttraumatic stress disorder ranged from 15% to 31% for samples of urban firefighters based on a traumatic exposure prevalence ranging from 85% to 91% (Beaton, Murphy, & Corneil, 1996).
- In a survey, it was found that 74% of PTSD cases last more than 6 months (Breslau et al., 1998).
- Symptoms of distress and PTSD are correlated with exposure to traumatic stressors (Weiss et al., 1995; Corneil, 1993; Wee et al., 1999).
- Clearly, trauma and stress are at epidemic proportions in the United States. It seems clear that such conditions represent a "clear and present danger" to the psychological health of American society.

Finally, reviews by Cohen and Herbert (1996), Baum and Posluszny (1999), Friedmam and Schnurr (1995), Harris (1991), Stoudemire (1995), and Williams (1995) point out the contribution that stress makes to a wide variety of physical diseases.

Contained within the Surgeon General's report, *Healthy People* (U.S. Public Health Service, 1979), was the most significant indication ever that stress and its potentially pathological effects are considered serious public health factors. More recently, the Surgeon General's report on mental health (U.S. Department of Health and Human Services, 1999) extended those observations made 20 years earlier and even sought to quantify the burden that mental illnesses represent as a disease entity. If, indeed, the aforementioned appraisals are credible, then what has emerged is a powerful rationale for the study of the nature and treatment of the human stress response. To that end, this book is written.

DEFINING STRESS

In this book written for clinicians, the focus is on the treatment of pathogenic stress. Yet it may be argued that effective treatment emerges from an understanding of the phenomenology of the pathognomonic entity itself. In this first chapter, the reader will encounter some of the basic foundations and definitions upon which the treatment of pathognomonic stress is inevitably based.

It seems appropriate to begin a text on stress with a basic definition of the stress response itself.

The term *stress* was first introduced into the health sciences in 1926 by Hans Selye. As a second-year medical student at the University of Prague, he noted that individuals suffering from a wide range of physical ailments all seemed to have a common constellation of symptoms, including loss of appetite, decreased muscular strength, elevated blood pressure, and a loss of ambition (Selye, 1974). Wondering why these symptoms seemed to appear commonly, regardless of the nature of the somatic disorder, led Selye to label this condition as "the syndrome of just being sick" (Selye, 1956).

In his early writings, Selye used the term *stress* to describe the "sum of all nonspecific changes (within an organism) caused by function or damage" or, more simply, "the rate of wear and tear in the body." In a more recent definition, the Selyean concept of stress is "the nonspecific response of the body to any demand" (Selye, 1974, p. 14).

Paul Rosch (1986) provides an interesting anecdote. Recognizing that the term stress was originally borrowed from the science of physics, he relates how Selye's usage of the term did not conform to original intent:

> In 1676, Hooke's Law described the effect of external stresses, or loads, that produced various degrees of "strain," or distortion, on different materials.
>
> Selye once complained to me that had his knowledge of English been more precise, he might have labeled his hypothesis the "strain concept," and he did encounter all sorts of problems when his research had to be translated. (Rosch, 1986, ix)

Indeed, confusion concerning whether stress was a "stimulus," as used in physics, or a "response," as used by Selye, has plagued the stress literature. As Rosch (1986) describes:

> The problem was that some used stress to refer to disturbing emotional or physical stimuli, others to describe the body's biochemical and physiologic response ... and still others to depict the pathologic consequences of such interactions. This led one confused British critic to complain, 35 years ago, that stress in addition to being itself was also the cause of itself and the result of itself. (p. ix)

To summarize the discussion so far, the term *stress* used in the Selyean tradition, refers to a response, whereas in its original usage, within the science of physics, it referred to a stimulus, and the term *strain* referred to the response.

Using the term *stress* to denote a response left Selye without a term to describe the stimulus that engenders a stress response. Selye chose the term *stressor* to denote any stimulus that gives rise to a stress response.

In summary, drawing upon historical precedent, and consistent with Selye's original notion, the term *stress* is used within this volume to refer to a physiological reaction, or response, regardless of the source of the reaction. The term *stressor* refers to the stimulus that serves to engender the stress response.

With this fundamental introduction to the concept of stress, let us extend the conceptualization a bit further.

TEN KEY CONCEPTS IN THE STUDY OF STRESS

1. The stimulus that evokes a stress response is referred to a *stressor*. There are two primary forms of stressors (Girdano, Everly, & Dusek, 2001): (a) psychosocial stressors (including personality-based stressors) and (b) biogenic stressors.

2. *Psychosocial stressors* become stressors by virtue of the cognitive interpretation of the event, that is, the manner in which they are interpreted, the meanings they are assigned (Ellis, 1973; Lazarus, 1966, 1991; Lazarus & Folkman, 1984; Meichenbaum, 1977). Selye once noted, "It's not what happens to you that matters, but how you take it." Epictetus is credited with saying, "Men are disturbed, not by things, but the views which they take of them." For example, a traffic jam is really a neutral event; it only becomes a stressor by virtue of how the individual interprets the event (i.e., as threatening or otherwise undesirable). If the individual views the traffic jam as neutral or positive, no stress response ensues. Some stressors are inherently more stressful than others and leave less potential variation for cognitive interpretation (e.g., objective external threats to one's safety or well-being, grief, guilt, etc.). But even in these cases, cognitive interpretation will play a role in the adjustment to the stressor and serve to augment or mitigate the resultant stress response.

Phenomenological research conducted by Smith, Everly, and Johns (1992, 1993) evaluated the credibility of this notion of a mediating role for psychological variables in the relationship between stressor stimuli and the signs and symptoms of distress. Using structural mathematical modeling, exploratory and confirmatory factor analyses, they demonstrated that psychosocial environmental stressors exert their pathogenic effect upon the human organism primarily through cognitive processes. More specifically, evidence of cognitive–affective discord predicted signs and symptoms of physical ill-health as well as maladaptive coping behaviors. This notion of a mediating role for cognitive–affective processes in the stressor-to-illness paradigm is explored further in Chapter 2.

3. *Biogenic stressors,* on the other hand, require no cognitive appraisal in order to assume stressor qualities; rather, biogenic stimuli possess an inherent stimulant quality. This stimulant characteristic, commonly referred to as a sympathomimetic characteristic, is found in substances such as tea, coffee, ginseng, guarana, ginkgo biloba, yohimbine, amphetamines, and cocaine. Extremes of heat and cold, and even physical exercise exert sympathomimetic effects. Biogenic stressors directly cause physiological arousal without the necessity of cognitive appraisal (Ganong, 1997; Katzung, 1992).

The inclusion of the biogenic sympathomimetic category of stressors in no way contradicts the work of Lazarus and others who have studied the critical role that interpretation plays in the formation of psychosocial stressors. Such an inclusion merely extends the stressor concept to recognize that stimuli that alter the normal anatomical or physiological integrity of the individual are also capable of activating many of the same psychoendocrinological mechanisms that we refer to as the *stress response.* Thus, even if a patient convincingly reports that he or she really enjoys drinking 15 cups of caffeinated coffee per day, the clinician must be sensitive to the fact that those 15 "enjoyable" cups of coffee can serve as a powerful stressor activating an extraordinary systemic release of stress-response hormones such as epinephrine and norepinephrine, and in doing so can be a contributing factor in cardiac conduction abnormalities, for example. Similarly, individuals who belong to "Polar Bear" clubs and voluntarily immerse themselves in frigid waters during the winter undergo an extraordinary stress response characterized by massive sympathetic nervous system (SNS) arousal. Thus, even though the consumption of caffeine and the immersion of oneself into frigid bodies of water may truly be reinforcing, that person still experiences a form of physiological arousal that is accurately described as a stress response and may pose some risk to health, depending upon the intensity and chronicity of the exposure to the stressors. These issues are reiterated once again in Chapter 2.

In general, it is important for the clinician to understand that by far the greater part of the excessive stress in the patient's life is self-initiated and self-propagated, owing to the fact that it is the patient who interprets many otherwise neutral stimuli as possessing stress-evoking characteristics. Kirtz and Moos (1974) suggest that social stimuli do not directly affect the individual. Rather, the individual reacts to the environment in accordance with his or her interpretations of the environmental stimuli. These interpretations are affected by such variables as personality components or status and social-role behaviors. These cognitive–affective reactions are also subject to exacerbation through usually self-initiated exposures to sympathomimetic stimuli, such as excessive caffeine consumption, and the like. Having the patient realize and accept reasonable responsibility for the cause and reduction of excessive stress can be a major crossroads in the therapeutic intervention. Therefore, we also discuss this issue in greater detail in Chapter 3.

4. Stress is a response, or reaction, to some stimulus. The stressor–stress response notion is illustrated in Figure 1.1.

5. The stress response represents a physiological reaction, as defined in the Selyean tradition (Cannon, 1914; Selye, 1956); Everly (1985a; Everly & Sobelman, 1987) has extended this concept somewhat and conceptualizes the stress response as a "physiologic mechanism of mediation," that is, a medium to bring about a result or effect. More specifically, the stress response may be viewed as the physiological link between any given stressor and its target-organ effect. This then will be the working definition of stress used in this volume: *Stress is a physiological response that serves as a mechanism of mediation linking any given stressor to its target-organ effect or arousal.* This notion is captured in Figure 1.2.

When communicating with patients or simply conceptualizing the clinical importance of the stress response, however, Selye's (1974, 1976) notion that stress is the "sum total of wear and tear" on the individual seems useful.

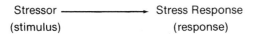

Stressor ———————————→ Stress Response
(stimulus)   (response)

Figure 1.1. A basic stress response model.

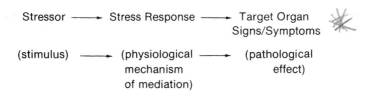

Stressor ———→ Stress Response ———→ Target Organ
                                                    Signs/Symptoms

(stimulus) ———→ (physiological ———→ (pathological
                        mechanism   effect)
                        of mediation)

Figure 1.2. The stress response as a mechanism of mediation.

6. The stress response, as a physiological mechanism of mediation, can be characterized by a widely diverse constellation of physiological mechanisms (Cannon, 1914; Makara, Palkovits, & Szentagothal, 1980; Mason, 1972; Selye, 1976) that may be categorized as (1) neurological response pathways, (2) neuroendocrine response mechanisms, and (3) endocrine response pathways. These potential response mechanisms will be reviewed in detail in Chapter 2.

Although the mechanisms of the stress response are processes of arousal, and the target-organ effects are usually indicative of arousal, the stress response has been noted as entailing such forms of arousal as to cause actual slowing, inhibition, or complete stoppage of target-organ systems (Engel, 1971; Gellhorn, 1968, 1969; Gray, 1985; Selye, 1976). These inhibiting or depressive effects are typically a result of the fact that, upon occasion, stress arousal constitutes the activation of inhibitory neurons, inhibitory hormones, or simply an acute hyperstimulation that results in a nonfunctional state (e.g., cardiac fibrillation). This seeming paradox is often a point of confusion for the clinician; hence, its mention here.

7. Selye (1956, 1976) has argued for the "nonspecificity" of the stress response. Other authors (Everly, 1972; Humphrey & Everly, 1980; Mason, 1971; Harris, 1991; Mason et al., 1976) have argued that the psychophysiology of stress may be highly specific with various stressors and various individuals showing different degrees of stimulus or response specificity, respectively. Current evidence strongly supports the existence of highly specific neuroendocrine and endocrine efferent mechanisms. Whether there exists another way of collectively categorizing stress-response mechanisms may be as much a semantic as a physiological issue (Everly, 1985a; Selye, 1980).

8. A vast literature argues that when stress arousal becomes excessively chronic or intense in amplitude, target-organ (the organ affected by the stress response) disease and/or dysfunction will result (Everly, 1986; Selye, 1956; Harris, 1991; Stoudemire, 1995). When stress results in *organic* biochemical and/or structural changes in the target organ, these results are referred to as a *psychophysiological disease* (American Psychiatric Association, 1968) or a *psychosomatic disease* (Lipowski, 1984). Psychosomatic diseases were first cogently described by Felix Deutsch in 1927. However, it was Helen Dunbar (1935) who published the first major treatise on psychosomatic phenomena. In 1968, in the *Diagnostic and Statistical Manual of Mental Disorders*, second edition (American Psychiatric Association, 1968), the term *psychophysiological disorder* was used to define a "group of disorders characterized by physical symptoms that are caused by emotional factors" (p. 46). Thus, we see the terms *psychosomatic* and *psychophysiological* used interchangeably to refer to organically based physical conditions resulting from excessive stress.

Sometimes these terms are confused with the development of neurotic-like physical symptoms without any basis in organic pathology. The terms *conversion hysteria* or *somatoform disorders* are usually used to designate such nonorganic physical symptomatology.

The *Diagnostic and Statistical Manual of Mental Disorders*, fourth edition, used the designation "Psychological Factors Affecting Medical Condition" to encompass stress-related physical disorders (see Stoudemire, 1995). By virtue of its multiaxial diagnostic schema, this nosological manual allowed clinicians to assess levels of stress and environmental support as they may affect not only physical symptoms but also psychiatric symptoms. Physical symptoms without a basis in or manifestation of organic pathology are subsumed under the somatoform category.

In the context of this volume, it is recognized that stress can be directed toward discrete anatomical or physiological target organs and therefore can lead to physical disorders characterized by organic pathology (i.e., psychophysiological or psychosomatic disorders); yet we must also recognize that the human mind can serve as a target organ. Thus, in addition to somatic stress-related disorders, it seems reasonable to include psychiatric-stress-related disorders as potential target-organ effects as well.

In summary, the terms *psychosomatic* and *psychophysiological* disorders are considered in this book as terms that refer to disorders characterized by physical alterations initiated or exacerbated by psychological processes. If tissue alterations are significant enough, and if the target organ is essential, then psychosomatic disorders could be life threatening. Neurotic-like somatoform disorders, on the other hand, involve only functional impairments of the sensory or motor systems and therefore cannot threaten life. Like the psychosomatic disorder, somatoform disorders are psychogenic; unlike psychosomatic processes, somatoform disorders entail no real tissue pathology. Confusion between the psychosomatic concept, on one hand, and the somatoform concept, on the other, is easily understandable. Yet, such confusion may lead to an underestimation of the potential severity of the disorder, thereby affecting treatment motivation and compliance.

9. Although recent reports emphasize the negative aspects of stress, there do exist positive aspects as well.

Previous writers have viewed the stress response as an innate preservation mechanism, which in earlier periods of evolutionary development allowed us to endure the challenges to survival. Numerous researchers (Cannon, 1953; Chavat, Dell, & Folkow, 1964; also see Henry & Stephens, 1977, for a brief review) have concluded, and we shall see in later chapters, that the nature of the psychophysiological stress response is that of apparent preparatory arousal—arousal in preparation for physical exertion. When used in such a way, it is easy to see the adaptive utility of the stress response. Yet stress arousal in modern times under circumstances of strictly psychosocial stimulation might be viewed as inappropriate arousal of primitive survival mechanisms, in that the organism is aroused for physical activity but seldom is such activity truly warranted and, therefore, seldom does it follow (see Benson, 1975).

Selye (1956, 1974) further distinguishes constructive from destructive stress, clearly pointing out that not all stress is deleterious. He argues that stress arousal can be a positive, motivating force that improves the quality of life. He calls such positive stress "eustress" (prefix *eu* from the Greek meaning "good") and debilitating, excessive stress "distress." Figure 1.3 depicts the relationship between stress and health/performance. As stress increases, so does health/performance and general well-being. However, as stress continues to increase, a point of maximal return is reached. This point may be called the *optimal stress level,* because it becomes deleterious to the organism should stress arousal increase.

The point at which an individual's optimal stress level is reached, that is, the apex of one's tolerance for stress as a productive force, seems to be

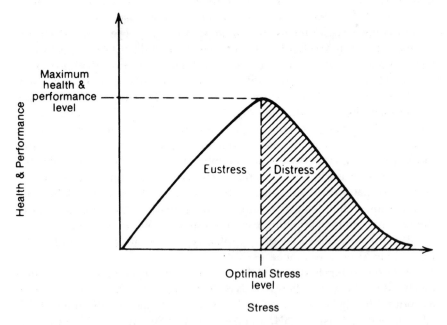

Figure 1.3. The graphic relationship between stress arousal (horizontal axis) and performance (vertical axis). As stress increases, so does performance (eustress). At the optimal stress level, performance has reached its maximum level. If stress continues to increase into the "distress" region, performance quickly declines. Should stress levels remain excessive, health will begin to erode as well.

a function of genetic, biological, acquired physiological, and behavioral factors.

10. Last in this series of assumptions about what stress is and is not, is the point that confusion exists regarding the role of the nonmedical clinician in the treatment of the stress response. This is so primarily because the target-organ effects or pathologies that result from excessive stress are mistakenly thought of as the psychophysiological stress response itself. It is important to remember the distinction that stress is a process of psychophysiological arousal (as detailed in Chapter 2), whereas the effects and pathologies (such as migraine headache, peptic ulcers, etc.) are the manifestations of chronically repeated and/or intense triggerings of the psychophysiological stress response (see Chapter 3). Treating the end-organ pathologies is clearly within the realm of the physician or nonmedical specialist in behavioral medicine. However, the traditional psychologist, counselor, physical therapist, social worker, or health educator can effectively intervene in the treatment of the stress arousal process itself. This includes treating the excessive stress/anxiety that accompanies, and often exacerbates, chronic infectious and degenerative diseases.

It is important to understand that this text addresses the clinical problem of excessive psychophysiological arousal—that is, the excessive stress-response process itself. It is not a detailed guide for psychotherapeutic intervention in the psychological trauma or conflict that may be at the root of the arousal (although such intervention can play a useful role). Nor does this text address the direct treatment of the pathologies' target organs that might arise as a result of excessive stress. We shall limit ourselves to a discussion of the clinical treatment of the psychophysiological stress-response process itself.

Based on a review of the literature, we may conclude that treatment of the process of excessive psychophysiological stress arousal may take the form of three discrete interventions (see Girdano, Everly, & Dusek, 2001):

1. Helping the patient develop and implement strategies by which to avoid/minimize/modify exposure to stressors, thus reducing the patient's tendency to experience the stress response (Ellis, 1973; Lazarus, 1966, 1991; Meichenbaum, 1985).

2. Helping the patient develop and implement skills that reduce excessive psychophysiological functioning and reactivity (Benson, 1975; Emmons, 1978; Gellhorn & Kiely, 1972; Girdano et al., 2000; Jacobson, 1938, 1970, 1978; Stoyva, 1976, 1977; Stoyva & Budzynski, 1974).

3. Helping the patient develop and implement techniques for the healthful expression, or utilization, of the stress response (see

Chavat et al., 1964; Gevarter, 1978; Kraus & Raab, 1961; Pennebaker, 1999).

Finally, it has been suggested that the clinicians who are the most successful in treating the stress response have training not only in the psychology of human behavior, but also medical physiology (Miller, 1978; Miller & Dworkin, 1977). Our own teaching and clinical observations support this conclusion. If indeed accurate, this conclusion may be due to the fact that stress represents the epitome of mind–body interaction. As Miller (1979) suggests, mere knowledge of therapeutic techniques is not enough. The clinician must understand the nature of the clinical problem as well. Therefore, the reader will find that the treatment section of this text is preceded by a basic discussion of the functional anatomy and physiology of the stress response.

PLAN OF THE BOOK

The purpose of this text is to provide an up-to-date discourse on the phenomenology and treatment of pathogenic human stress arousal. As noted earlier, once target-organ signs and symptoms have been adequately stabilized, or ameliorated, the logical target for therapeutic intervention becomes the pathogenic process of stress arousal that engendered the target-organ signs and symptoms in the first place. To treat the target-organ effects of stress arousal while ignoring their pathogenic, phenomenological origins is palliative at best, and often predicts a subsequent relapse.

The unique interaction of psychological and physiological phenomena that embodies the stress response requires a unique therapeutic understanding, as Miller has noted. Therefore, this volume is divided into three sections: Part I addresses the anatomical and physiological nature of stress arousal. Also discussed are measurement considerations. Part II offers a practical clinical guide for the actual treatment of the human stress response and addresses a multitude of various technologies. Finally, Part III discusses several aspects of clinical practice that warrant special consideration. Also included in this volume is an appendix that provides a series of brief discussions on "special" topics and innovations relevant to the treatment of human stress arousal.

2

The Anatomy and Physiology of the Human Stress Response

It is highly dishonorable for a Reasonable Soul to live in so Divinely built a Mansion as the Body she resides in, altogether unacquainted with the exquisite structure of it.

ROBERT BOYLE

In the first chapter, we provided the following working definition of the stress response: "Stress is a physiological response that serves as a mechanism of mediation linking any given stressor to its target-organ effect." By viewing the phenomenology of stress within the context of a "linking" mechanism, we can answer one of the most critical questions in psychosomatic medicine, that is, through what mechanisms can stressor stimuli, such as life events, lead to disease and dysfunction? The response to that query will be addressed within the next two chapters.

This chapter describes, within the boundaries of current findings and speculation, the anatomical and physiological foundations of the human stress response by (1) addressing basic neuroanatomical structures and (2) tracing the psychophysiological effector mechanisms that actually represent the stress response, as currently defined. To assist in the pedagogical process, a basic model of the human stress response is constructed to serve as a unifying thread for better understanding of not only the phenomenology of human stress but also its measurement and treatment. Chapter 3 will pursue the logical extension by reviewing several models of pathogenesis, that is, the process by which stress arousal leads to disease.

NEUROLOGICAL FOUNDATIONS

In order to understand the stress response, we must first understand its foundations, which reside in the structure and function of the human nervous systems.

The basic anatomical unit of the nervous systems is the *neuron* (see Figure 2.1). Indeed the smallest functional unit of the nervous system, the neuron serves to conduct sensory, motor, and regulatory signals throughout the body. The neuron consists of three basic units: (1) the *dendrites* and their outermost membranes—the postsynaptic dendritic membranes; (2) the *neural cell body*, which contains the nucleus of the cell; and (3) the *axon*, with its branching projections called the *telodendria* and their end points, the presynaptic membranes.

Neural Transmission

An incoming signal is first received by the postsynaptic membranes of the dendrites. Chemical (metabotropic) or electrical (ionotropic) processes are initiated upon stimulation of the postsynaptic dendritic membranes, which cause the neuron to conduct the incoming signal through the dendrites and the cell body. Finally, a neural impulse relayed to the axon travels down the axon until it reaches the telodendria and ultimately the presynaptic membranes. It is the task of the presynaptic membrane to relay the signal to the subsequent postsynaptic membrane of the next neuron.

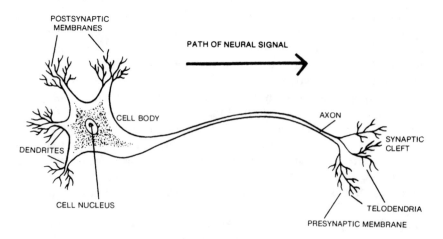

Figure 2.1. A typical neuron.

This is not easily achieved, however, because the neurons do not actually touch one another. Rather, there exists a space between neurons called the *synaptic cleft*.

In order for a signal to cross the synaptic cleft, chemical substances called *neurotransmitters* are called into play. Residing in storage vesicles in the telodendria, chemical neurotransmitters await the proper cues to migrate toward the presynaptic membrane. Once there, they are ultimately discharged into the synaptic cleft to stimulate (or inhibit) the postsynaptic membrane of the next neuron. Table 2.1 contains a list of major neurotransmitters and their anatomical loci.

Having completed a basic overview of the anatomy of neural transmission, it is necessary to return to a brief discussion of the dynamics of intraneuronal communication. For clinicians, this phenomenon is extremely important because it serves as the basis for electrophysiological events such as electromyography, electrocardiography, and electroencephalography.

Table 2.1. Major Neurotransmitters and Their Loci

Neurotransmitter	Neuronal pathways
Norepinephrine (NE) (a major excitatory neurotransmitter)	Locus ceruleus Limbic system, especially Amygdala Hippocampus Septum And interconnecting pathways Postganglionic sympathetic nervous system Cerebellum
Serotonin (5-HT)	Brain stem Limbic system
Acetylcholine (Ach)	Neuromuscular junctions Preganglionic sympathetic nervous system Preganglionic parasympathetic nervous system Postganglionic parasympathetic nervous system Septal–hippocampal system
Gamma amino butyric acid (GABA) (a major inhibitory neurotransmitter)	Hippocampus Substantia nigra Limbic system—general
Dopamine (DA)	Mesolimbic system Nigrostriatal system

Shortly after the incoming signal passes the postsynaptic dendritic membrane and moves away from the cell body toward the axon, it becomes a measurable electrical event that serves as the basis for electrophysiological techniques such as electrocardiography. The foundations of these electrical events are based upon the dynamics of ionic transport.

The neuron at rest has ions both within the boundaries of its membranes and outside, around its membranes. Sodium (Na^+) is the positively charged ion that makes up the majority of the ionic constituency outside the neuron. In addition to the sodium concentration outside the neuron (about 0.142 M) there resides another ion, chloride (Cl^-). Chloride is a negatively charged ion that makes up the second largest ionic constituency outside the neuron (about 0.103 M). Whereas Na^+ and Cl^- predominate in the extraneural space, negatively charged protein anions dominate the internal milieu of the neuron along with potassium (K^+). Thus, relatively speaking, the outside of the neuron possesses a positive charge and the inside, a negative charge. This resting status is called a polarized state (*polarization*). The relative intensity of the negatively charged intraneuronal constituency is about -70 mV and is called the *resting electrical potential.*

When a neuron is in the act of transmitting a neural signal, the resting status of the neuron is altered. Ionically, Na^+ rushes across the membrane of the neuron and enters the intraneuronal space. This influx of Na^+ pushes the electrical gradient to about $+50$ mV (from the resting -70 mV). This process of sodium ion influx is called *depolarization* and represents the actual firing, or discharge, of the neuron. Depolarization lasts about 1.5 msec. Depolarization moves longitudinally along the axon as a wave of ionic influx. After 1.5 msec, however, the neuron begins to repolarize. *Repolarization* occurs as K^+ and Na^+ are pumped out of the neuron and any remaining Na^+ is assimilated into the neuron itself. The result of repolarization is the return of the $+50$ mV to a resting -70 mV, ready for subsequent discharge. This process is captured in Figure 2.2.

Basic Neuroanatomy

From the preceding discussion of basic neural transmission, the next step to be undertaken is an analysis of the fundamental anatomical structures involved in the human stress response.

The nervous systems, the functional structures within which millions upon millions of neurons reside, may be classified from either an anatomical or a functional perspective. For the sake of parsimony, we describe the nervous systems from an anatomical perspective.

From an anatomical perspective, there are two fundamental nervous systems: *the central nervous system* (CNS) and *the peripheral nervous system* (PNS) (see Figure 2.3).

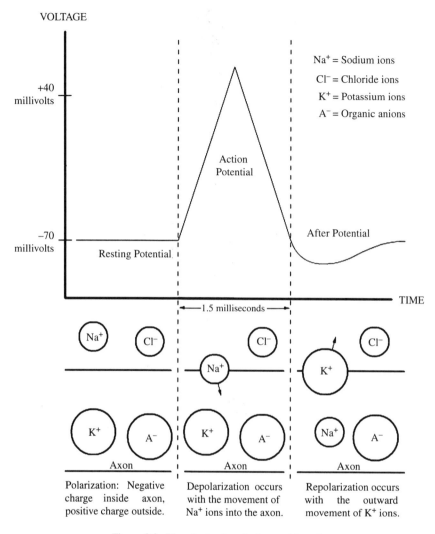

VOLTAGE

Na⁺ = Sodium ions
Cl⁻ = Chloride ions
K⁺ = Potassium ions
A⁻ = Organic anions

Figure 2.2. The electrochemical neural impulse.

The CNS. The CNS consists of the brain and the spinal cord (see Table 2.2). MacLean (1975) has called the human brain the "triune brain" because it can be classified as having three functional levels (see Figure 2.4). The *neocortex* represents the highest level of the triune brain and is the most sophisticated component of the human brain. Among other functions, such as the decoding and interpretation of sensory signals, communications, and gross control of motor (musculoskeletal) behaviors, the neocortex

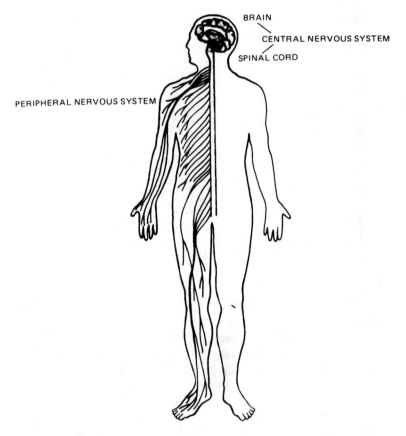

Figure 2.3. Nervous systems (adapted from Lachman, 1972).

Table 2.2.   The Human Nervous Systems

   I. The central nervous system (CNS)
      A. Brain
      B. Spinal cord
  II. The peripheral nervous systems (PNS)
      A. The somatic branch
      B. The autonomic branches (ANS)
         1. Sympathetic (SNS)
         2. Parasympathetic (PSNS)

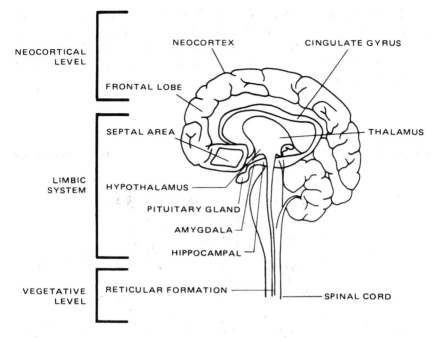

Figure 2.4. The human brain.

(primarily the *frontal lobe*) presides over imagination, logic, decision making, memory, problem solving, planning, and apprehension.

The *limbic system* represents the major component of the second level of the triune brain. The limbic brain is of interest in the discussion of stress because of its role as the emotional (affective) control center for the human brain. The limbic system is believed to be just that, that is, a *system*, consisting of numerous neural structures, for example, the *hypothalamus, hippocampus, septum, cingulate gyrus*, and *amygdala*. The *pituitary gland* plays a major functional role in this system in that *it is a major effector* endocrine gland. The limbic system is examined in greater detail in Chapter 9.

The *reticular formation* and the *brain stem* represent the lowest level of the triune brain. The major functions of this level are the maintenance of vegetative functions (heart beat, respiration, vasomotor activity) and the conduction of impulses through the reticular formation and relay centers of the *thalamus* en route to the higher levels of the triune brain.

The spinal cord represents the central pathway for neurons as they conduct signals to and from the brain. It is also involved in some autonomically regulated reflexes.

The PNS. The PNS consists of all neurons exclusive of the CNS. Anatomically, the PNS may be thought of as an extension of the CNS in that the functional control centers for the PNS lie in the CNS. The PNS may be divided into two networks: the *somatic* (SNS) and the *autonomic nervous systems* (ANS).

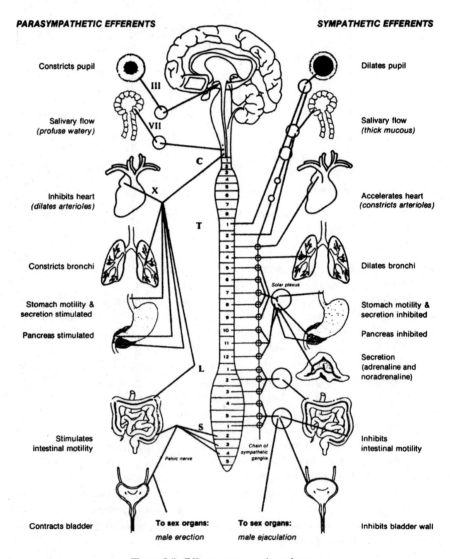

Figure 2.5. Efferent autonomic pathways.

The somatic branch of the PNS carries sensory and motor signals to and from the CNS. Thus, it innervates sensory organs as well as the striate musculature (skeletal musculature).

The autonomic branches carry impulses that are concerned with the regulation of the body's internal environment and the maintenance of the homeostasis (balance). The autonomic network, therefore, innervates the heart, the smooth muscles, and the glands.

The ANS can be further subdivided into two branches, the *sympathetic* and the *parasympathetic* (see Figure 2.5 for details of autonomic innervation). The sympathetic branch of the ANS is concerned with preparing the body for action. Its effect on the organs it innervates is that of generalized arousal. The parasympathetic branch of the ANS is concerned with restorative functions and the relaxation of the body. Its general effects are those of slowing and maintenance of basic bodily requirements. The specific effects of sympathetic and parasympathetic activation on end organs are summarized later in this chapter (see Table 2.3).

To this point, we have briefly described the most basic anatomical and functional aspects of the human nervous system. We are now ready to see how these elements become interrelated as constituents of the human stress-response process.

A SYSTEMS MODEL OF THE HUMAN STRESS RESPONSE

The human stress response is perhaps best described within the context of the dynamic "process" it represents. This process may then be delineated from a "systems" perspective, that is, one of interrelated multidimensionality. Figure 2.6 details a systems perspective brought to bear upon the phenomenology of the human stress response. This model, which has evolved significantly in recent years, will serve as a unifying theme to assist in gaining a better understanding of not only the phenomenology of human stress but also its measurement and treatment. These latter themes will be expanded upon later in the text.

An analysis of Figure 2.6 reveals the epiphenomenology of the human stress response to be that of a multidimensional, interactive process possessing several key elements:

1. Stressor events (real or imagined)
2. Cognitive appraisal and affective integration
3. Neurological triggering mechanisms (e.g., locus ceruleus, limbic nuclei, hypothalamic nuclei)
4. The stress response (a physiological mechanism of mediation)
5. Target-organ activation
6. Coping behavior

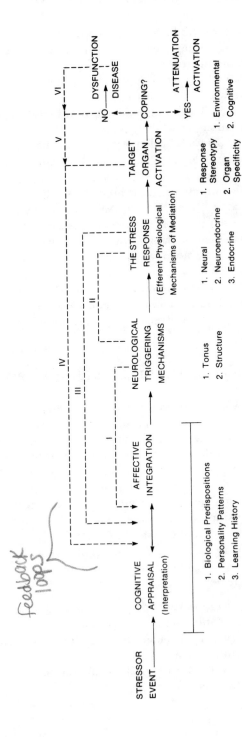

Figure 2.6. A systems model of the human stress response.

A detailed analysis of each of these elements is appropriate at this point.

Stressor Events

Because Selye used the term *stress* to refer to a "response," it was necessary to employ a word to delineate the stimulus for the stress response—that word is *stressor*. Stressor events, as noted earlier, fall in one of the two categories: (1) psychosocial stressors and (2) biogenic stressors (Girdano et al., 2001).

Psychosocial stressors are either real or imagined environmental events that "set the stage" for the elicitation of the stress response. They cannot directly "cause" the stress response but must work through cognitive appraisal mechanics. Most stressors are, indeed, psychosocial stressors. For this reason, one may argue that "stress, like beauty, resides in the eye of the beholder."

Biogenic stressors, however, actually "cause" the elicitation of the stress response. Such stimuli bypass the higher cognitive appraisal mechanisms and work directly on affective and neurological triggering nuclei. Thus, by virtue of their biochemical properties, they directly initiate the stress response without the usual requisite cognitive–affective processing. Examples of such stimuli include the following:

- Ginseng
- Ginkgo biloba
- Amphetamine
- Phenylpropanolamine
- Caffeine
- Theobromine
- Theophylline
- Nicotine
- Certain physical factors such as pain-evoking stimuli, extreme heat, and extreme cold
- Guarana
- Yohimbine

As just mentioned, however, most stressors are not biogenic stressors. Therefore, in clinical practice, therapists will most likely be treating patients who are plagued by environmental events—real, imagined, anticipated, or recalled—that are perceived in such a manner as to lead to activation of the stress response. To better understand this process we move now to the second step in the model: the cognitive–affective integration stage.

Cognitive–Affective Domain

Practically speaking, there is simply no such thing as "reality" without considering the human perspective that might be brought to bear upon it. The cognitive–affective domain is delineated within this model in order to capture that notion.

Cognitive appraisal refers to the process of cognitive interpretation, that is, the meanings that we assign to the world as it unfolds before us. *Affective integration* refers to the blending and coloring of felt emotion into the cognitive interpretation. The resultant cognitive–affective complex represents how the stressors are ultimately perceived. In effect, this critical integrated perception represents the determination of whether psychosocial *stimuli* become psychosocial *stressors* or not. Such a perceptual process, however, is uniquely individualized and vulnerable to biological predispositions (Millon & Everly, 1985; Strelau, Farley, & Gale, 1985), personality patterns (Millon, 1981), learning history (Lachman, 1972), and available resources for coping (Lazarus & Folkman, 1984; Ray, Lindop, & Gibson, 1982).

Although Figure 2.6 portrays a reciprocity between cognitive and affective mechanisms, it should be noted that there exists substantial evidence supporting the cognitive primacy hypothesis (see Chapter 9); that is, cognition determines affect (felt emotion) and thus assumes a superordinate role in the process of restructuring human behavior patterns. Let us explore this important notion further.

Perhaps the earliest recognition that cognition is superordinate to affect has been credited by Albert Ellis to the fifth-century Greco-Roman philosopher Epictetus, who reportedly said, "Men are disturbed not by things, but by the views which they take of them." The science of physiology follows in kind. Hans Selye, also known as the father of modern endocrinology, has summarized over 50 years of research into human stress with the conclusion, "It is not what happens to you that matters, but how you take it." Similarly, the noted neurophysiologist Ernest Gellhorn (Gellhorn & Loofbourrow, 1963) recognized the preeminent role of the prefrontal lobe cognitive processes in felt and expressed emotion in his research spanning the 1950s, 1960s, and 1970s. Influential authors such as Arnold (1970, 1984), Cassel (1974), Lazarus (1966, 1982, 1991), Meichenbaum (1985; Meichenbaum & Jaremko, 1983), and Selye (1976) strongly support the cognitive primacy position as it relates to human stress.

More recently, Smith, Everly, and Johns (1992, 1993) assessed the role of cognitive processes in the determination of stress-related illness. "Stressors, like beauty, lie in the eye of the beholder," is the assertion. Using a sample of 1,618 adults, these authors employed structural modeling, exploratory, and confirmatory factor analyses to investigate the relative roles of environmental stressors compared to cognitive processes as predictors of physiological symptoms of stress-related illness or dysfunction. The role of coping mechanisms was also investigated. The results of this investigation indicated that, consistent with the speculations of Epictetus and even Selye, environmental stressors exert their pathogenic effect only indirectly. Rather, environmental stressors act "through their ability to cause psychological discord. In fact, psychological discord had the strongest influence on maladaptive coping behaviors and stress-related illness" (Smith et al., 1993, p. 445). Psychological discord, as assessed by these authors, reflects the cognitive interpretations of the environmental events.

An extended physiological perspective may be of value at this point. If a given, nonsympathomimetic stimulus is to engender a stress response, it must first be received by the receptors of the PNS. Once stimulated, these receptors send their impulses along the PNS toward the brain. According to Penfield (1975), once in the CNS, collateral neurons diverge from the main ascending pathways to the neocortical targets and innervate the reticular formation. Snyder has noted that "via these collaterals, events perceived in the environment may be integrated with...emotional states encoded in the hypothalamus and limbic system" (p. 221). These collaterals diverge and pass through limbic constituents, but seldom are such afferent diversions sufficient to generate full-blown emotional reactions. Rather, such diversions may account for nonspecific arousal (startle or defense reflexes) or subtle affective coloration ("gut reactions"). Cognitive theorists do not regard these momentary acute, ontogenetically primitive events as emotions (Lazarus, 1982).

These divergent pathways ultimately reunite with the main ascending pathways and innervate the primary sensory and appraisal loci. Arnold (1984) has written that "the sheer experience of things around us cannot lead to action unless they are appraised for their effect on us" (p. 125). She has hypothesized the anatomical locus of such appraisal to be the cingulate gyrus and the limbic–prefrontal neocortical interface (see Aggleton, 1992).

Arnold (1984) notes that the granular cells of the limbic–prefrontal interface contain relay centers that connect all sensory, motor, and association areas. She states:

> These connections would enable the individual to appraise information from every modality: smells, via relays from the posterior orbital cortex; movement and movement impulses, via relays from frontal and prefrontal cortex; somatic sensations can provide data via relays from parietal association areas; and things seen could be appraised over relays from occipital association areas. Finally, something heard can be appraised as soon as relays from the auditory association area reach the hippocampal gyrus. (pp. 128–129)

As noted in Figure 2.6, appraisal is a function of any existing biological predispositions, personality patterns, learning history, and available coping resources. Once appraisal is made, efferent impulses project so as to potentiate the stimulation of two major effector systems:

1. Impulses project back to the highly sensitive emotional anatomy in the limbic system (Arnold, 1984; Cullinan et al., 1995; Gellhorn & Loufbourrow, 1963; Gevarter, 1978; Nauta, 1979), especially the hippocampus (Reiman et al., 1986), for the experience of stimulus-specific felt emotion and the potential to trigger visceral effector mechanisms.
2. Impulses similarly project to the areas of the neocortex concerned with neuromuscular behavior where, through pyramidal and extrapyramidal systems, muscle tone (tension) is increased and the intention to act can be potentially translated to actual overt motor activity (Gellhorn, 1964).

Thus far, we have seen that psychosocial stimuli, once perceived, excite nonspecific arousal and cognitive appraisal mechanisms. If the appraisal of the stimulus is ultimately one of threat, challenge, or aversion, then emotional arousal will likely result.

In most individuals, activation of the limbic centers for emotional arousal leads to expression of the felt emotion in the form of visceral activation and neuromuscular activity. Such visceral and neuromuscular activation represents the multiaxial physiological mechanisms of mediation Selye called the "stress response." Thus, in the final analysis, it can be seen that physiological reactions to psychosocial stimuli result from the cognitive interpretations and emotional reactions to those stimuli, *not* the stimuli themselves. Stressors are, indeed, in the eye of the beholder!

Before turning to a discussion of the multiaxial nature of the stress response, we must first discuss a mechanism that prefaces activation of the stress response axes. Research in the last several years has necessitated specific consideration of mechanisms that serve to "trigger" the elicitation of the multiaxial stress response. These mechanisms are referred to as *neurological triggering mechanisms*.

Neurological Triggering Mechanisms

The next step in the model depicted in Figure 2.6 is the neurological triggering mechanisms consisting of the locus ceruleus (LC), limbic system, and hypothalamic efferent triggering complex. Linked through ventral and dorsal adrenergic as well as serotonergic projections (among others), this complex appears to consist of the LC, the hippocampus, the septal–hippocampal–amygdaloid complexes, and the anterior and posterior hypothalamic nuclei (Nauta & Domesick, 1982; Reiman et al., 1986). These structures appear to be the anatomical epicenters for the visceral and somatic efferent discharges in response to emotional arousal (Aggleton, 1992; Gellhorn, 1964, 1965, 1967; MacLean, 1949; Nauta, 1979; Redmond, 1979); that is, these structures appear to give rise to the multiaxial stress response. Indeed, these centers even seem capable of establishing an endogenously determined neurological tone that is potentially self-perpetuating (Gellhorn, 1967; Weil, 1974). This notion of a positive feedback loop is initially depicted in Figure 2.6 by the dotted line labeled I. Subsequent dotted lines are labeled with Roman numerals to show other feedback mechanisms that maintain what Gellhorn (1957) has called a state of "egotropic tuning," what Everly (Everly & Benson, 1989) calls "limbic hypersensitivity" (discussed in Chapter 3), and what Weil (1974) has called a "charged arousal system." Each of these terms is indicative of a predisposition for physiological arousal.

More specifically, these terms describe a preferential pattern of SNS (and related arousal mechanism) responsiveness. Such a chronic tonic status may, over time, serve as the basis for a host of psychiatric and psychophysiological disorders (Gellhorn, 1967). The mechanisms by which such neurological tone can exert an effect upon a given target organ is the subject of the next phase of the system's model: the stress response— a physiological mechanism of mediation.

The Stress Response

Recall the question that has plagued psychosomatic research: Through what mechanisms of pathogenic mediation can a stressor and its subsequent appraisal ultimately affect a target organ to such a degree as to result in dysfunction and disease? Although a definitive answer on *all* levels has yet to be found, research in applied physiology has yielded considerable insight into the mechanisms of pathogenesis by which stressors cause disease. This section details three such physiological pathways known to demonstrate extraordinary responsiveness with respect to psychosocial stimuli: (1) the neural axes, (2) the neuroendocrine axis, and (3) the endocrine axes (see Figure 2.7).

The Neural Axes—Stress Response via Neural Innervation of Target Organs. Three neural axes comprise the neural stress response: (1) the sympathetic nervous system, (2) the parasympathetic nervous system, and, (3) the neuromuscular nervous system. These neural pathways are the first

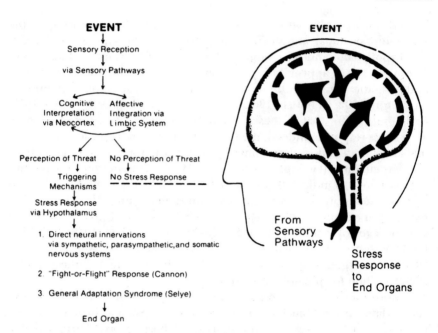

Figure 2.7. The stress response.

of all stress response axes to become activated during stress arousal. This phenomenon is based upon the fact that the structure of these pathways, from origination to target-organ innervation, are completely neural, and therefore quickest.

It is clear that ANS activation occurs during states of emotional arousal in human beings (Duffy, 1962; Johnson & Spalding, 1974; Lindsley, 1951). These neural axes are the most direct of all stress pathways. Following the complex neocortical and limbic integrations that occur in the interpretation of a stimulus as "threatening," neural impulses descend to the posterior hypothalamus (in the case of a sympathetic activation) and the anterior hypothalamus (in the case of a parasympathetic activation). From here, sympathetic neural pathways descend from the anterior hypothalamus through the cranial and sacral spinal cord regions. Parasympathetic nerves then innervate the end organs.

Generally speaking, the release of the neurotransmitter norepinephrine from the sympathetic telodendria is responsible for changes in most end-organ activity. Acetylcholine is the neurotransmitter in the remaining cases and in parasympathetic postganglionic transmissions as well (see Ganong, 1997).

The effects of neural activation via the sympathetic system are those of generalized arousal within the end organs—what Hess (1957) referred to as an "ergotropic" response. The effects of activation via the parasympathetic system are inhibition, slowing, and "restorative" functions—what Hess called a "trophotropic" response. The specific end-organ effects of the sympathetic and the parasympathetic nervous systems are summarized in Table 2.3 (see Ganong, 1997).

Although the most common form of neural autonomic stress responsiveness in human beings is in the form of the ergotropic response (Johnson & Spalding, 1974), simultaneous trophotropic responses have been observed in human beings as well (Gellhorn, 1969). The trophotropic stress response may be perceived by some clinicians as paradoxical, owing to the expectation of manifestations of somation "arousal." However, the important work of Gellhorn (1968, 1969) and Williams (1986), in addition to the clinical observations of Carruthers and Taggart (1973), and Karasarsky (1969), have demonstrated that sympathetic stress arousal can be accompanied by parasympathetic trophotropic activation.

Finally, there is evidence (Gellhorn, 1967, 1958a,b, 1964b; Malmo, 1975; Williams, 1986) that the skeletal muscular is also a prime target for immediate activation during stress and emotional arousal. Such activation, if excessive, may lead to a host of neuromuscular dysfunctions as well as increased limbic excitation (Gellhorn, 1958b; Malmo, 1975; Weil, 1974) and therefore heightened emotional arousal.

Although neuromuscular activation may last virtually indefinitely—hence, the proliferation of various neuromuscular dysfunction syndromes—the major effects of autonomic neural activation on target organs are immediate but not potentially chronic. This is because of the limited ability of the sympathetic telodendria to continue to constantly release neurotransmitting substances under chronically high stimulation (LeBlanc, 1976). Therefore, in order to maintain high levels of stress arousal for prolonged periods, an additional physiological stress axis must be activated. This axis is the neuroendocrine "fight-or-flight" response axis.

The "Fight-or-Flight" Response—The Neuroendocrine Axis. In 1926, the same year that Selye first described the "syndrome of just being sick," physiologist Walter Cannon first wrote about a phenomenon that he termed *homeostasis,* described as the effort of the physiological systems within the body to actively maintain a level of functioning, within the limits of tolerance of the systems, in the face of ever-changing conditions. Homeostasis was the adaptational effort of the body to stay in balance. From his early efforts, it was clear that the work of Cannon was to parallel and augment that of Selye in terms of understanding the psychophysiological stress response.

Table 2.3. Responses of Effector Organs to Autonomic Nervous System Impulses

	SNS	PSNS
Function	Ergotropic; catabolism	Trophotropic; anabolism
Activity	Diffuse	Discrete
Anatomy		
Emerges from spinal cord	Thoracolumbar	Craniosacral
Location of ganglia	Close to spinal cord	Close to target organ
Postganglionic neurotransmitter	Noradrenalin[a] (adrenergic)	Acetylcholine (cholinergic)
Specific actions		
Pupil of eye	Dilates	Constricts
Lacrimal gland	—	Stimulates secretion
Salivary glands	Scanty, thick secretion	Profuse, water secretion
Heart	Increases heart rate	Decreases heart rate
	Increases contractility	Decreases metabolism
	Increases rate of idiopathic pacemakers in ventricles	
Blood vessels		
Skin and mucosa	Constricts	—
Skeletal muscles	Dilates	—
Cerebral	Constricts	Dilates
Renal	Constricts	—
Abdominal viscera	Mostly constricts	—
Lungs: Bronchial tubes	Dilates	Constricts
Sweat glands	Stimulates[a]	Constricts
Liver	Glycogenolysis for release of glucose	Expels bile
Spleen	Contracts to release blood high in erythrocytes	—
Adrenal medulla	Secretes adrenaline (epinephrine) and noradrenaline (norepinephrine)[a]	—
Gastrointestinal tract	Inhibits digestion	Increases digestion
	Decreases peristalsis and tone	Increases peristalsis and tone
Kidney	Decreases output of urine	?
Hair follicles	Piloerection	—
Male sex organ	Ejaculation	Erection

[a]Postganglionic SNS neurotransmitter is acetylcholine for most sweat glands and some blood vessels in skeletal muscles. Adrenal medulla is innervated by cholinergic sympathetic neurons. Partially adapted from Hassett (1978).

Cannon wrote extensively on one particular aspect of the ANS's role in the stress response—the neuroendocrine process. He researched what he termed the "fight-or-flight" response. The pivotal organ in this response is the adrenal medulla—thus giving this response both neural ANS and endocrine characteristics (Cannon, 1914, 1953; Cannon & Paz, 1911).

The "fight-or-flight" response is thought to be a mobilization of the body to prepare for muscular activity in response to a perceived threat. This mechanism allows the organism either to fight or to flee from the perceived threat (Cannon, 1953).

Research has demonstrated that the homeostatic, neuroendocrine "fight-or-flight" response can be activated in human beings by numerous and diverse psychological influences, including varied psychosocial stimuli (Ametz, Fjeliner, Eneroth, & Kaliner, 1986; Froberg, Karlsson, Levi, & Lidberg, 1971; Levi, 1972; Mason, 1968a, 1972; Roessler & Greenfield, 1962).

The dorsomedial amygdalar complex appears to represent the highest point of origination for the "fight-or-flight" response as a functionally discrete psychophysiological axis (Lang, 1975; Roldan, Alvarez-Palaez, & de Molina, 1974). From that point, the downward flow of neural impulses passes to the lateral and posterior hypothalamic regions (Roldan et al., 1974). From here, neural impulses continue to descend through the thoracic spinal cord, converging at the celiac ganglion, then innervating the adrenal gland, or more specifically, the adrenal medulla.

The adrenal gland in mammals consists of two functionally and histologically discrete constituents: the adrenal medulla and the adrenal cortex. The adrenal medulla consists of chromaffin cells (pheochromoblasts) that lie at the core, or center, of the adrenal gland (*medulla* means stalk). Chromaffin cells are responsible for the creation and secretion of adrenal medullary catecholamines. This process is referred to as *catecholaminogenesis*.

The hormonal output of the neuroendocrine stress-response axis is the secretion of the adrenal medullary catecholamines. There are two adrenal medullary catecholamines: norepinephrine (noradrenaline) and epinephrine (adrenaline). These two hormones are collectively referred to as adrenal medullary catecholamines because of their origin and the chemical nature; that is, these hormones are secreted by the two adrenal medullae that lie at the superior poles of the kidneys. Furthermore, the biochemical structure of these hormones is related to a group of organic compounds referred to as *catechols* (or pyrocatechols).

The adrenal medullary cells are divided into two types: A cells, which secrete epinephrine, and N cells, which secrete norepinephrine. About 80% of the medullary catecholamine activity in humans is accounted for by epinephrine (Harper, 1975). It is critical to note at this juncture that norepinephrine is secreted by not only the adrenal medulla but also the adrenergic neurons of the CNS and the SNS. The biosynthesis and actions are the same regardless of whether the norepinephrine originates in the medulla or in the adrenergic neurons of the CNS or SNS (see Appendix F).

Upon neural stimulation, the adrenal medulla releases the medullary catecholamines as just described. The effect of these medullary catecholamines is an increase in generalized adrenergic somatic activity in human beings (Folkow & Neil, 1971; Maranon, 1924; Wenger et al., 1960). The effect, therefore, is functionally identical to that of direct sympathetic innervation (see Table 2.3), except that the medullary catecholamines require a 20- to 30-sec delay of onset for measurable effects and display a 10-fold increase in effect duration (Usdin, Kretnansky, & Kopin, 1976). Also, the catecholamines only prolong the adrenergic sympathetic response. Cholinergic responses, such as increased electrodermal activity and bronchiole effects, are unaffected by medullary catecholamine release (Usdin et al., 1976).

The "fight-or-flight" response has been somewhat reformulated by writers such as Schneiderman (McCabe & Schneiderman, 1984), who view this system as an "active coping" system. This active coping system has been referred to as the "sympathoadrenomedullary system" (SAM).

Specific somatic effects that have been suggested or observed in humans as a result of activation of this axis in response to psychosocial stressor exposure are summarized in Table 2.4.

This brings us to a discussion of the third and final stress response mechanism—the endocrine axes.

Table 2.4. Effects of Adrenal Medullary Axis Stimulation[a]

Increased arterial blood pressure
Increased blood supply to brain (moderate)
Increased heart rate and cardiac output
Increased stimulation of skeletal muscles
Increased plasma free fatty acids, triglycerides, cholesterol
Increased release of endogenous opioids
Decreased blood flow to kidneys
Decreased blood flow to gastrointestinal system
Decreased blood flow to skin
Increased risk of hypertension
Increased risk of thrombosis formation
Increased risk of angina pectoris attacks in persons so prone
Increased risk of arrhythmias
Increased risk of sudden death from lethal arrhythmia, myocardial ischemia, myocardial fibrillation, myocardial infarction

[a]See Brod, 1959, 1971; Froberg, Karlsson, Levi, & Lidberg, 1971; Henry & Stephens, 1977; Ametz, Fjellner, Eneroth, & Kallner, 1986; Axelrod & Reisine, 1984; McCabe & Schneiderman, 1984, for reviews.

Endocrine Axes. The most chronic and prolonged somatic responses to stress are the result of the endocrine axes (Mason, 1968b). Four well-established endocrine axes have been associated with the stress response:

1. The adrenal cortical axis
2. The somatotropic axis
3. The thyroid axis
4. The posterior pituitary axis

These axes not only represent the most chronic aspects of the stress response but also require greater intensity stimulation to activate (Levi, 1972).

Reviews by Axelrod and Reisine (1984), Levi (1972), Makara et al. (1980), Mason (1968c, 1972), Mason et al. (1995), McCabe and Schneiderman (1984), McKerns and Pantic (1985), Selye (1976), and Yehuda et al. (1995) demonstrate that these axes can be activated in humans by numerous and diverse psychological stimuli, including varied psychosocial stimuli.

The Adrenal Cortical Axis. The septal–hippocampal complex appears to represent the highest point of origination for the adrenal cortical axis as a physiologically discrete mechanism (Henry & Ely, 1976; Henry & Stephens, 1977). From these points, neural impulses descend to the median eminence of the hypothalamus. The neurosecretory cells in the median eminence release corticotropin-releasing factor (CRF) into the hypothalamic–hypophyseal portal system (Rochefort, Rosenberger, & Saffran, 1959). The CRF descends the infundibular stalk to the cells of the anterior pituitary. The chemophobes of the anterior pituitary are sensitive to the presence of CRF and respond by releasing adrenocorticotropic hormone (ACTH) in the systemic circulation. At the same time, the precursor to the various endogenous analgesic opioids (endorphins) is released. This precursor substance, beta lipotropin, yields the proliferation of endogenous opioids during human stress (Rossier, Bloom, & Guillemin, 1980).

ACTH is carried through the systemic circulation until it reaches its primary target organ: an endocrine gland, the adrenal cortex. The two adrenal cortices are wrapped around the two adrenal medullae (neuroendocrine axis) and sit at the superior poles of the kidneys.

ACTH appears to act upon three discrete layers, or zona, of the adrenal cortex. It stimulates the cells of the zona reticularis and zona fasciculata to release the glucocorticoids cortisol and corticosterone into the systemic circulation. The effects of the glucocorticoids in apparent response to stressful stimuli are summarized in Table 2.5.

Table 2.5. The Effects of the Glucocorticoid Hormones[a] and HPAC Activation

Increased glucose production (gluconeogenesis)
Exacerbation of gastric irritation
Increased urea production
Increased release of free fatty acids into systemic circulation
Increased susceptibility arteherosclerotic processes
Increased susceptibility to nonthrombotic myocardial necrosis
Thymicolymphatic atrophy (demonstrated in animals only)
Supression of immune mechanisms
Exacerbation of herpes simplex
Increased ketone body production
Appetite supression
Associated feelings of depression, hopelessness, helplessness, and a loss of control

[a]See Henry & Stephens (1977), Selye (1976), Yates & Maran (1972), Yuwiler (1976), MaCabe & Schneiderman (1984), and Makara, Palkovitz, & Szentagothal (1980) for reviews.

Similarly, ACTH allows the zona glomerulosa to secrete the mineralo-corticoids aldosterone and deoxycorticosterone into the systemic circulation. The primary effects of aldosterone release are an increase in the absorption of sodium and chloride by the renal tubules and a decrease in their excretion by the salivary glands, sweat glands, and gastrointestinal tract. Subsequent fluid retention is noted as a corollary of this process. Although cortisol does exhibit some of these properties, aldosterone is about 1,000 times more potent as an electrolyte effector. As the prepotent mineralocorticoid, aldos-terone may effect other physiological outcomes, among them increasing glycogen deposits in the liver and decreasing circulating eosinophils.

Excessive activation of mineralocorticoid secretion in human beings has been implicated in the development of Cushing's syndrome (hyper-adrenocorticism) by Gifford and Gunderson (1970) and in high blood pressure and myocardial necrosis by Selye (1976).

As a tropic hormone, the main function of ACTH is to stimulate the synthesis and secretion of the glucocorticoid hormones from the adrenal cor-tex, yet ACTH is known to cause the release of cortical adrenal androgenic hormones such as testosterone as well. Finally, there is evidence that ACTH affects the release of the catecholamines described earlier in this chapter. Its effect on the catecholamines epinephrine and norepinephrine appears to be through a modulation of tyrosine hydroxylase, which is the "rate-limiting" step in catecholamine synthesis. This effect is a minor one, however, com-pared with other influences on tyrosine hydroxylase. Thus, adrenal medullary and cortical activities can be highly separate, even inversely related, at times (Kopin, 1976; Lundberg & Forsman, 1978). See Axelrod and Reisine (1984) for an excellent review of hormonal interaction and regulation.

The adrenal cortical response axis has been referred to by various authors (e.g., McCabe & Schneiderman, 1984), as the hypothalamic–pituitary–adrenal cortical system (HPAC). Activation of this system in the aggregate has been associated with the helplessness/hopelessness depression syndrome, passivity, the perception of no control, immunosuppression, and gastrointestinal symptomatology. Behaviorally, the HPAC system appears to be activated when active coping is not possible; thus, it has been called the "passive coping" system. Considering the HPAC system with respect to the SAM, Frankenhauser (1980) has concluded:

1. Effort without distress → activation of the SAM response system.
2. Distress without effort → activation of the HPAC response system.
3. Effort with distress → activation of both SAM and HPAC.

The most extreme variation of the human stress response is, arguably, posttraumatic stress. The codified variant of this response is posttraumatic stress disorder (PTSD), the subject of a specialized review in Chapter 20. Nevertheless, we believe it warrants mention in this discussion of physiological mechanisms because of complex and often contradictory findings. In PTSD, both the adrenal medullary catecholamine axis and the HPAC pathways are implicated in PTSD. Given the aforementioned discussion, one would expect increased glucocorticoid secretion in PTSD given the intensity, chronicity, and overall severity of PTSD as a clinical synrome. While enhanced cortisol secretion is, indeed, evidenced in PTSD patients, there is also evidence of decreased cortisol secretion. Yehuda et al. (1995) provide a useful review and reformulation of this issue. PTSD patients evidence enhanced CRF activity but lower overall cortisol levels in many instances. These authors summarize as follows:

> The study of PTSD, whose definition rests on being the sequelae of stress, represents an opportunity to express the effects of extreme stress…from a unique perspective. The findings suggest that…individuals who suffer from PTSD show evidence of a highly sensitized HPA axis characterized by decreased basal cortisol levels, increased number of lymphocyte glucocorticoid receptors, a greater suppression of cortisol to dexamethasone, and a more sensitized pituitary gland. (p. 362)

Thus, in summary, in addition to the more "classic" Selyean observation of increased cortisol as a constituent of extreme stress, PTSD may represent an extension of the Selyean formulation characterized by an increase in CRF, a hypersensitized pituitary, and a resultant down-regulation of the HPAC system via an enhanced negative feedback system. As Yehuda et al. (1995) note, "The findings challenge us to regard the stress response as diversified and varied, rather than as conforming to a simple, unidirectional pattern" (pp. 362–363).

The Somatotropic Axis. The somatotropic axis appears to share the same basic physiological mechanisms from the septal–hippocampal complex through the hypothalamic–hypophyseal portal system as the previous axis, with the exception that somatotropin-releasing factor (SRF) stimulates the anterior pituitary within this axis. The anterior pituitary responds to the SRF by releasing growth hormone (somatotropic hormone) into the systemic circulation (see Makara et al., 1980; Selye, 1976).

The role of growth hormone in stress is somewhat less clearly understood than that of the adrenal cortical axis. However, research has documented its release in response to psychological stimuli in human beings (Selye, 1976), and certain effects are suspected. Selye (1956) has stated that growth hormone stimulates the release of the mineralocorticoids. Yuwiler (1976), in his review of stress and endocrine function, suggests that growth hormone produces a diabetic-like insulin-resistant effect, as well as mobilization of fats stored in the body. The effect is an increase in the concentration of free fatty acids and glucose in the blood.

The Thyroid Axis. The thyroid axis is now a well-established stress response mechanism. From the median eminence of the hypothalamus is released thyrotropin-releasing factor (TRF). The infundibular stalk carries the TRF to its target—the anterior pituitary. From here, the tropic thyroid-stimulating hormone (TSH) is released into the systemic circulation. TSH ultimately stimulates the thyroid gland to release two thyroid hormones: triiodothyronine (T3) and thyroxine (T4). Once secreted into the systemic circulation system, these hormones are bound to specific plasma protein carriers, primarily thyroxin-binding globulin (TBG). A small amount of the thyroid hormones remains as "free" unbound hormones. About .04% of T4 and about .4% of T3 remain unbound. Proper evaluation of thyroid function is best based upon an assessment of free thyroid hormones. At the level of target-cell tissue, only free hormone is metabolically active.

The T3 and T4 hormones serve to participate in a negative feedback loop, thus suppressing their own subsequent secretion.

In humans, psychosocial stimuli have generally led to an increase in thyroidal activity (Levi, 1972; Makara et al., 1980; Yuwiler, 1976). Levi (1972) has stated that the thyroid hormones have been shown to increase general metabolism, heart rate, heart contractility, peripheral vascular resistance (thereby increasing blood pressure), and the sensitivity of some tissues to catecholamines. Hypothyroidism has been linked to depressive episodes. Levi therefore concludes that the thyroid axis could play a significant role as a response axis in human stress. See Mason et al. (1995) for a comprehensive review.

The Posterior Pituitary Axis and Other Phenomena. Since the early 1930s, there has been speculation on the role of the posterior pituitary in the stress response. The posterior pituitary (neurohypophysis) receives neural impulses from the supraoptic nuclei of the hypothalamus. Stimulation from these nuclei results in the release of the hormones vasopressin (antidiuretic hormone, or ADH) and oxytocin into the systemic circulation.

ADH affects the human organism by increasing the permeability of the collecting ducts that lie subsequent to the distal ascending tubules within the glomerular structures of the kidneys. The end result is water retention.

Corson and Corson (1971), in their review of psychosocial influences on renal function, note several studies that report significant amounts of water retention in apparent response to psychological influences in human beings.

Although there seems to be agreement that water retention can be psychogenically induced, there is little agreement on the specific mechanism. Corson and Corson (1971) report studies that point to the release of elevated amounts of ADH in response to stressful episodes. On the other hand, some studies conclude that the antidiuretic effect is due to decreased renal blood flow. Some human subjects even responded with a diuretic response to psychosocial stimuli.

Nevertheless, Makara et al. (1980), in their review of 25 years of research, found ample evidence for the increased responsiveness of ADH during the stress response. ADH is now seen as one of the wide range of diverse, stress-responsive hormones.

Oxytocin, the other major hormone found in the posterior pituitary axis, is synthesized in the same nuclei as ADH, but in different cells. Its role in the human stress response is currently unclear but may be involved in psychogenic labor contractions (Omer & Everly, 1988) and premature birth.

Various investigations have shown that both interstitial cell-stimulating hormone (Sowers et al., 1977), also known as luteinizing hormone, and testosterone (Williams, 1986) have been shown to be responsive to the presentation of various stressors.

Finally, the hormone prolactin has clearly shown responsiveness to psychosocial stimulation as well (see Makara et al., 1980). The role of prolactin in disease or dysfunction phenomena, however, has not been well established. Attempts to link prolactin with premenstral dysfunction have yet to yield a clear line of evidence. The specific role of prolactin in stress-related disease needs further elucidation.

The "General Adaptation Syndrome".   As a means of integrating his psychoendocrinological research, Hans Seyle (1956) proposed an integrative model for the stress response, known as the "General Adaptation Syndrome" (GAS).

The GAS is a triphasic phenomenon. The first phase Selye refers to as the "alarm" phase, representing a generalized somatic shock, or "call to arms" of the body's defense mechanisms. The second phase is called the "stage of resistance," in which there is a dramatic reduction in most alarm stage processes and the body fights to reestablish and maintain homeostasis. Stages 1 and 2 can be repeated throughout one's life. Should the stressor persist, however, eventually the "adaptive energy," that is, the adaptive mechanisms in the second stage, may become depleted. At this point, the body enters the third and final stage, the "stage of exhaustion," which, when applied to a target organ, is indicative of the exhaustion of that organ, and the symptoms of disease and dysfunction become manifest. When the final stage is applied to the entire body, life itself may be in jeopardy. The three stages of the GAS are detailed in Table 2.6.

The Stress Response: A Summary

In this section, we have presented a unifying perspective from which to view the complex psychophysiological processes that have come to be

Table 2.6. The General Adaptation Syndrome

Alarm Stage
    Sympathetic nervous system arousal
    Adrenal medullary stimulation
    ACTH release
    Cortisol release
    Growth hormone release
    Prolactin release
    Increased thyroid activity
    Gonadotropin activity increased
    Anxiety
Resistance Stage
    Reduction in adrenal cortical activity
    Reduction in sympathetic nervous system activity
    Homeostatic mechanisms engaged
Exhaustion Stage
    Enlargement of lymphatic structures
    Target organ disease/dysfunction manifest
    Increased vulnerability to opportunistic disease
    Psychological exhaustion: depression
    Physiological exhaustion: disease → death?

known as the stress response. The intention was to provide clinicians with an understandable interpretation of the complexities of the stress-response process that they often find themselves treating. Because effective treatment of the stress phenomenon is related to comprehension of the nature of the problem (Miller, 1978, 1979), it is our hope that this discussion will prove useful for the clinician.

The unifying thread throughout this discussion has been the temporal sequencing of the stress-response process. We have shown that the most immediate response to a stressful stimulus occurs via the direct neural innervations of end organs. The intermediate stress effects are due to the neuroendocrine "fight-or-flight" axis. The reaction time of this axis is reduced by its utilization of systemic circulation as a transport mechanism. However, its effects range from intermediate to chronic in duration and may overlap with the last stress-response system to respond to a stimulus—the endocrine axes. The endocrine axes are the final pathways to react to stressful stimuli, owing primarily to the almost total reliance on the circulatory system for transportation, as well as the fact that a higher intensity stimulus is needed to activate this axis. The GAS provides an additional schema to extend the endocrine response axis in the adaptation of the organism to the presence of a chronic stressor (see Selye, 1956, for a discussion of diseases of adaptation). Figure 2.8 summarizes the sequential activation of the stress-response axes.

It is important to understand that there is a potential for the activation of each of these axes to overlap. The most common axes to be simultaneously active are the neuroendocrine and endocrine axes—both of which have potential for chronic responsivity (Mason, 1968a,c).

On the other hand, it is clear that all mechanisms and axes detailed cannot possibly discharge each and every time a person is faced with a stressor. Perhaps clearest of all is the fact that each sympathetic and parasympathetic effect is not manifest to all stressors. Therefore, what determines which stress-response mechanisms will be activated by which stressors in which individuals? The answer to this question is currently unknown. However, some evidence suggests the existence of a psychophysiological predisposition for some individuals to undergo stress-response pattern specificity (see Sternbach, 1966). We expand on this topic in Chapter 3.

These, then, are the stress-response axes and the various mechanisms that work within each. They represent the potential response patterns result each time the human organism is exposed to a stressor. As to when each responds and why, we are unsure at this time. Current speculations are reviewed in Chapter 3. Despite this uncertainty, the clinician should gain useful insight into the treatment of the stress response by understanding the psychophysiological processes involved once the stress

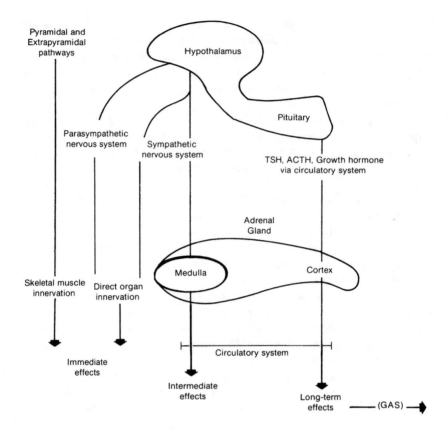

Figure 2.8. Temporal relationship between primary stress axes.

response becomes activated. To assist the reader in putting the picture together, Figure 2.9 provides a unique "global" perspective into the multi-axial nature of psychophysiological stress.

As a final note, returning to Figure 2.6, feedback loops II and III simply indicate the ability of the physiological stress response to further stimulate the cognitive–affective domain as well as the neurological triggering mechanisms, so as to further promulgate the stress response. Such a feedback mechanism may provide the potential for a psychophysiologically self-sustaining response. This, then, is the physiology of human stress as currently understood.

Target-Organ Activation

The term *target-organ activation* as used in the present model refers to the phenomenon in which the neural, neuroendocrine, and endocrine

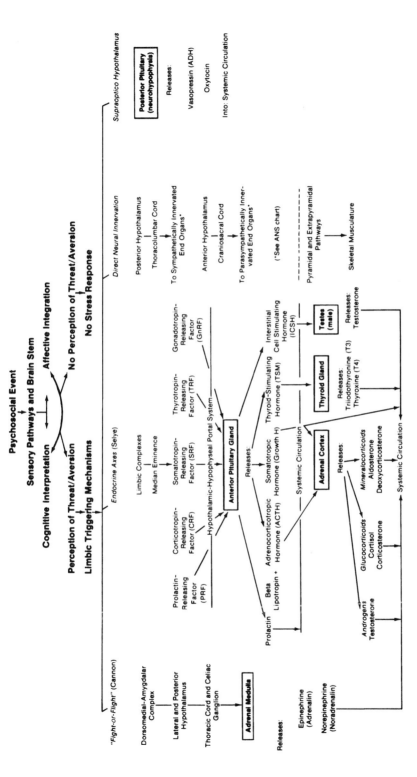

Figure 2.9. The multiaxial nature of the stress response.

constituents of the stress response just described (1) activate, (2) increase or (3) inhibit normal activation, or (4) catabolize some organ system in the human body. Potential target-organ systems for the stress response include the cardiovascular system, the gastronintestinal system, the skin, the immune system, and even the brain and its mental status, to mention only a few. It is from activation of the target organs and the subsequent emergence of various clinical signs and symptoms that we often deduce the presence of excessive stress arousal.

As for which target organs are most likely to manifest stress-related disease or dysfunction, it appears that two major biogenic factors assist in that determination: response mechanism stereotypy (Sternbach, 1966) and target-organ specificity (Everly, 1978). *Response mechanism stereotypy* refers to a preferential pattern of stress-related neural, neuroendocrine, or endocrine activation. The more consistent such activation, the greater the likelihood of a stress-related disease (Stoyva, 1977). Target-organ specificity refers to a predisposing vulnerability of the target organ to experience pathogenic arousal (Everly, 1986). Genetic, prenatal, neonatal, and traumatic stimuli may all play a role in such a determination.

Finally, feedback loop IV (in Figure 2.6) indicates that target-organ activation and subsequent signs and symptoms of disease may affect the patient's cognitive–affective behavior and, therefore, further neurological triggering and continued stress-response activity. In some cases (e.g., agoraphobic patients, obsessive patients, and hysteria-prone patients), a hypersensitive awareness to target-organ symptoms can create a self-sustaining pathogenic feedback loop.

We elaborate upon the issue of target-organ disease in the next chapter.

COPING

The preceding two sections went into great detail in an attempt to describe what many phenomenologists have called the "missing link" in psychosomatic phenomena, that is, the physiological mechanisms of mediation by which cognitive–affective discord could result in physical disease and dysfunction. It is an understanding of these physiological mechanisms of mediation that allows us to see stress-related disorders as the quintessential intertwining of "mind and body" as opposed to some anomaly of hysteria. Yet we know that the manifestations of human stress are highly varied and individualistic. Whereas biological predisposition certainly plays a role in this process, a major factor in determining the impact of stress on the patient is his or her perceived ability to cope.

Coping is defined as

> efforts, both action-oriented and intrapsychic, to manage (that is, master, tolerate, reduce, minimize) environmental and internal demands, and conflicts among them, which tax or exceed a person's resources. Coping can occur prior to a stressful confrontation, in which case it is called anticipatory coping, as well as in reaction to a present or past confrontation with harm. (Cohen & Lazarus, 1979, p. 219)

More recently, coping has been defined as "constantly changing cognitive and behavioral efforts to manage specific … demands that are appraised as taxing or exceeding the resources of the person" (Lazarus & Folkman, 1984, p. 141).

From the perspective of the current model (Figure 2.6), coping may be thought of as environmental or cognitive tactics designed to attenuate the stress response. The present model views coping as residing subsequent to the physiological stress response and target-organ activation. Thus, coping is seen as an attempt to reestablish homeostasis. Anticipatory coping, as mentioned by Lazarus and other theorists, is subsumed, in the present model, in the complex interactions of the cognitive–affective domain.

To further refine the notion of coping, we suggest that coping strategies can be either adaptive or maladaptive (Girdano, Everly, & Dusek, 2001). Adaptive coping strategies reduce stress while at the same time promoting long-term health (e.g., exercise, relaxation, proper nutrition). Maladaptive coping strategies, on the other hand, do indeed reduce stress in the short term but serve to erode health in the long term (alcohol/drug abuse, cigarette smoking, interpersonal withdrawal) (see Everly, 1979a).

Figure 2.6 reflects the belief that when coping is successful, extraordinary target-organ activation is reduced or eliminated and homeostasis is reestablished. If coping strategies are unsuccessful, target-organ activation is maintained and the chances of target-organ disease are increased.

Feedback loops V and VI once again reflect the interrelatedness of all components included in Figure 2.6.

The model depicted in Figure 2.6 reflects an integration of recent research and critical thought concerning human stress. It is presented as nothing more than a pedagogical tool designed to facilitate the clinician's understanding of the phenomenology of the stress response. If it has sensitized the clinician to the major components of the stress response and shown their interrelatedness, it has served its purpose. This phenomenological model is used as a common reference in subsequent chapters to facilitate better understanding of the topics of measurement and treatment of the human stress response.

SUMMARY

Our purpose has been to provide a somewhat detailed analysis of the psychophysiological nature of the human stress response. Let us review the main points of this chapter.

1. The nervous systems serve as the foundation of the stress response. The neuron is the smallest functional unit within any given nervous system. Communications between neurons, and therefore within nervous systems, are based upon electrical (ionic transport) and chemical (neurotransmitter mobilization) processes.

Nervous systems are anatomically arranged in the following schema:
  I. Central nervous system
     A. Brain
     B. Spinal
  II. Peripheral nervous systems
     A. Somatic (to skeletal musculature)
     B. Autonomic (to glands, organs, viscera)
        1. Sympathetic
        2. Parasympathetic

2. Figure 2.6, which represents an integrative epiphenomenological model of the stress response, is reproduced once again here as Figure 2.10 for review purposes. Let us summarize its components.

3. Environmental events (stressors) may either "cause" the activation of the stress response (as in the case of sympathomimetic stressors) or, as is usually the case, simply "set the stage" for the mobilization of the stress response.

4. The cognitive–affective domain is the critical "causal" phase in most stress reactions. Stress, like beauty, appears to be in the eye of the beholder. One's interpretation of the environmental event is what creates most stressors and subsequent stress responses.

5. The locus ceruleus, limbic complexes, and the hypothalamic nuclei trigger efferent neurological, neuroendocrine, and endocrine reactions in response to higher cognitive–affective interactions.

6. The actual stress response itself is the next step in the system's analysis. Possessing at least three major efferent axes—neurological, neuroendocrine, and endocrine—this "physiological mechanism of mediation" represents numerous combinations and permutations of efferent activity directed toward numerous and diverse target organs (see Figure 2.9).

The most rapid of the physiological stress axes are the neurological axes. They consist of mobilization of the sympathetic, parasympathetic, and neuromuscular nervous systems. The neuroendocrine axis, sometimes called the sympathoadrenomedullary system (SAM), but better known as

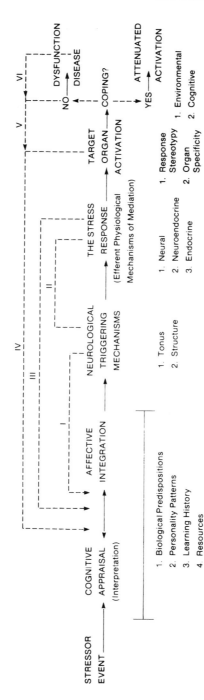

Figure 2.10. A systems model of the human stress response.

Cannon's "fight-or-flight" response, is next to be mobilized. Activation leads to the extraordinary release of epinephrine and norepinephrine. Finally, the endocrine axes, researched primarily by Hans Selye, are potential response mechanisms. Consisting of the adrenal cortical axis (HPAC system), the somatotropic axis, the thyroid axis, and the posterior pituitary axis, these axes play a major role in chronic disease and dysfunction. Selye's notion of the General Adaptation Syndrome is an attempt to unify these axes (see Table 2.6).

7. As a result of the stress response axes being extraordinarily mobilized, target-organ activation is realized.

8. The final step before pathogenic target-organ activation is coping. Here, the patient has the opportunity to act environmentally or cognitively, or both, so as to reduce or mitigate the overall amplitude and level of activation that reaches the target organs.

9. Should stress arousal be excessive in either acute intensity or chronicity, target-organ dysfunction and/or pathology will result.

10. As a final note, remember that the aforementioned axes are always activated at some level of functioning. Inclusion in this chapter simply reflects their potential for pathogenic arousal in response to stressor stimuli and thus their aggregate designation as the physiological mechanisms of the stress response.

11. In summary, this chapter was designed to provide the reader with a reasonable approximation of the mechanisms that serve to link the stressor stimulus with target-organ activation. Chapter 3 extends this examination into the link between stress arousal and subsequent disease.

3

The Link from
Stress Arousal to Disease

The notion that one's psychosocial environment, lifestyle, and attitudes are linked to disease is by no means a new idea, as discussed in Chapter 1. In a scholarly meta-analysis, Tower (1984) reviewed 523 published reports investigating the relationship between psychosocial factors and disease. Ultimately selecting 60 of those studies on the basis of design considerations, she then submitted the data to a meta-analysis. The results supported the conclusion that there exists a strong relationship between psychosocial factors and illness. She notes, "Psychological well-being appeared to be most strongly associated with coronary heart disease and infectious processes ... although it was significantly associated with all diseases [investigated] except complications of pregnancy" (p. 51). To assess the power of her findings, Tower calculated the number of fugitive studies required to reject the findings of her meta-analysis. The results of this analysis of outcome tolerance revealed that over 28,000 fugitive studies would be required to reject the conclusion that psychosocial factors are related to disease.

In the tradition of Pasteur, however, in order for a stimulus to be recognized as being a credible cause or contributor to disease, the pathophysiological processes that culminate in target-organ disease and dysfunction (sometimes called *mechanisms of mediation*) must be understood. Chapter 2 reviewed a model by which a *stressor* may activate *stress-response mechanisms*. That chapter further detailed potential stress-response effector mechanisms that might undergird such pathogenic relationships as confirmed by Tower (1984). The chapter offered evidence that an aggregation of neural, neuroendocrine, and endocrine response axes, collectively referred to as the *stress response*, were indeed vulnerable to extraordinary activation upon exposure to psychosocial stimuli. This chapter examines the logical extension of stress physiology by reviewing several noteworthy models of target-organ pathogenesis, that is, those proposed factors that link *stress arousal* mechanisms, once they are activated, to *target-organ disease.*

Although the literature in psychosomatic phenomenology as a global concept is voluminous, relatively few models exist that concern themselves more directly with the link between extraordinary arousal of the stress axes and the ultimate manifestations of stress-related disease. Let us take this opportunity to review several of those models.

SELYE'S "GENERAL ADAPTATION SYNDROME"

In Chapter 2, Selye's General Adaptation Syndrome (GAS) was introduced as a means of integrating the manifestations of the stress response as a sequential series of physiological events. Its triphasic constituency was described at that point: (1) the alarm stage, (2) the stage of resistance (adaptation), and (3) the exhaustion stage. The GAS is mentioned in the present chapter because, not only does it serve to integrate, from a temporal perspective, many of the stress axes described earlier, but it also serves to explain the link from stress arousal to disease. As described by Selye (1956), Stage 1 of the GAS involves a somatic "shock" and initial "alarm reaction" for biological sources within the body following exposure to a stressor. The insult to the bodily tissues during this acute alarm phase could be so great as to deprive the target organ of its ability to compensate. If this happens, as might occur in cases of burns, electrical shock, or acute psychological trauma, the target organ may simply cease to function (e.g., in the case of cardiac fibrillation). Thus the target organ will have been traumatically exhausted and rendered incapable of further functioning. Serious illness or death may then result.

If, however, the resources of the body are not completely compromised as a result of the "alarm" phase, then the stage of resistance is entered. Here the body's resources are mobilized to reestablish homeostasis. This is what usually occurs in most stress-related conditions. Yet, in order to maintain homeostasis in the face of a persistent stressor, there is a chronic drain of "adaptive energy," that is, physiological resources. Should the stressor persist indefinitely (even in the form of cognitive rumination) or should Stages 1 and 2 recycle themselves too frequently, eventual exhaustion of the target organ is predicted. This is the third and final stage in Selye's schema, the exhaustion phase. Thus stress-related disease manifestation would occur as a result of a depletion of adaptive physiological resources and the subsequent target-organ exhaustion would be considered a result of excessive "wear and tear" (Selye, 1974). This then is the GAS as it attempts to define the stress-to-disease process. The GAS has been criticized for its global generality and lack of sensitivity for physiological response specificity (Mason, 1971).

In Selye's original exposition, he states, "It seems to us that more or less pronounced forms of this three-stage reaction represent the usual response of the organism to stimuli such as temperature changes, drugs, muscular exercise, etc., to which habituation or inurement can occur" (1936, p. 32). Yet subsequent researchers such as Mason (1971) argued that the stress response and subsequent target-organ pathology may indeed be rather specific, rather than generalized, pathogenic processes. This was a point with which Selye would have to contend for the rest of his career.

Given that Selye's important formulations were from the perspective of an endocrinologist more interested in pathogenic mechanisms than target-organ pathology per se, later writers in the emerging field of psychosomatic medicine would greatly elaborate upon the link from stress arousal to stress-related disease. Those mechanisms we consider most important are summarized below.

LACHMAN'S MODEL

In a "behavioral interpretation" of psychosomatic disease, Lachman (1972) proposes an "autonomic learning theory" that emphasizes

> ... the role of learning in the development of psychosomatic aberrations without minimizing the role of genetic factors or of nongenetic predisposing factors. The essence of the theory proposed is that psychosomatic manifestations result from frequent or prolonged or intense ... reactions elicited via stimulation of receptors. (pp. 62–63)

Lachman argues that a major source of frequent, prolonged, or intense emotional and physiological reactions is a *learned* pattern of emotional and autonomic responsiveness. More specifically, he notes with regard to the stress-to-disease phenomenon, "In order for emotional reactions to assume pathological significance such reactions must be intense or chronic or both" (p. 70). He goes on to state that which end-organ structure will be affected pathologically depends on the following:

1. Genetic factors that biologically predispose the organ to harm from psychophysiological arousal.
2. Environmental factors that predispose the organ to harm from psychophysiological arousal, including such things as nutritional

influences, infectious disease influences, physical trauma influences, and so on.

3. The specific structures involved in the physiological reactivity.
4. The magnitude of involvement during the physiological response, which he has defined in terms of intensity, frequency, and duration of involvement of the organ.

Lachman (1972) concludes that the determination of which structure is ultimately affected in the psychosomatic reaction depends on "the biological condition of the structure" (whether a function of genetic or environmental influences), "on the initial reactivity threshold of the organ, and on ... learning factors" that affect the activation of the organ. He goes on to note that the "magnitude of the psychosomatic phenomenon" appears to be a function of the frequency, intensity, and chronicity of the organ's activation.

STERNBACH'S MODEL

In a somewhat more psychophysiologically oriented model, Sternbach (1966) provides another perspective on the stress-to-disease issue, which is considered a variation on the diathesis–stress model of Levi and Andersson (1975).

The first step in Sternbach's model is *response stereotypy*. This term generally refers to the tendency of an individual to exhibit characteristically similar patterns of psychophysiological reactivity to a variety of stressful stimuli. Sternbach views it as a "predisposed response set." That such a response stereotypy phenomenon does indeed exist has been clearly demonstrated in patient and normal populations (Lacey & Lacey, 1958, 1962; Malmo & Shagass, 1949; Moos & Engel, 1962; Schnore, 1959).

Response stereotypy may be generally thought of as a form of the "weak-link" or "weak-organ" theory of psychosomatic disease. Whether the weak organ is genetically determined, a function of conditioning, or acquired through disease or physical trauma is unclear.

The second step in the Sternbach model entails the frequent activation of the psychophysiological stress response within the stereotypical organ. As Stoyva (1977) notes, the mere existence of response stereotypy is not enough to cause disease. It is obvious that the organ must be involved in frequent activation in order to be adversely affected.

Finally, Sternbach's model includes the requirement that homeostatic mechanisms fail; that is, once the stereotypical organ has undergone psychophysiological arousal, that stress-responsive organ must now evidence slow return to baseline level of activity. Such homeostatic failure has been implicated in the onset of disease since the work of Freeman (1939). Freeman advanced the theory that autonomic excitation that is slow to deactivate from an organ system does increase the strain on that system. Malmo, Shagass, and Davis (1950) empirically demonstrated that such a phenomenon exists. Lader's (1969) review on this issue implicates it as a potential precursor to disease.

Sternbach (1966) has then put forward these conditions as prerequisites for the development of a stress-related disorder. The reader is referred to the work of Stoyva for further commentary on the Sternbach model, as well as other theories of psychosomatic illness (Stoyva, 1976, 1977; Stoyva & Budzynski, 1974).

KRAUS AND RAAB'S "HYPOKINETIC DISEASE" MODEL

In their treatise on exercise and health, Kraus and Raab (1961) argue that many stress-related diseases are induced not so much by the direct physiology of the stress response, but by the lack of subsequent somato-motor expression of that physiology. They argue that a little over 100 years ago, vigorous physical labor was a way of life that actually served as a protective mechanism against diseases commonly referred to today as "diseases of civilization." These authors suggest that modern sedentary lifestyles have put that protective mechanism "all but out of commission." Kraus and Raab (1961) conclude:

> The system that has been put all but out of commission, the striated musculature ... has an important role which exceeds the mere function of locomotion. Action of the striated muscle influences directly and indirectly circulation, metabolism, and endocrine balance. ... Last but not least the striated muscle serves as an outlet for our emotions and nervous responses. ... Obliteration of [this] important safety valve ... might well upset the original balance to which the bodies of primitive man have been adapted. (p. 4)

Therefore Kraus and Raab coined the term "hypokinetic disease" (*hypo* = under; *kinetic* = motion/exercise) to refer to a wide array of diseases that as a result of the lack of healthful expression/utilization of the physiological mechanisms of the stress response. The notion of the lack of physical activity serving as a risk factor for disease and dysfunction has been supported by the World Health Organization (Chavat et al., 1964), which conclude that suppression of somatomotor activity in response to stress arousal is likely to lead to increased cardiovascular strain.

SCHWARTZ'S "DISREGULATION" MODEL

Gary Schwartz, working at Yale University (1977, 1979), devised a general systems model of stress-related pathogenesis that revolves around homeostatic disregulation as its pathogenic core (see Figure 3.1). He notes, "It follows directly from cybernetic and systems theory that a normally self regulatory system can become disordered when communication... between specific parts of the system is... disrupted" (1979, p. 563).

Schwartz (1977) describes his model:

> When the environment (Stage 1) places demands on a person, the brain (Stage 2) performs the regulatory functions necessary to meet the specific demands. Depending on the nature of the environmental demand on stress, certain bodily systems (Stage 3) will be activated, while others may be simultaneously inhibited. However, if this process is sustained to the point where the tissue suffers deterioration or injury, the negative feedback loops (Stage 4) of the homeostatic mechanism will normally come into play, forcing the brain to modify its directives to aid the afflicted organ. (p. 76)

Thus the negative feedback loops described by Schwartz dominate the normal physiological milieu and are necessary to effective, adaptive functioning. Yet Schwartz argues that it is a *disregulation* in Stage 4 homeostatic mechanisms that may lead to a host of stress-related diseases through target-organ overstimulation. Overstimulation may occur by the creation of positive, self-sustaining feedback mechanisms or the blockage of natural

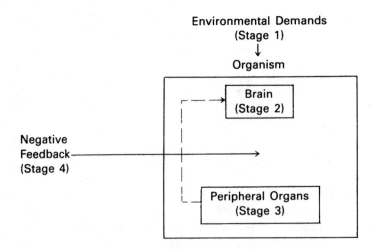

Figure 3.1. Schwartz's model.

inhibitory processes. Schwartz argues that disconnection of any feedback mechanism, from a systems view, is capable of leading to disregulation and thus to disease.

Congruent with the aforementioned model, therapeutic interventions would entail reestablishing homeostasis (homeostatic regulation). Consistent with this is Greengard's (1978) perspective based on the observation of physiological systems: "It seems probable that derangements of homeostatic processes are responsible for many disease states. Conversely, it seems likely that the effects of many therapeutic ... agents are exerted on such homeostatic systems" (p. 146). Therefore, as one might expect, Schwartz sees biofeedback and other autoregulatory therapies as useful agents for the treatment of stress-related disorders.

CONFLICT THEORY OF PSYCHOSOMATIC DISEASE

Spawned in the formulative years of psychosomatic medicine, Alexander (1950) postulated that specific types of conflicts lead to specific types of physical illnesses. More specifically, specific psychical conflicts engendered specific mechanisms of physiological pathogenesis. The result was a specific target-organ illness. Several specific conflict–illness relationships were suggested:

Guilt   → vomiting
Alienation   → constipation
Repressed hostility   → migraine headaches
Dependence   → asthma

More recently, Harris (1991), using a specially designed psychometric instrument, the Life Events and Difficulties Schedule (LEDS), empirically investigated the relationship between life events and illness. The following relationships emerged:

Long-term threat and loss → depression
Danger   → anxiety
Goal frustration   → gastrointestinal disorders and
                            coronary artery disease
Major challenge   → amenorrhea or dysmenorrhea

With the possible exception of Rosenman and Friedman's (1974) Type A behavior pattern and its predictive relationship with premature coronary artery disease, the specific conflict approach to psychosomatic illness has not proven very predictive of any specific physical or psychological disorder.

EVERLY AND BENSON'S "DISORDERS OF AROUSAL" MODEL

The "disorders of arousal" model of pathogenesis (Everly & Benson, 1989) is a direct result of an integration of efforts from Harvard University to understand the mechanisms of pathogenesis in psychosomatic disorders (Everly, 1986) and the mechanisms active in the amelioration of such psychosomatic disorders (Benson, 1975, 1987, 1996).

It has been observed for over four decades that various technologies that could be used to induce a hypoarousal relaxation response were able to ameliorate, or at least diminish, the severity of a wide and diverse variety of diseases. Despite data supporting specific clinical and experimental effects for various stress-management methods (Lehrer, Carr, Sargunaraj, & Woolfolk, 1994), it also seems that the initiation of what Herbert Benson (1975) has called the "relaxation response" has virtually a generic applicability across a wide spectrum of stress-related, psychosomatic diseases. That observation led to an investigation of the source of the broad-spectrum therapeutic effect of the relaxation response as a way of understanding the disorders it was useful in treating. The investigation culminated in an analysis of common phenomenological mechanisms, that is, common denominators (latent), occurring across anxiety and stress-related diseases that would serve to homogenize such disorders.

Based upon an integration of the work of Goddard on "kindling" (Goddard & Douglas, 1976), Post on "sensitisation" (Post & Ballenger, 1981), Gellhorn on "ergotropic tuning" (1967), and Gray (1982) on the limbic system, it has been proposed by Everly that the phenomenology of many chronic anxiety- and stress-related diseases is undergirded by the existence of a latent, yet common denominator, existing in the form of a neurological hypersensitivity for excitation (or arousal) residing within the subcortical limbic circuitry (Everly, 1985b). This limbic hypersensitivity phenomenon (LHP) may be understood as an unusually high propensity for neurological arousal/excitation with the potential to lead to, or exist as, a pathognomonic state of excessive arousal within the limbic system. "Hyperstartle reaction," "autonomic hyperfunction," and "autonomic lability" are diagnostic terms commonly used to capture such a notion. The LHP is believed to develop as a result of either acutely traumatic or repeated extraordinary limbic excitation and is credited with the potential to ignite a cascade of extraordinary arousal of numerous and varied neurological, neuroendocrine, and endocrine efferent mechanisms (as discussed in Chapter 2) and, therefore, the potential to give rise to a host of varied psychiatric and somatic disorders. The subsequent disorders are then referred to as "disorders of arousal." This concept is captured in Figure 3.2.

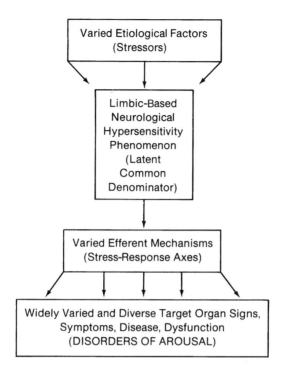

Figure 3.2. Limbic hypersensitivity phenomenon: the latent taxon in stress-related "disorders of arousal."

Figure 3.2 depicts the notion that, responsive to a host of widely disparate etiological factors (stressors) including environmental events, cognitive–affective dynamics, personologic predispositions, and the like, there exists a subtle, latent mechanism of pathogenesis: a neurological hypersensitivity for pathogenic arousal located within the limbic circuitry. Such arousal is believed to be capable of triggering a subsequent variety of physiological effector mechanisms (stress-response axes) within existing patterns of response predisposition (response stereotypy), so as to ultimately give rise to a wide and diverse spectrum of target-organ disorders (disorders of arousal). Included in the disorders of arousal taxonomy would be most anxiety and adjustment disorders, including some forms of depression, as well as virtually any and all stress-related physical disorders. The disorders of arousal will be enumerated in greater detail later in this volume. The reader may also refer to Everly and Benson (1989), Doane (1986), and Post (1986).

The natural corollary of the disorders of arousal model of pathogenesis is the notion that effective treatment of such disorders is highly related to reducing the subcortical hypersensitivity through the use of some "antiarousal" therapy. In addition to various pharmacological interventions, Benson's concept of the relaxation response represents a natural antiarousal phenomenon that appears antithetical to the mechanisms that undergird the disorders of arousal. Thus it may well be that a major source of the broad-spectrum therapeutic effect exhibited by the relaxation response resides in the homeostasis-seeking, antiarousal phenomenology of the relaxation response, which serves to inhibit the mechanism of limbic hypersensitivity believed to exist as a common denominator among the various disorders of arousal.

In summary, the disorders of arousal model of stress-induced pathology recognizes the influences of environmental factors, cognitive–affective dynamics, patterns of previous learning, and patterns of preferential psychophysiological excitation as described in previous models and summarized elsewhere (Everly, 1986). Yet it focuses upon the limbic system proper, its efferent influences on cognitive processes, and its effector mechanisms through the hypothalamus. More specifically, it focuses upon a proposed LHP, developed as a result of extraordinary limbic excitation, as key constituents in linking the stress response to stress-related disease formation, especially chronic manifestations of such diseases.

Several different theories have been enumerated here to explain how psychophysiological arousal can be channeled to affect target organs adversely. Despite the disparity between the theories mentioned, there does appear to be one element, either directly stated or implied, that is common to all. That commonality pertains to how the target organs ultimately become dysfunctional or pathological—simply stated, if any given target organ is subjected to psychophysiological overload (overstimulation) for a long enough period, that organ will eventually manifest symptoms of dysfunction or pathology due to excessive "wear and tear," be it biochemically induced trauma or toxicity, or actual visceromotor fatigue or exhaustion. According to Stoyva (1976) in his review of stress-related disorders, "A number of investigators have hypothesized that if the stress response is evoked too often, or sustained for too long, then disorders are likely to develop" (p. 370). In a "behavioristic interpretation" of psychosomatic disorders, Lachman (1972) states, "The longer a given structure is involved in an ongoing emotional reaction pattern, the greater is the likelihood of it being involved in a psychosomatic disorder" (pp. 69–70). Lachman concludes, "Theoretically, any bodily structure or function can become the end focus of psychosomatic phenomena—but especially those directly innervated and regulated by the autonomic nervous system" (p. 71).

Perhaps of greater interest to the clinician than the theory concerning what causes a target-organ symptom to be overloaded is the widely accepted conclusion that target-organ stress-related diseases result from excessively frequent, intense, and/or prolonged activation, that is, overstimulation (see Everly, 1986; Everly & Benson, 1989; Kraus & Raab, 1961; Lachman, 1972; Sternbach, 1966; Stoyva, 1976; Stoyva & Budzynski, 1974). See Table 3.1.

Table 3.1. From Stress to Disease: Theories of Psychosomatic Pathogenesis

Theory	Pathogenic mechanisms	Result
Selye's "General Adaptation Syndrome"	Triphasic fluctuation of neuroendocrine and endocrine mechanisms, especially ACTH. The chronic maintenance of the stage of resistance yields a depletion of adaptive energy.	Depletion of adaptive physiological energy → exhaustion → disease, due to excessive wear and tear.
Lachman's "behavioral" model	Biological and learned factors interact to establish predisposing patterns of target-organ arousal and disease from excessively frequent stress arousal. Emotional and autonomic learning play a major role in repeated target-organ excitation.	Excessively intense or excessively chronic activation of target organs → stress-related disease (excessive wear and tear).
Sternbach's model	Response stereotypy. Frequent stress arousal. Homeostatic recovery failure.	Frequent target-organ activation → organ fatigue and pathology.
Kraus and Raab's "hypokinetic disease" model	Suppression of somatomotor behavior. Failure to ventilate and utilize the stress response once activated. Increased pathogenic risk.	Target-organ overload and pathology.
Schwartz's "disregulation" model	Failure in homeostatic feedback mechanisms following stressor exposure.	Target-organ overload and pathology.
Conflict theory	Specific psychic conflicts lead to specific physical illnesses.	Target-organ overload and pathology.
Everly and Benson's "disorders of arousal" model	Limbic hypersensitivity phenomenon causing extraordinary arousal of stress response axes.	Excessively intense and/or excessively frequent or chronic activation of stress response axes → target-organ overstimulation and pathology.

SUMMARY

Chapter 2 described a mechanism by which psychosocial factors could serve to ignite extraordinary arousal of the physiological stress-response axes through cognitive–affective integrations and limbic–hypothalamic neurological mechanisms. This chapter pursued the logical extension of stress–axis arousal by reviewing the pathogenic mechanisms that are postulated to link the stress response to subsequent target-organ disease. Let us review the main points covered in this review.

1. All major theories agree that target-organ pathology ultimately results when the specific target organ is overstimulated. Overstimulation may occur as a result of excessively frequent, chronic, or intense stimulation. Pathological states emerge from excessive "wear and tear" on the target organ and can be caused by biochemical toxicity or trauma (e.g., necrosis) as well as structural alteration and visceromotor fatigue or exhaustion.

2. The GAS of Selye presents a triaphasic model by which acute "shock" or chronic excitation could ultimately deplete the physiological constituents that normally allow target organs to continue to function in the face of stress arousals. The results would be target-organ exhaustion and perhaps even death.

3. Lachman's behavioral model emphasizes the point that emotional and autonomic responses could be learned. Interacting with other biological factors that are not learned, emotional and autonomic learning can cause repeated target-organ excitation. Excessively prolonged, frequent, or intense target-organ stimulation may then lead to disease.

4. Sternbach's psychophysiological model cites response stereotypy, frequent arousal of stress-response axes, and homeostatic recovery delay as factors that serve to exhaust target organs and lead to disease. Once again, the theme of overutilization emerges as the key pathogenic constituent.

5. Kraus and Raab's model emphasizes the role of suppressed somatomotor expression in the etiology of stress-related pathology. Such suppression leads to target-organ overstimulation, exhaustion, and ultimately disease.

6. Schwartz's "disregulation" model also accepts the overload/overstimulation concept, but emphasizes the role of faulty negative feedback mechanisms in the pathological etiology.

7. The conflict theory postulates that specific psychological conflicts lead to specific physical and/or psychological disorders. This is clearly the weakest of the major psychosomatic theories.

8. Finally, Everly and Benson propose a model that serves to unite stress-related illnesses on the basis of a LHP, that is, a sensitization (increased

propensity for activation) of cognitive, affective, and stress-response efferents in the formulation of stress-related disease. It is proposed that excessively frequent, chronic, or intense activation of target organs based upon the limbic hypersensitivity could ultimately exhaust the target organ and lead to a stress-related disease.

9. Thus, we see that all theories of pathogenesis, while emphasizing different phenomenological aspects as to why target-organ overstimulation occurs, agree that, indeed, overstimulation and excessive wear of target organs lead to stress-related dysfunction and disease.

Chapter 4 will review specific stress-related diseases commonly encountered in clinical practice.

4

Stress-Related Disease
A Review

I'm at the mercy of any rogue who cares to annoy and tease me.
JOHN HUNTER, *18th-century physician*

There has been skepticism that emotions aroused in a social context can so seriously affect the body as to lead to long-term disease or death. But the work, such as that of Wolf, shows that machinery of the human body is very much at the disposal of the higher centers of the brain. ... Given the right circumstances, these higher controls can drive it mercilessly, often without awareness on the part of the individual of how close he is to the fine edge. (Henry & Stephens, 1977, p. 11)

To review what we have covered so far, Chapter 2 proposed a model of how psychosocial factors can activate a complex myriad of neurological, neuroendocrine, and endocrine response axes. Similarly, Chapter 2 reviewed the physiological constituents of these stress axes in considerable detail. Chapter 3 reviewed the link from stress arousal to disease by summarizing several noteworthy models constructed to elucidate how stress arousal can lead to disease and dysfunction, that is, mechanisms of pathogenesis that link causally stress arousal to target-organ pathology. The goal of this chapter is to review some of the most common clinical manifestations of excessive stress, and more specifically, to familiarize the clinician with some of the most frequently encountered target-organ disorders believed to be related to excessive stress arousal.

GASTROINTESTINAL DISORDERS

Excessive stress and the diseases of the gastrointestinal (GI) system have been thought to be related for decades. The most commonly encountered stress-related GI disorders are peptic ulcers, ulcerative colitis, irritable bowel syndrome, and esophageal reflux.

Gastrointestinal Physiology

Before reviewing specific disorders, let us briefly review the basic physiology of the GI system. As described by Weinstock and Clouse (1987), the GI system involves a series of sequentially arranged tubular organs separated by sphincters. This system includes the esophagus, the stomach, the duodenum, the small intestine, and the large intestine (colon). See Figure 4.1.

The esophagus provides a tubular canal for the connection of the mouth and the stomach. The activity of the esophagus is primarily under vagal control and neural mechanisms are primarily responsible for esophageal motility. The upper border of the esophagus is the cricopharyngeus (upper esophageal sphincter). The lower border is the lower esophageal sphincter, the gateway to the stomach.

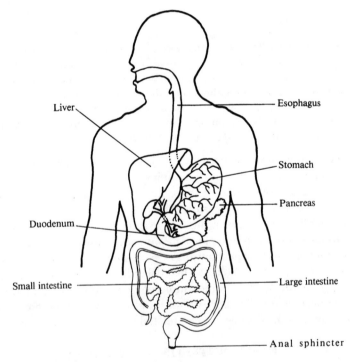

Figure 4.1. The gastrointestinal system. (SOURCE: Daniel A. Girdano and George S. Everly, Jr. (1986). *Controlling Stress and Tension: A Holistic Approach*, 2nd ed., pp. 36, 39. Reprinted by permission of Prentice-Hall, Inc., Englewood Cliffs, NJ.)

The basic functions of the stomach are to receive, pulverize, nutritionally regulate, and temporarily store the food one consumes. The stomach is lined with a mucosal tissue that serves to protect it from its own digestive processes. Under the influence of factors such as gastrin, histamine, and vagal and sympathetic stimulation, intragastric dynamics involving the release of hydrochloric acid, pepsin, and mucus, as well as muscular contractions, act upon food that has been delivered to the stomach from the esophagus.

From the stomach, the food passes through the pyloric sphincter to the duodenum. The gallbladder is responsible for releasing bile into the duodenum.

The small intestine and its specialized mucosal lining serves as the primary location for digestion and nutrient absorption.

Finally, the large intestine is designed for the absorption and orderly evacuation of concentrated waste products (Weinstock & Clouse, 1987).

Let us now review several common stress-related GI disorders.

Peptic Ulcers

Peptic ulcers are usually further classified by their location in the GI system: gastric, or stomach, ulcers, and duodenal ulcers. The incidence of peptic ulcer disease is about 18 in 10,000, with duodendal ulcers accounting for about 75% of those cases.

It was demonstrated many years ago that emotions of anger and rage are related to increased secretion of acid and pepsin by the stomach and that this secretion decreased with depression (Mahl & Brody, 1954; Mittelman & Wolff, 1942; Wolf & Glass, 1950). Although it might be concluded that what one sees in gastric ulcers, that is, an erosion of the wall of the stomach by the acid and enzyme it produces, is simply an exaggeration of a normal physiological response; actually it is not quite so simple. Certainly, emotions can raise gastric acid secretion and exacerbate an already existing ulcer, but normally the stomach wall is protected from the acid within it by a lining of mucus secreted by other cells in its wall. How this protective system breaks down and what predisposes a person to such an event remain elusive.

There seems to be a combination of emotional and genetic factors involved in the pathogenesis of gastric ulcers, and such studies as that of Weiner, Thaler, Reiser, and Mirsky (1957) have demonstrated this quite well. These investigators were able to predict which individuals in a group of recruits in basic training in the army would develop gastric ulcers on the basis of serum pepsinogen levels—a genetic trait that is apparently a necessary but not sufficient factor in the formation of gastric ulcers. Gastric ulcers were also of interest to Selye (1951), who described ulcers apparently in response to chronic arousal of the endocrine stress axes in the general adaptation syndrome. One could thus conceive of a mechanism whereby stress, through the intermediation of neural or hormonal mechanisms, could result in significant irritation. In individuals who are so predisposed, ulceration of the stomach would occur given sufficient time and continued exposure to the stress. The picture is less clear-cut, however, in that it has been suggested that the duodenal ulcer results from changes in the mucosal wall "associated with sustained activation and a feeling of being deprived" (Backus & Dudley, 1977, p. 199).

Therefore, strongly implicated in the stress response, the specific causal mechanisms involved in peptic ulcer formation are probably multifactorial. Vagus-stimulated gastric hypersecretion as well as glucocorticoid anti-inflammatory activity on the mucous lining have been implicated. Yet conclusive data are lacking at present with regard to the selective activation of each mechanism. Bacteriological infections have most recently been implicated in ulcer formation, but a primary main effect seems doubtful. Rather, some complex interaction effect between arousal and bacteria seems more likely in instances where bacteria are, indeed, implicated.

Ulcerative Colitis

Ulcerative colitis is an inflammation and ulceration of the lining of the colon. Research by Grace, Seton, Wolf, and Wolff (1949) and Almy, Kern, and Tulin (1949) produced evidence that the colon becomes hyperactive and hyperemic with an increase in lysozyme levels (a proteolytic enzyme that can dissolve mucus) under stress. The emotions of anger and resentment are reported to create observable ulcerations of the bowel (Grace et al., 1950). "Sustained feelings of this sort might be sufficient to produce enough reduction in bowel wall defenses to the point that the condition becomes self-sustaining" (Backus & Dudley, 1977, p. 199).

The predominant symptom of ulcerative colitis is rectal bleeding, although diarrhea, abdominal cramping and pain, and weight loss may also be present. Ulcerative colitis is sometimes associated with disorders of the spine, liver, and immune system. Rosenbaum (1985) has stated, "The frequency with which emotional precipitating-factors are identified varies, being as high as 74% in adults and 95% in children" (p. 79). Personologic investigations of colitis patients commonly find them to possess an immature personality structure often demonstrating extreme compulsive traits.

Irritable Bowel Syndrome

Mitchell and Drossman (1987) refer to irritable bowel syndrome (IBS) as the most common of the functional disorders. It is viewed as a syndrome of dysfunctional colonic motility; that is, the colon proves to be overreactive to psychological as well as physiological stimuli.

The diagnostic criteria for IBS include atypical abdominal pain, altered bowel habits, symptomatic duration of 3 months or more, and disruption of normal lifestyle (Latimer, 1985). Abdominal distention, mucus in the stools, fecal urgency, nausea, loss of appetite, and even vomiting are other IBS symptoms.

The pathophysiology of IBS is clearly multifactorial, with abnormal myoelectric phenomena, altered gut opiate receptors, abnormal calcium channel activity, and increased alpha-adrenergic activity. Personality characteristics of IBS patients often include compulsiveness, overly conscientious behavior, interpersonal sensitivity, and nonassertiveness (Latimer, 1985). White head et al. (1992) found stress to be related to acute IBS exacerbation and disability.

Esophageal Reflux

Before leaving this section on GI disorders it would be prudent to mention gastroesophageal reflux and its frequent corollary, esophagitis. Dotevall (1985) has indicated that these syndromes are common stress-related disorders. According to Young, Richter, Bradley, and Anderson (1987):

> Heartburn, a common GI symptom, generally is experienced as a painful substernal burning sensation. However, sensations can radiate into the arms or jaw and mimic pain associated with coronary artery disease. Heartburn [esophageal reflux] symptoms typically occur after eating, when lying down, or during bending or straining. The symptoms result from frequent irritation of the sensitive mucosal lining of the esophagus by the usually acidic gastric contents. (p. 8)

Although the primary physiological cause of esophageal reflux and esophagitis is a weakened lower esophageal sphincter, psychological factors are known to contribute to the reflux phenomenon (Dotevall, 1985).

In his superb review of GI physiology and stress, Dotevall (1985) listed the known effects of varied emotional reactions on GI activity. These are summarized in Table 4.1.

CARDIOVASCULAR DISORDERS

The cardiovascular system is thought by many researchers and clinicians to be the prime-target end organ for the stress response. The cardiovascular disorders most often associated with excessive stress are essential hypertension, migraine headache, and Raynaud's disease.

Table 4.1. Psychological Stimuli and Gastrointestinal Responses

Psychological state	GI response
Anxiety	Increased esophageal motility
	Increased colonic contractions
	Increased intraluminal pressure of the colon
Hostility, resentment, aggression	Increased colonic contractions
(without somatomotor expression)	Increased gastric acid
	Increased contractile activity of stomach
Depression	Decreased gastric acid
	Decreased colonic contractions
Wish to be rid of trouble	Rapid colonic transit with diarrhea

Cardiovascular Physiology

Before reviewing those specific disorders, a brief review of cardiovascular physiology is appropriate. Figure 4.2 details the cardiovascular system.

The heart is the key component in the cardiovascular system. It pumps nutrient-rich, oxygenated arterial blood to the cells of the body while at the same time pumping venous blood, which carries the various metabolic waste products.

The heart is divided into two halves: a right heart and a left heart. The circulatory cycle begins with blood entering the right heart. This blood supply is waste-filled venous blood. It has traveled throughout the venules and veins once it left the capillary beds, where the nutrient and gaseous exchanges initially took place within the body. The venous blood enters the resting heart and fills a small feeder chamber called the right atrium. Blood then passively moves through the tricuspid valve into the pumping chamber of the right heart, the right ventricle. Once the right ventricle is almost completely filled, an electrical impulse begins in the sinoatrial conducting node so as to contract the right atrium. This action forces any remaining blood into the right ventricle.

More specifically, the electrical impulse transverses the atrium until it reaches the atrioventricular node, where there is a fraction-of-a-second delay completing the filling of the right ventricle. Then the electrical impulse is sent through the ventricle, forcing it to contract and pump the venous blood through the pulmonary valve toward the lungs via the pulmonary artery. Once the blood arrives in the lungs, waste products such as carbon dioxide are exchanged for oxygen and the blood is returned to the heart.

The left heart receives the fresh, oxygenated blood from the lungs via the pulmonary vein. This blood enters the left heart at the point of the left atrium. From here the blood is moved through the mitral valve into the left heart's pumping chamber, the left ventricle. Once again, when the heart

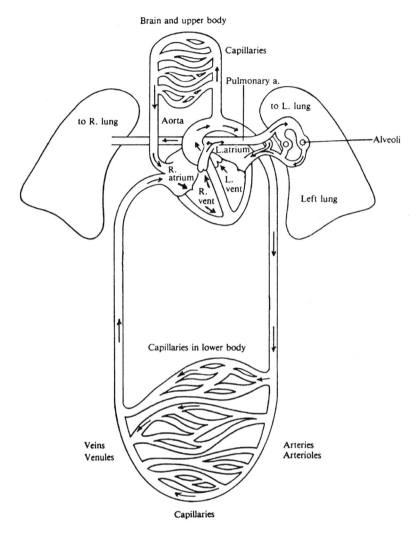

Figure 4.2. The cardiovascular system. (SOURCE: Daniel A. Girdano and George S. Everly, Jr. (1986). *Controlling Stress and Tension: A Holistic Approach,* 2nd ed., pp. 36, 39. Reprinted by permission of Prentice-Hall, Inc., Englewood Cliffs, NJ.)

beats, it sends the electrical impulse from the sinoatrial node through the left atrium to the atrioventricular node, ultimately culminating in the contraction of the left ventricle. Blood pumped from the left ventricle passes through the aortic valve through the aorta into the arterial system, including the coronary arteries. The arteries narrow into arterioles, which feed the capillary beds where the cells exchange gases and nutrients. Then the capillaries feed the venules, which feed the veins, and the cycle is repeated.

Both the right and left hearts pump simultaneously; therefore, blood is being pumped to the lungs at the same time it is being pumped out to the body.

The cardiovascular system is a closed-loop system. As such, pressure within the system is a necessary driving force. The arterial system, including the left heart, is a high-pressure system driven by the contraction of the left ventricle. The venous system, including the right heart, is a low-pressure system, assisted in venous return by the contraction of the skeletal muscles during movement. Blood pressure, as it is typically measured and expressed, relates to the arterial system pressures. Blood pressure is measured in millimeters of mercury (mm Hg) and is expressed in terms equivalent to the amount of pressure required to raise a column of mercury so many millimeters. Blood pressure is expressed in terms of the systolic pressure (the pressure within the arteries during the contraction of the ventricles—called *systole*) and the diastolic pressure (the pressure within the arteries when the ventricles are filling at rest—called *diastole*).

Essential Hypertension

According to current estimates, 24% of adult Americans suffer from "the silent killer," cardiovascular hypertension. Cardiovascular hypertension is usually defined as arterial pressures over 140 mm Hg systolic pressure and/or 90 mm Hg diastolic pressure, although many authorities will adjust these figures upward (especially the systolic pressure) if the patient is advanced in age.

There are basically two types of cardiovascular hypertension: secondary and essential. Secondary cardiovascular hypertension represents a status of elevated blood pressure due to some organic dysfunction, for example, a pheochromocytoma (tumor of the adrenal gland). Essential hypertension has been loosely interpreted as being related to stress and such factors as diet. The term "essential" reflects the once-held notion that with advancing age one always acquired elevated blood pressure. This notion has been refuted (Henry & Stephens, 1977).

In a review of the pathophysiology of hypertension, Eliot (1979) states that in less than 10% of the cases, organic disorders explain hypertension. However, he suggests that both the SAM and the anterior pituitary–adrenocortical stress axes are capable of increasing blood pressure in response to psychosocial factors alone. This may occur through a wide range of diverse mechanisms (see also Selye, 1976). With chronic activation, he concludes, the deterioration of the cardiovascular system may be irreversible.

Henry and Stephens (1977), in a useful review of psychosocial stimulation and hypertension, present evidence similar to that of Eliot. In their review of animal and human studies, they point to the ability of the psychophysiological stress mechanisms to effect an increase in blood pressure. They point to the role of medullary norepinephrine as a vasoconstrictive force capable of increasing blood pressure. In addition, they point to the notion that increased sympathetic tonus (apparently regardless of origin) will lead to further increased sympathetic discharge. The end result may well be the tendency for the carotid sinus and aortic baroreceptors to "reset" themselves at a higher level of blood pressure. The normal effect of the baroreceptors is to act to moderate blood pressure elevations. However, if they are reset at higher levels, they will tolerate greater blood pressure before intervening. Therefore, resting blood pressure may be allowed to rise slowly over time. Finally, these authors point to the role of the adrenocortical response in the elevation of blood pressure, perhaps through some arterial narrowing or sodium-retaining mechanism. They suggest that psychosocial disturbance can play a major role in blood pressure elevations that could become chronic in nature (see Steptoe, 1981).

Weiner (1977), however, states that "psychosocial factors do not by themselves 'cause' essential hypertension" (p. 183). They do, however, "interact with other predispositions" to produce high blood pressure (p. 185). He concludes that the available data point toward the conclusion that hypertension essentially can be caused by a wide variety of influences and that psychological and sociological factors "may play a different etiological, pathogenetic, and sustaining role in its different forms" (p. 185).

Vasospastic Phenomena

Stress-related vasospastic phenomena include migraine headaches and Raynaud's disease. These disorders involve vascular spasms; more specifically, their phenomenology involves spasms of the arterial vasculature induced by excessive neurological tone (usually SNS activity) (see Ganong, 1997).

Migraine headaches may affect as many as 17 million Americans. There are two basic subtypes: classical migraine and common migraine. Although both are characterized by vasomotor spasms, the classical migraine is accompanied by a prodrome. The prodrome is often manifest in the form of visual disturbances, hearing dysfunction, expressive aphasia, and/or GI dysfunction. The most common form of prodrome is the visual prodrome, for example, the development of an acute visual scotoma. The prodrome is a symptom of severe arterial vasoconstriction. The pain that accompanies migraine headaches occurs on the "rebound," that is, the point at which the arterial vasculature vasodilates in response to the original vasoconstriction. It is unclear whether the pain actually results from the physical dystension of the arterial vasculature or from associated biochemical processes (see Raskin, 1985; Wolff, 1963).

Raynaud's disease is another vasospastic disorder characterized by episodic pallor and cyanosis of the fingers and/or toes. Upon rebound vasodilation, there can be extreme pain characterized by sensations of aching and throbbing. Both exposure to cold and psychosocially induced stress can induce an attack of Raynaud's (Taub & Stroebel, 1978) (see Appendices C and D).

Myocardial Ischemia and Coronary Artery Disease

Myocardial ischemia is a condition wherein the heart muscle endures a state of significantly reduced blood flow. "Myocardial ischemia occurs frequently in patients with coronary artery disease (CAD) and is a significant predictor of future cardiac events" (Gullette, et al., 1997, p. 1521). Using a case-crossover design, Gullette and her colleagues demonstrated that mental stress can induce myocardial ischemia. Electrocardiogram (ECG) data were gathered with specific foci upon the emotions of negative tension, sadness, and frustration. Results of this investigation indicated that these negative emotions during daily life can more than double the risk of myocardial ischemia in the subsequent hour. Such ischemic findings were not in evidence subsequent to the states of happiness and feeling in control.

Previous studies have shown a significant correlation between myocardial episodes and the emotion of anger (Mittleman et al., 1995). Other studies have shown a significant relationship between the stress associated with mass disasters (Leor, Poole, & Kloner, 1996) and even missile attacks (Kark, Goldman, & Epstein, 1995), and subsequent cardiac death. Yet the Gullette et al. (1997) study is important in that the mechanisms of pathogenesis were observed rather than inferred.

Finally, the relationship between stress and CAD has been vigorously debated. In a review of investigations, Niaura and Goldstein (1995) conclude, "Our review of sociocultural and interpersonal factors... has identified evidence for a positive association among the following factors and CAD: occupational factors (e.g., job strain, low control, few possibilities for growth, low social support, life stress, and social isolation" (pp. 45–46). An important paper by Manuck and his colleagues (1995) that reviewed animal research concluded that psychosocial variables and social stress are associated with the promotion of coronary atherogenesis, impaired vasomotor responses of the coronary arteries, coronary lesions, and specific injury to arterial endothelium.

While more research is clearly needed, the argument in support of a significant role for stress in the etiology of CAD appears to be growing.

RESPIRATORY DISORDERS

Allergy

An allergy is a hypersensitivity that some people develop to a particular agent. The patient's body reacts with an exaggerated immunodefensive response when it encounters the agent (antigen).

One of the most familiar forms of allergy is hay fever. In this condition, the individual is sensitive to some forms of plant pollen, and when these are inhaled from the air, mucous membranes swell, nasal secretion becomes excessive, and nasal obstruction can occur. Because other particles in the air do not seem to elicit such a response, this is clearly an overreaction to a stimulus. However, hay fever has been generally thought to be a phenomenon related only to the body, as opposed to the mind. Yet the mind–body dualism is once again questioned by the finding that some subject with hay fever may respond minimally, if at all, when challenged with the allergenic substance in an environment in which he or she feels secure and comfortable, whereas in other, more stressful situations, the same challenge is met with the usual nasal hypersecretion, congestion, and the like (Holmes, Trenting, & Wolff, 1951).

Bronchial Asthma

Although sharing some similarities with allergy, asthma is a more complex and potentially serious disorder. In asthmatic patients, bronchial secretions increase, mucosal swelling takes place and, finally, smooth muscle surrounding the bronchioles contracts, leading to a great difficulty in expiring air from the lungs. This "inability to breath" is, of course, anxiety-producing, and this stress itself leads to a need for more oxygen, thus exacerbating the stress response caused by the original stimulus no matter what its nature. That bronchial asthmatic attacks can be caused by or at least exacerbated by psychosocial stimulation is no longer in question. Research reviewed by Lachman (1972) warrants such a conclusion, as does the work of Knapp (1982). Stress-related asthma appears to be related to activation of the parasympathetic nervous system (Moran, 1995).

Hyperventilation

Hyperventilation may be considered an example of an acute stress response. However, episodic hyperventilation can become a long-standing problem that goes undiagnosed for long periods of time in patients presenting vague problems that do not fit any particular pattern, such as vague aches and pains, nausea, vomiting, chest pains, and the like. The clinician must be on guard for this particular manifestation of the stress response, in order to protect the individual from unnecessary suffering and expense while searching for the cause. This, again, is a part of the fight-or-flight response in which the body is readied for action by increasing O_2 and decreasing CO_2; however, no action takes place. It has been suggested that any time a patient presents such vague problems that seem elusive, the clinician should maintain a high degree of suspicion regarding hyperventilation. Consideration may then be given to asking the patient to hyperventilate in the office. If the symptoms are reproduced, much time and effort of both physician and patient may be saved. For methods and cautions, refer to articles by Campernolle, Kees, and Leen (1979) and Lum (1975); see also Knapp (1982).

MUSCULOSKELETAL DISORDERS

This system comprises, as its name implies, all the body's muscles and bony support. It is thus the system that is responsible for the body's mobility and therefore plays one of the more obvious roles in a fight-or-flight type of response. At such a time, the muscles tense, blood flow is increased to them, and the very word "tension" associated with emotions such as anger or anxiety relates to this state of the musculoskeletal system (Tomita, 1975).

The stress-related disorders here are quite predictable. Low back pain may often be produced in a situation in which there is contraction of the back muscles as if to keep the body erect for fleeing a situation. If the contraction continues but there is no associated action (and therefore the stress situation remains), blood flow to the muscles decreases, metabolites increase, and pain is produced (Dorpat & Holmes, 1955; Holmes & Wolff, 1952).

Tension headache is a similar situation. The muscles of the head and neck are kept in prolonged contraction, resulting in pain by the same mechanism. This is to be differentiated from the pain of vascular headaches, which seems to begin in periods *following* tension.

There have even been some studies that indicate a possible role for stress in the development or influence of the course of the inflammatory joint disease, rheumatoid arthritis (Amkraut & Solomon, 1974; Heisel, 1972; Selye, 1956).

SKIN DISORDERS

The skin is thought to be a common target end organ for excessive arousal (Musaph, 1977). Common stress-related disorders include eczema, acne, urticaria, psoriasis, and alopecia areata (patchy hair loss) (Lachman, 1972, Engels, 1985). According to Medansky (1971), 80% of dermatological patients have a psychological overlay. Supporting such a conclusion is empirical evidence that various neurodermatological syndromes have either been initiated or exacerbated through the controlled manipulation of psychosocial variables (Engels, 1985; Lachman, 1972). The specific mechanisms of pathogenesis have yet to be satisfactorily detailed in most instances, however. Folks and Kinney (1995) provide a useful review of the role of psychological factors and various dermatological conditions.

PSYCHOLOGICAL MANIFESTATIONS OF THE STRESS RESPONSE

The final category of disease to be discussed in this chapter is the psychological manifestations of the stress response. The psychological disturbances most associated with excessive stress are diverse, and for the first time are in some instances being officially recognized as resulting from excessive stress.

Acute and chronic stress episodes are implicated in the development of both diffuse anxiety, and manic behavior patterns that are without defined direction or purpose. Gellhorn (1969) argues that high levels of sympathetic activity can result in anxiety reactions. This anxiety may occur as a result of SNS and proprioceptive discharges at the cerebral cortical level. Thus, generalized ergotropic tone may then lead to conditions of chronic and diffuse anxiety. Guyton (1982), in apparent agreement with Gellhorn, notes that general sympathetic discharge and proprioceptive feedback may contribute to arousal states such as mania, anxiety, and insomnia. Greden (1974) and Stephenson (1977) have both found that the consumption of methylated xanthines (primarily caffeine) can create signs of diffuse anxiety as well as insomnia and may lead to a diagnosis of anxiety neurosis. The action of the methylated xanthines rests on their ability to stimulate a psychophysiological stress response primarily through sympathetic activation. Finally, Jacobson (1938, 1978) has argued that proprioceptive impulses as such would be found in conditions of high musculoskeletal tension and can contribute to anxiety reactions (see also Everly, 1985b).

Physiologically, in each of the cases just cited, it may be suggested that an ascending neural overload via the reticular activating system to the limbic and neocortical areas may be responsible for creating unorganized and dysfunctional discharges of neural activity that are manifested in clients' presenting symptoms of insomnia, undefined anxiety, and in some cases manic behavior patterns lacking direction or apparent purpose (see Everly, 1985b; Guyton, 1982).

In each of the three examples, activation of the psychophysiological stress response preceded the manifestation of diffuse, undefined anxiety, often diagnosed as generalized anxiety disorder or atypical anxiety
disorder.

It is interesting to note that one link between anxiety and sympathetic
stress arousal, specifically, striate muscle tension (Gellhorn, 1969; Jacobson,
1938, 1978), has prompted the development of techniques designed to
reduce anxiety through the reduction of muscle tension. We review such
techniques later in this text.

Another psychological manifestation of excessive stress is thought to be
depressive reactions. Stressor events that lead the patient to the interpretation that his or her efforts are useless, that is, that he or she is in a helpless
situation, are clearly associated with arousal of the psychophysiological
stress response (Henry & Stephens, 1977). The affective manifestation
that typically follows is depression. Henry and Stephens have compiled an
impressive review that points to the reactivity of the anterior pituitary–
adrenocortical axes during depressive episodes.

In addition to physiological evidence, there is psychological evidence
to support the notion that excessive stress can precipitate a depressive reaction. Sociobehavioral research with depressed patients (see Brown, 1972;
Paykel et al., 1969) produced somewhat similar evidence that social stressors can lead to major affective syndromes. Rabkin (1982), in her review
of stress and affective disorders, states, "Overall, it seems justifiable to conclude that life events do play a role in the genesis of depressive disorders"
(p. 578). Indeed, depressed patients report more stressful life events than
do normal controls. This was especially true for a 3-week period immediately preceding the onset of the depression (Rabkin, 1982).

Evidence supports a link between stress and schizophrenia as well.
One behavioral interpretation of schizophrenia views the illness as a maladaptive avoidance mechanism in the face of an anxiety-producing environment (Epstein & Coleman, 1970). Serban (1975) found in a study of
125 acute and 516 chronic schizophrenics that excessive stress did play a
role in the precipitation of hospital readmission. A more far-reaching view
of psychopathology and stress is presented by Eisler and Polak (1971). In a
study of 172 psychiatric patients, they concluded that excessive stress could
contribute to a wide range of psychiatric disorders, including depression
and schizophrenia, as well as personality disturbance—depending on the
predisposing characteristics of the individual (see Millon & Everly, 1985).
Rabkin (1982) concludes that stress may well be associated with schizophrenic relapse and subsequent hospitalization.

Most important, however, with the advent of the multiaxial DSM, came
the identification of psychiatric disorders that were, by definition, a result

**Table 4.2. Psychological Disorders
and Excessive Stress**

Brief reactive psychosis
Posttraumatic stress disorder
Adjustment disorders
Various anxiety disorders
Various affective disorders
Some forms of schizophrenia

of stressful life events. Thus, for such categories, mental status, that is, the mind, need no longer be seen as a viable target organ only by inference. Both the diagnoses of *brief reactive psychosis* and *posttraumatic stress disorder* are viewed diagnostically as being a *direct* consequence of a "recognizable stressor." So, too, would be the diagnostic categories of *adjustment disorders.* Diagnoses such as adjustment disorder with anxious mood, adjustment disorder with depressed mood, and adjustment disorder with mixed emotional features demonstrate an official nosological acceptance of the wide spectrum of psychiatric manifestations that can result directly from stress.

Thus, we see that in the last several years, the "mind" has been officially recognized as a potential target organ for pathogenic stress arousal. Table 4.2 summarizes diagnostic categories that serve as psychological target-organ manifestations of excessive stress.

SUMMARY

The purpose of this chapter has been to briefly review some of the more common disorders seen in clinical practice that potentially possess a significant stress-related component. Let us review some of the main points addressed in this chapter:

1. There is a well-established literature linking the GI system to the stress response. The most commonly encountered stress-related GI disorders are peptic ulcers (gastric and duodenal), ulcerative colitis, irritable bowel syndrome, and esophageal reflux. There appear to be two major pathogenic mechanisms in these disorders: vagus-induced hypersecretion of digestive acids and glucocorticoid (cortisol)-induced diminution of the protective mucosal lining of the GI system. Gastric acid hypersecretion has been shown to be related to anger and rage (Wolfe & Glass, 1950), whereas alterations in mucosal integrity have been shown to be related to depression and feelings of deprivation (Backus & Dudley, 1977).

2. The cardiovascular system is believed by many to be the prime target organ of the stress response, especially in males (Humphrey & Everly, 1980). The cardiovascular disorders most commonly associated with excessive stress are essential hypertension, migraine headaches, and Raynaud's disease. Essential hypertension is clearly a multifactorial phenomenon. Although stress may not be the solitary etiological factor in the majority of cases of essential hypertension, it appears to be a contributory factor in the majority of cases in a nonobese population. Mechanisms within the stress response that may contribute to the acute and chronic elevation of blood pressure include SNS activity and adrenomedullary activity, as well as cortisol and aldosterone hyperactivity (refer to Chapter 2).

3. Vasospastic phenomena such as migraine headaches and Raynaud's disease seem to be primarily a function of excessive SNS activity, as are myocardial ischemia and coronary endothelial injury.

4. There is evidence that the respiratory system can also be a target organ for the stress response. Bronchial asthma, hyperventilation syndrome, and even some forms of allergies may be stress related. Mechanisms of mediation may include excessive parasympathetic activation, excessive sympathetic activation, and extraordinary adrenomedullary activity, respectively.

5. According to Jacobson (1938, 1970), Gellhorn (1967), and Tomita (1975), the striated neuromuscular system is an underestimated yet prime target for excessive stress arousal. Stress-response efferent mechanisms of mediation include alpha-motoneuron innervation, adrenomedullary activity, and perhaps even SNS activity.

6. The skin serves as a target for excessive stress. Disorders such as eczema, acne, psoriasis, and alopecia areata have been implicated as stress-related disorders. Specific mechanisms of mediation are unclear.

7. A final yet important target organ for the stress response must be the "mind," that is, psychological status. Mental disorders such as brief reactive psychosis, posttraumatic stress disorder, adjustment disorders, certain anxiety and affective disorders, and even some forms of schizophrenia may possess significant stress-related components.

8. In closing this chapter, it should be noted that the concept of stress-related psychosomatic diseases has been far broadened with the advent of the multiaxial DSM. Now, via such diagnostic perspectives, the clinician can indicate the degree to which stress may have contributed to the primary Axis I diagnosis through the use of Axis III, Axis IV, and Axis V. Finally, data from the field of psychoneuroimmunology cogently suggest that even infectious and degenerative diseases may have significant stress-related components in their initiation or exacerbation. In the next chapter we explore and review this notion that stress may affect the body's most fundamental disease protection system—the immune system.

5

Psychoneuroimmunology

An unexamined life is not worth living.
SOCRATES

Whereas the preceding chapter familiarized the clinician with some of the most frequently encountered organic manifestations related to excessive stress arousal, the purpose of this chapter is to expand this inquiry to investigate the proposed effects of excessive stress on the immune system. Selye (1976) and Amkraut and Solomon (1974) presented early reviews that support the conclusion that excessive stress can exert a generalized immunosuppressive effect. Selye (1976) reported that "the immunosuppressive effect of stress and glucocorticoides is probably one of the characteristic consequences of thymicolymphatic involution and lymphopenia which have long been recognized as typical stress effects" (p. 712). If excessive stress can exert generalized immunosuppressive effects, then it must be considered as a potential influence in the initiation and propagation not only of psychosomatic diseases but also of infectious and degenerative diseases (Jemmott, 1985).

Since the early speculations of Solomon and Moos (1964), research efforts have been undertaken for more than 35 years to advance the field of psychoneuroimmunology (Ader, 1981; Ader, Felten, & Cohen, 1991), which is "the study of interactions among behavior, neural and endocrine function, and immune processes" (Ader & Cohen, 1993, p. 53). Before addressing the proposed links and interactions between psychological factors such as stress and immunosuppression, we provide a brief overview

We would like to thank Dr. Wayne Campbell, Chief of Infectious Diseases at the Union Memorial Hospital, for his early review of this chapter.

of the fundamentals of the immune system. This cursory review is followed by the suggested interactions between the central nervous system (CNS), the immune system, and the stress response. A summary of some of the prominent animal and human stress research related to psychoneuroimmunology concludes the chapter.

IMMUNE SYSTEM

The immune system basically serves to protect the body from invading toxins and microorganisms that may damage organs and tissues. Some of the protective functions of the immune system are to eliminate bacteria and to reject foreign substances, known as antigens, that have entered the body. In addition, the immune system possesses a "memory" for encounters with foreign substances, such that a subsequent encounter induces a more rapid and potent response (Borysenko, 1987). The immune system is often conceptually divided into innate or nonspecific immunity, which provides a general defense, and specific or acquired immunity, which acts against particular threatening antigens.

Innate Immunity

As the term implies, *innate immunity* refers to processes that are apparent from birth and provide a general or nonspecific defense by acting against anything identified as foreign or *not self* (Thibodeau & Patton, 1993). There are many variations of innate immunity. For example, species-resistant, innate immunity makes the human body unsuitable to some potentially lethal animal diseases such as distemper. Conversely, dogs and cats are resistant to human diseases such as mumps or measles. Other non-specific types of immunity include physical barriers, such as the skin's outer keratin layer, which limits entry into the body, and biochemical substances, such as tears, saliva, and perspiration, which contain enzymes that digest or weaken the walls surrounding bacterial cells (Parslow, 1994). These anatomical and chemical barriers serve as the body's *first line of defense* against invading toxins (Thibodeau & Patton, 1993).

If bacteria or other microorganisms penetrate this first line of defense, the body has a second, nonspecific or general line of innate protection that incorporates phagocytosis, natural killer (NK) cells, interferon, and inflammation. Phagocytosis, which involves the destruction and absorption of microorganisms, utilizes cells known as phagocytes to eliminate pathogens (any organism causing disease). Nearly all tissues and organs possess inhabitant phagocytes. There are a variety of phagocytic cells, including (1) neutrophils, the most numerous type, accounting for one-half to two-thirds of circulating white blood cells (which are primarily involved in destroying pathogens); (2) monocytes, which are relatively large cells produced in the bone marrow and released into the blood for about 1 day before settling in a selective tissue; and (3) macrophages, the settled or mature monocytic cells, which are large, avid eliminators of foreign particles and debris (Thibodeau & Patton, 1993).

In addition to phagocytes, the body possesses natural killer (NK) cells, which are lymphocytes (one type of white blood cell) that kill various tumor cells and cells infected by viruses. One of the common ways NK cells function is by breaking down or lysing cells by damaging their plasma membrane. NK cells are currently considered to be an initial or frontline protective response that is utilized before a more specific response can be exhibited (Imboden, 1994). Therefore, although probably related to cytotoxic T lymphocytes (see acquired immunity below), NK cells serve a broad surveillance-like function that, unlike T cells, do not require prior antigen interaction (McDaniel, 1992). Therefore, NK cells are often included as part of the nonspecific immune functions.

About 40 years ago, it was discovered that some cells exposed to viruses produce a secretory protein known as interferon, which, as the name implies, "interferes" with the ability of viruses to produce diseases. Basically, interferon works by producing an antiviral state within the host that prevents viruses from replicating in cells. Interferon has also been associated with the modulation of immune responses.

Inflammation, or the inflammatory response, is also considered part of the body's second line of defense and characterizes the complex manner in which tissues and cells react to an insult or microbial invasion. Immediately after an injury, there is a brief constriction, followed by dilation, of blood vessels. Injured tissues then release a number of chemical mediators, such as histamine, kinins, and prostaglandins (Thibodeau & Patton, 1993). The factors involved in the inflammatory response characteristically results in redness, warmth, swelling, and pain. Although the inflammatory response is considered beneficial, it can be detrimental if it permanently injures the host tissues and/or impedes normal functioning.

Acquired Immunity

Contrary to nonspecific immunity described earlier, acquired or specific immune mechanisms attack certain agents that the body recognizes as *not self.* Therefore, specific immunity may be considered the body's *third line of defense* (Thibodeau & Patton, 1993). Acquired immunity develops in late fetal and neonatal life, and is part of the body's lymphatic system. The lymphatic system, a part of the circulatory system, consists of a vast network of vessels and organs that drains excess fluid and provides a defense for the body (Moore, 1992). Lymphocytes, which circulate in the body's fluids, are the major cells controlling the immune response. They are found most extensively in the lymph nodes, which are glands composed of composites of lymphoid tissues, but are also located in special lymphoid tissues such as the spleen, bone marrow, and gastrointestinal tract (Moore, 1992). Lymphoid tissue is strategically disseminated throughout the body, and allows for rapid interception and filtering of invading organisms and toxins. Two major types of lymphocytes involved in acquired immunity are T (thymus-derived) cells that form activated lymphocytes and are primarily involved in the slower acting cell-mediated immunity, and B (bone-marrow derived) cells that form circulating antibodies and are primarily involved in the more rapidly responding humoral immunity. Although these two types of lymphocytes are structurally similar, T and B cells are functionally distinct in their reaction to antigens.

Cell-Mediated Processes

In cell-mediated immunity, each T lymphocyte, or T cell, operates by having a precisely distinctive surface receptor that allows it to recognize and bind to only one invading antigen. Thus, a T cell may have numerous receptor sites; however, all of them will be specific for only a certain antigen. T cells, which account for 70–80% of disseminated lymphocytes, circulate in the blood in an inactive form and are incapable of recognizing antigens without assistance. Therefore, when an antigen invades the body, it is typically first identified and then ingested by macrophages, which initiate the process of digestion. The T cells, whose surface receptors match the antigens, then travel to the now inflamed tissues and bind to the antigen.

Once in contact with the antigen, the sensitized T cell begins to divide repeatedly to form a clone of identical, activated T cells (Thibodeau & Patton, 1993). The antigen-bound, sensitized T cells then release lymphocyte-derived chemical messengers, commonly called cytokines, into the inflamed tissue to facilitate the immune response (Dunn, 1989). Several variations of T lymphocytes, or T cells, include, for example, helper cells (T-4). The T-helper cell, once activated by the cytokine interleukin-1 (IL-1), releases interleukin-2 (IL-2), which fosters the maturation and marshals the subsequent immune response, including the promotion and multiplication of cytotoxic cells used to combat the invading antigen. There are also suppressor cells (T-8), which inhibit the immune response in order to regulate it, memory T cells, which initiate a rapid response if the antigen is encountered again, and cytotoxic or killer cells, which release a powerfully destructive cytokine called lymphotoxin (Borysenko, 1987).

A distinguishing characteristic of cell-mediated immunity is that specifically sensitized or activated lymphocytes are employed to pursue and contact the invading antigen. Typically, these antigen cells are foreign to the body, malignant, or have been transplanted into the tissue. Therefore, cell-mediated immunity, which requires a localized response that may require several days to detect the invader and to employ the necessary cells to battle it, not only defends us from viruses and cancer but also is directly involved in the rejection of organ and tissue transplants.

Humoral Responses

Comparable to T lymphocytes, B lymphocytes, or B cells, are also initiated by macrophage stimulation. In humoral immunity, an encounter with an antigen activates the B lymphocytes, which, after being released from the bone marrow, circulate to the lymph nodes, spleen, and other lymphoid tissues. Whereas cytotoxic T cells, as described earlier, exit lymphoid tissue to encounter an antigen directly, B cells produce their effects indirectly (McDaniel, 1992). When an antigen binds to antigen receptors on the B cell, the activated B cell divides to form a clone or group of identical B cells. Some of the offspring of these B cells become differentiated to form plasma cells known as antibodies that circulate in the lymph and the blood, and combine selectively with the triggering antigen (Thibodeau & Patton, 1993). Thus, antibodies are produced within a species to fit part of the antigen (Kendall, 1998). The binding of the antigen to the antibodies forms a complex that may (1) render the toxic antigens innocuous, (2) facilitate a bundling of antigens that allows phagocytes and macrophages to dispose of them rapidly, or (3) slightly alter the contour of the antibody, allowing the destruction of the foreign cells.

Antibodies belong to a group of proteins called globulins and are, therefore, referred to as immunoglobulins. The five different classes of antibodies or immunoglobulins known to exist in humans are designated as IgG, IgA, IgM, IgD, and IgE. Each immunoglobulin has a unique structure and function, and as mentioned earlier, generally defends the host by neutralizing toxins, blocking attachment of viruses to cells, or inducing phagocytosis of bacteria or other microorganisms. IgG is the most common immunoglobulin, accounting for around 70% of the circulating antibodies (Goldsby, Kindt, & Osborne, 2000). Therefore, immunoglobulins "not only serve as surface receptors for foreign substances, but also can be released to search out and bind their targets at a considerable distance from the cell" (Parslow, 1994, p. 26).

Activated B cells that do not differentiate into plasma cells are known as memory B cells. Memory B cells do not produce or secrete antibodies.

However, if they are exposed at some later time to the antigen responsible for their initial formation, then memory B cells convert into plasma cells that secrete antibodies (Thibodeau & Patton, 1993). Because there are many more memory cells than the initial B lymphocyte that was cloned, subsequent exposure to the same antigen will produce a more rapid and formidable antibody response (Guyton, 1996).

Different antigens stimulate distinct B cells to develop into plasma cells and memory B cells. Most antigens activate both T and B lymphocytes concurrently, and there is in fact a cooperative relationship between the two (Guyton, 1996). The primary difference between the T and B cells is that B cells release antibodies, whereas whole T cells are activated and released into the lymph. Therefore, these latter cells may last for months to years in the body fluid.

Also of note, the effects of circulating antibodies and cellular immunity are influenced by a component of blood plasma enzymes known as the complement system, which entails different protein compounds. This system can be initiated by specific or nonspecific immune mechanisms and is closely involved in destroying various foreign tissues in a process known as cytolysis.

Because there is no easy access to the organs containing immune cells, and given that components of the immune system circulate in blood, it is not surprising that psychneuroimmunological research often involves assessing the immune processes occurring in circulating peripheral blood. However, although peripheral blood is a key factor in immune responses and relatively easy to access (Herbert & Cohen, 1993), some researchers have questioned whether quantifying the typically variable and minute changes in the number or percentages of various white blood cells (neutrophils, monocytes, and lymphocytes) allows for a consistently reliable and completely valid detection of altered immune functioning (Cohen & Herbert, 1996).

Immune functioning has also been assessed by stimulating lymphocytes through incubation with mitogens, which produce nonspecific divergence of T or B cells. In this type of research, greater propagation of cells is usually equated with more effectiveness. Phytohemagglutinin (PHA), pokeweed mitogen (PWM), and concanavalin A (ConA) are the most commonly investigated mitogens. The procedures just described utilize what are known as *in vitro* tests, in which cells are removed from an organism and their function is then studied in a lab. There are also *in vivo* tests that study cellular function in living organisms. The quantification of antibodies to herpesviruses is an *in vivo* test frequently used in psychoneuroimmunology research. Basically, herpesviruses are common viruses that we have all been exposed to at some time in our lives. What makes them unique, however, is that after exposure, they usually remain present yet inactive in the body. When the immune system is threatened or challenged, this inactive virus may begin to replicate. Therefore, assessing and quantifying the level of antibodies to the herpesviruses provides evidence of immune function. More specifically, greater levels of herpesvirus antibodies indicate suppressed cellular immune function (Herbert & Cohen, 1996).

INTEGRATED RELATIONSHIP BETWEEN THE CENTRAL NERVOUS SYSTEM AND THE IMMUNE SYSTEM

Animal Lesion Studies

To further understand the field of psychoneuroimmunology, it is important to discern the potential connection or hypothesized direct link between the CNS and the immune system. Ballieux and Heijnen (1989) suggested that the CNS and the immune system are interconnected by two pathways, which they labeled the "wiring" and the "soluble" systems. Electrolytic lesioning studies on animals, primarily of various areas of the hypothalamus, have provided the principal method to investigate the possible wiring circuitry involved in brain–immune system communication. For example, studies investigating lesions in the anterior hypothalamus have demonstrated a decreased number of nucleated spleen cells (Brooks, Cross, Roszman, & Markesbery, 1982), decreased antibody production (Tyrey & Nalbandov, 1972), decreased NK cell activity (Cross, Brooks, Roszman, & Markesbery, 1984), and restricted progression of a lethal anaphylactic (immediate hypersensitivity when exposed to a specific antigen) response (Luparello, Stein, & Park, 1964). As summarized by Felten and his colleagues (1991), "The consensus ... is that the anterior hypothalamus is involved, either directly or indirectly, in the stimulation of both humoral and cell-mediated immune functions" (p. 7).

Although somewhat more equivocal, there are data suggesting that electrical lesions of the dorsal and medial hypothalamus in animals lead to depressed humoral and cell-mediated immunity, lethal anaphylaxis, and strengthened graft rejection (Dann, Wachtel, & Rubin, 1979; Katayama, Kobayashi, Kuramoto, & Yokoyama, 1987). Moreover, antigens injected directly into the brain have been located in cervical lymph, suggesting that they likely departed through the cranial nerves (Yamada, DePasquale, Patlak, & Cserr, 1991).

Lesions in the limbic forebrain, an area involved directly in emotional arousal (see Chapter 2), have also demonstrated alterations in immune function. Lesions of the hippocampus and amygdaloid complex revealed a temporary proliferation of T cells to a mitogen (Cross et al., 1982), and lesions of the lateral septal area, which has major connections to the hypothalamus, resulted in persistent alterations in T-cell responses (Nance, Rayson, & Carr, 1987).

It is important to note that these facilitory and inhibitory alterations in functioning are precluded by surgical removal or destruction of the pituitary gland. This procedure, known as an hypophysectomy, confirms the pituitary's mediative effect in hypothalamic functioning (Khansari, Murgo, & Faith, 1990). Moreover, direct lesioning of the pituitary gland has led to alterations in immune functioning, such as atrophy of lymphoid organs and general immunodeficiency (Berczi & Nagy, 1991).

Conditioning Studies (Animals)

Whereas lesioning studies have provided pertinent data regarding the relationship of the CNS and the immune system, some of the most compelling evidence for the functional interaction between the brain and the immune system comes from experiments in which immune responses in animals are classically conditioned. Utilizing a prototypical Pavlovian conditioning paradigm, Metal'nikov and Chorine (1926, 1928) performed what are considered to be the earliest studies of immune conditioning. In this seminal work, they paired a neutral conditioned stimulus (CS; e.g., heat or tactile stimulation) with injections of an antigen (unconditioned stimulus, UCS); subsequent presentation of the CS alone was sufficient to elicit increases in inflammatory responses and antibody levels.

Ader and Cohen (1975) are usually credited with initiating the modern studies of conditioned immune responses. Employing a taste aversion learning paradigm, they paired a distinctively flavored saccharin solution in Pavlovian fashion with an intraperitoneal injection of cyclophosphamide (an immunosuppressive drug), which produced an aversion to the flavored water and an attenuated antibody response in the injected antigen in the exposed animals. Nonconditioned and conditioned animals not reexposed to the CS did not demonstrate the responses.

In another notable study, Ader and Cohen (1982) demonstrated the clinical applicability of this type of work. Again, using a taste aversion learning paradigm, they were able to alter the progression of autoimmune disease in genetically susceptible, lupus-prone mice. The development of systemic lupus symptoms can be delayed, and survival enhanced, by weekly administration of cyclophosphamide, which is quite toxic; however, if it is not administered on a consistent weekly basis, it does not maintain therapeutic efficacy. Ader and Cohen, through the use of classical conditioning, demonstrated that pairing a saccharine-flavored solution (CS) with injections of cyclophosphamide (UCS) allowed the solution to be substituted for the drug every other week. Thus, the onset of autoimmune disease was shown to be delayed by using a cumulative dose of cyclophosphamide that was not, by itself, sufficient to modify the disease progression. Furthermore, in previously conditioned, lupus-prone, mice reexposure to the solution after discontinuation of the cyclophosphamide treatment enhanced survival (Ader, 1985; Maier, Watkins, & Flesher, 1994).

Although most contemporary research in this area has utilized a taste aversion paradigm, conditioned immunomodulatory results are not restricted to the use of taste as the CS or immunosuppressive drugs as the UCS (Ader & Cohen, 1993). This type of research has been extended and generalized across various types of conditioned and unconditioned stimuli, as well as to different measures of immune suppression and enhancement. For example, comparable results have been obtained using electric shock as the UCS (Zalcman, Kerr, & Anisman, 1991; Zalcman, Richter, & Anisman, 1989; for a comprehensive review, see Ader & Cohen, 1991). Moreover, taste aversions can be expressed without concurrent changes in immune function, and conditioned changes in immune response can be achieved without detecting conditioned avoidance taste responses (Ader et al., 1991). Furthermore, data revealing decreased antibody response from reexposure to the CS prior to injection of an immunosuppressive drug suggests that an antigen-activated immune system is not essential for the conditioned response (Kusnecov, Husband, & King, 1988; Schulze, Benson, Paule, & Roberts, 1988). These data suggest that different mechanisms are involved when conditioning is enacted on a currently resting or previously activated antigen system, or that the same UCS may have different effects on activated or nonactivated immune responses (Ader et al., 1991).

As Maier and colleagues (1994) suggested, current research should continue to explore the likely multiple mechanisms underlying the conditioned modulation of immunity, including whether the observed immune changes are directly conditioned, or whether some other conditioned reaction, such as neuroendocrine distribution, anxiety, or aversion, then accounts for the immune changes. Another future area of investigation will be to explore the interesting phenomenon of conditioned physiological effects induced by drugs typically producing conditioned responses (CRs) that mimic the drug instead of compensatory or conditioned responses in the opposite direction.

Conditioning Studies (Human)

While the preponderance of research on conditioned immune modulation has used animals, data on human beings suggest other clinical applications. Numerous older case studies, in which individuals exposed to stimuli such as artificial roses or pictures of hay fields, reportedly evince asthmatic symptoms or hay fever attacks (Mackenzie, 1896; Hill, 1930). More recently, Hegel and Ahles (1992) reported on a proposed case of interoceptive conditioning (classical conditioning of the mucosa of some internal organ) in a 52-year-old man with a history of alcoholism, who had a gagging and vomiting response to bladder sensations. Formal laboratory studies have also demonstrated that exposure to a nonallergenic stimulus (CS) paired with allergic reactions (UCS) can induce symptoms consistent with asthma in certain individuals (Dekker, Pelser, & Groen, 1957; Khan, 1977).

The area of human research most often associated with classically conditioned responding is the anticipatory nausea and vomiting that occurs in patients undergoing repeated exposure to cytotoxic drugs used in cancer treatment. Chemotherapeutic drugs, such as cyclophosphamide, are prescribed because they inhibit the proliferation of rapidly dividing cancer cells. However, their effects are also immunosuppressive in that they inhibit the replication of immune cells, which also divide rapidly (Maier et al., 1994). Conditioned stimuli, such as the thought of treatment, the site of the treatment setting, or a nurse's voice, have been considered to elicit the conditioned response of feelings of nausea (Carey & Burish, 1988). Moreover, data suggest that emotional distress relative to chemotherapy is higher in the treatment setting than in the home setting (Sabbioni, Bovbjerg, Jacobsen, Manne, & Redd, 1992), and that hospital stimuli can induce this conditioned response years after chemotherapy (Cella, Pratt, & Holland, 1986).

These findings have been expanded in nonexperimental designs to demonstrate that anticipatory anxiety, nausea, and immune suppression, as well as food and beverage aversions, can be developed in women undergoing chemotherapy for ovarian and breast cancer (Bovbjerg et al., 1990; Jacobsen, Bovbjerg, & Redd, 1993; Jacobsen, Bovbjerg, Schwartz et al., 1993). The results of a recent study of pediatric cancer patients who received the medication ondansetron to manage chemotherapy-induced nausea and vomiting revealed that despite taking the medication, anticipatory symptoms of nausea and vomiting were prevalent and consistent with Pavlovian conditioning (Tyc, Mulhern, Barclay, Smith, & Bieberich, 1997). For example, a positive relationship was found between the child's self-report ratings of intensity of postchemotherapy nausea and vomiting symptoms (the unconditioned response, UCR) and their reports of anticipatory nausea frequency and severity (the CR).

Recent formal experimental studies have randomly assigned patients to either an experimental or control condition to investigate whether patients undergoing repeated chemotherapy infusions can develop classically conditioned emotional distress to stimuli associated with the procedure.

Jacobsen and colleagues (1995) repeatedly paired lemon-lime Kool-Aid administered to patients in a distinctive clear cup with a bright orange lid (CS) and the infusion of the toxic chemotherapeutic agent (UCS); the control group received no such pairing. When the beverage was presented alone in a location not associated with the infusion procedure, the experimental subjects demonstrated significantly increased subjective emotional distress compared to the control group.

IMMUNE SYSTEM TO CENTRAL NERVOUS SYSTEM

Mediating mechanisms are considered to occur that underlie potential reciprocal communication, and bidirectional, or "cross talk," between the immune system and the CNS. In order for this mechanism to occur, the brain would need to receive information that an immune response is occurring (Maier et al., 1994). More than 25 years ago, Besedovsky, Sorkin, Keller, and Muller (1975) reported that glucocorticoid blood levels increased in rodents during the immune response following injection of an antigen. Recent researchers have begun to investigate the role of cytokines, which were addressed earlier. While it was originally believed that cytokines serve an exclusive communicative function within the immune system, evidence now suggests that they are inextricably linked to the CNS. For example, intraperitoneal injections of the cytokine interleukin 1 (IL-1) have been shown to cause an elevation in the hypothalamic setpoint leading to fever (Kelley, Johnson, & Dantzer, 1994). Also, humans injected with recombinant cytokines often experience neurological symptoms such as memory loss and weakness (Dantzer & Kelley, 1989). Moreover, specific antagonists to the IL-1 receptor block CNS changes (Dunn, 1993). There are several hypothesized ways that the cytokines may gain access to the CNS, such as through circumventricular organs of the brain that lack a true blood–brain barrier, through messenger glial cells, or by indirectly inducing their own synthesis (Kelley et al., 1994; Kent, Bluthé, Kelley, & Dantzer, 1992). Therefore, cytokines and other hormonal proteins released by immune cells, often referred to as "immunotransmitters," appear to complete the proposed bidirectional communication feedback loop by serving to inform the brain that a foreign agent has entered the body (Ballieux, 1994).

The Stress Response and the Immune System: A Soluble Link

The integrated regulatory feedback mechanisms between the brain and the immune system become more apparent when we consider the stress response more closely. As reviewed extensively in Chapters 2 and 3, corticotropin-releasing factor (CRF) is often considered the coordinator of the human stress response, and the peripheral physiological changes that make up this response have been termed the General Adaptation Syndrome (GAS).

The suggested soluble link between the brain and the immune system becomes increasingly plausible when we consider the functioning of the peripheral nervous system (PNS) during the human stress response (Maier et al., 1994). In particular, noradrenergic sympathetic innervation, originating in the posterior hypothalamus, has been documented to innervate both primary (bone marrow, thymus) and secondary (spleen and lymph nodes) immune organs (Black, 1994; Felten & Felten, 1992). Recall from Chapter 2 that norepinephrine is the catecholamine released by the nerve terminals of the SNS. Considering that immune organs and cells possess catecholamine receptors and "the terminals of sympathetic nerves in these immune organs make contacts with lymphocytes themselves" (Maier et al., 1994, p. 1006), then it is reasonable to conclude that there is a tangible connection between the brain and the immune system. Elaborating upon Table 2.5, glucocorticoid hormones, such as the corticosteroids, which are elevated during stress and released from the adrenal cortices, inhibit immune system functions such as lymphocyte and macrophage production. These hormones also decrease the production of particular cytokines and inflammatory molecules (Chrousos & Gold, 1992). Surgical removal or chemical inhibition of adrenal function eliminates many of the immunosuppressive effects of stress (Dantzer & Kelley, 1989). Moreover, corticotropin-releasing hormone (CRH) has been shown to induce human blood leukocytes to manufacture and secrete adrenocorticotropic hormone (ACTH) and B-endorphin (Ballieux, 1994).

Most of the literature on the human stress response has investigated the collective physiological arousal associated with the fight-or-flight response. The concurrent inhibition of vegetative functions has been much less explored; however, "during the adaptational response to stress... the systems regulating growth, reproduction, thyroid function, and immunity are down regulated" (Black, 1994, p. 2). Two immunoenhancing anterior pituitary hormones, growth hormone and prolactin, are required for ordinary immune functioning and resistance to infection. Both are elevated early in the human stress response (Khansari et al., 1990) and receptors for these hormones are located on lymphocytes and macrophages (Kelley, 1989).

Stress and Immune Functioning: Animal Studies

The primary interest in the field of psychoneuroimmunology has generally evolved from animal and human research investigating the link between biogenic and psychosocial stressors, immune functioning, and disease processes. The effects of humoral and cell-mediated immunity, as well as tumor growth and survival, have been used as outcome variables (Bohus & Koolhaas, 1991). In the animal literature, myriad stressors have been used to investigate the impact on immunological functioning. For example, Hans Selye's original description of the GAS was in response to exposing laboratory rats to diverse, nocuous agents, such as cold temperatures, severed spinal cords, excessive exercise, or drug injections. Following exposure to these stimuli, Selye (1936) documented decreased circulating lymphocytes; rapid decreased size of the thymus, spleen, lymph glands, and liver; formation of erosions in the stomach; and loss of muscle tone. He further noted that the animals often developed "resistance" with continued exposure to the stressors that mimicked normal functioning; however, with additional exposure of 1–3 months, the animals became "exhausted" and developed the symptoms described earlier.

The impact of environmental stressors on infectious disease processes has been reviewed extensively in the literature. Laboratory animals have been exposed to electric foot shocks, cold temperatures, loud noises, restraints, crowding, handling, and isolation. For example, restraint models that place rats or mice in narrow tubes or use adhesive substances placed on boards to maintain immobilization often prohibit their movement. These types of studies have often resulted in cellular and humoral suppression, as well as impaired NK-cell activity (Koolhaas & Bohus, 1995; Steplewski & Vogel, 1986). Studies examining the effects of handling, picking up, and holding laboratory animals for various lengths of time have shown a decrease in IgG antibody production and decreased T-cell function (Moynihan et al., 1994). However, additional data have shown that adding another stressor, such as an intraperitoneal injection, resulted in attenuated corticosterone and catecholamine responses in previously handled mice compared to unhandled mice. Thus, Moynihan and colleagues (1994) suggested that the psychosocial stressor of handling may result in habituation to the effects of the stress response.

The general immune responses of decreased IgG-antibody production, NK-cell activity, and lymphocyte generation have been fairly well established in response to electric shocks (Cunnick, Lysle, Armfield, & Rabin, 1988; Laudenslager et al., 1988). Other researchers have expanded these findings to include an investigation of psychosocial stressors such as decreased predictability and control. Despite equivocal data, evidence suggests that laboratory rats provided an opportunity to perform a response to avoid or eliminate electric shock developed less severe gastric ulceration and less rapid tumor growth formation than those exposed to the same amount of electric shocks without controllability (Weiss, 1968; Sklar &

Anisman, 1979). Foot shock as a physical stressor causes release of pheromones that are an important aspect of rodent communication. Moynihan and colleagues (1994) reported on the results of an investigation in which pheromones produced by foot-shocked mice changed immune functioning in those mice receiving the odor. Interestingly, they reported suppression in cell-mediated responses, and enhanced humoral responses in the odor-exposed mice. Other data have suggested that learning and memory circuits may be conditioned at the CNS level following acute exposure to electric shock, and that these conditioned responses may have both immunosuppressive and immunoenhancement effects (Koolhaas & Bohus, 1995).

Psychosocial stressors induced by crowding and isolation have also been widely studied for their modulating effects on immunity. The results of numerous studies of high-density crowding have generally demonstrated increased disease susceptibility and decreased survival. In one of the original studies of this phenomenon, Vessey (1964) reported that placing typically isolated male mice in a group setting for 4 hours a day resulted in lower antibody responses to a mitogen. Of particular interest, the dominant male mouse in the group had the highest antibody production. Other studies have shown that physically dominant or aggressive male rats in a social colony have higher antibody generation, whereas submissive or defeated rats and mice have demonstrated increased immunosuppression (Bohus & Koolhaas, 1991; Koolhaas & Bohus, 1989). Fleshner, Laudenslager, Simons, and Maier (1989) have also shown that engaging in submissive behaviors, as compared to continuing to react aggressively and receiving multiple bites, correlated with reduced antibody formation to an injected antigen. These data suggest that animals may evidence individual differences in coping styles to given stressors. The active coping style has been associated with high SNS reactivity, whereas passive coping has been considered to be affiliated with increased reactivity of the pituitary–adrenocortical axis. As noted by Koolhaas and Bohus (1995), "This interaction between environment and individual is ... crucial to understanding the relationship between stress and immunity" (p. 78).

Stress and Immune Function: Human Studies

If the data exploring stress and immunity in animals alerts investigators to the interactive effects between the environment and the individual, then it should be apparent that this type of modulation also applies to humans. Indeed, investigators need to consider the subtle, selective, multifaceted nature of the precipitants (e.g., age, gender, emotional status, and genetic factors) and physical consequences of stress, in addition to the complex and often lengthy duration of immune responses before generating broadly

93

conclusive causal statements about how stress directly alters immune function (Zeller, McCain, McCann, Swanson, & Colletti, 1996; see Maier et al., 1994, for a detailed discussion on this topic). As the eminent Paul Rosch (1995) noted, "These and other caveats must be considered when evaluating sweeping statements and conclusions about the effect of 'stress' on 'immune function' or therapeutic triumphs based on psychoneuroimmunological approaches" (p. 214).

These precautionary notes are not intended to diminish the outstanding advancements and notable influence of stress-induced immunomodulation research or the unequivocal impact that emotions such a stress have on immunity. Instead, they are intended to inform the reader that exploring, uncovering, and externally validating generally accepted tenets between psychological variables such as stress and immunity involve a complex process that continues to evolve. For example, it is worth considering that many of the proposed relations between psychosocial stressors (e.g., loss of a spouse) and disease (e.g., depression) that are often credited to immune changes may be strongly affected by behavioral health changes such as alcohol or drug consumption, noncompliance with medications, decreased sleep, and poorer diets that occur following the stressor (Cohen & Herbert, 1996).

Bereavement.   The preponderance of early evidence relating psychological components of human health and disease has been anecdotal, and, of course, ethical considerations have usually precluded the type of controlled experimental research conducted on animals. Correlational designs have primarily been used to examine the impact of stressors such as negative life events on illness and immune function. For example, bereavement studies have consistently demonstrated differences between unmarried and married individuals in terms of physical health. Immune functioning in the form of lymphocyte production was shown to be decreased in several prospective studies of bereaved and nonbereaved men and women who had lost a spouse due to illnesses such as breast and lung cancer (Bartrop, Luckhurst, Lazarus, Kiloh, & Penny, 1977; Irwin, Daniels, Smith, Bloom, & Weiner, 1987; Schleifer, Keller, Camerino, Thornton, & Stein, 1983). In a separate but related study, Linn, Linn, and Jensen (1984) suggested that reduction in lymphocytes was more influenced by level of depression than by bereavement. A meta-analysis demonstrated that clinically depressed individuals have a poorer response to mitogens PHA, ConA, and PWM, and lowered NK- and helper T-cell activity (Herbert & Cohen, 1993). Irwin, Lacher, and Caldwell (1992) have provided longitudinal data suggesting that with successful treatment of depression, decreased NK activity is abrogated. However, the data on immune correlates of depression are not universally supportive (Ravindran, Griffiths, Merali, & Anisman, 1995), and discrepant findings have led researchers to suggest that compromised immune functioning may be more evident in elderly, severely depressed, and hospitalized patients (Houldin, Lev, Prystowsky, Redei, & Lowery, 1991).

Schizophrenia. With regard to another major psychiatric disorder, researchers have also long noted the heterogenous pathophysiology of schizophrenia. Although not conclusive, studies examining immunoglobulin (IgG) in cerebrospinal fluid (CSF) in some patients have shown raised levels that may be due to impaired permeability of the blood–brain barrier (Muller & Ackenheil, 1995). Other studies in a subgroup of schizophrenic patients have revealed additional immunological abnormalities such as increased occurrence of autoimmune diseases and decreased lymphocyte (IL-2) production, among other immune changes. Muller and Ackenheil have proposed that schizophrenic patients should be classified as those with and without immune alterations. Moreover, preliminary epidemiological evidence utilizing maternal recall has demonstrated an association between second-trimester gestational influenza infections, obstetrical complications (e.g., anemia, emergency cesarean section, breech presentation), and low birth weights in newborns who later developed schizophrenia (Wright, Takei, Rifkin, & Murray, 1995).

Personal Relationships. Studies examining the link between personal relationships (e.g., marital conflict, divorce, and separation) and immune function have provided some notable findings. In a study of 32 women, the 16 women who had been separated 1 year or less showed poorer immune function on immunological blood assays compared to matched controls (Kiecolt-Glaser et al., 1987).

In a study of 64 men, Kiecolt-Glaser and associates (1988) found that the 32 men who had been separated or divorced reported feeling more lonely and described more recent illnesses. Evidence suggests, however, that subjects who initiate the separation and those who have less preoccupation with their ex-spouse may experience less distress and have better immune functioning (Keicolt-Glaser et al., 1988; Weiss, 1975). Using rigorous selection criteria, Kiecolt-Glaser and her colleagues (1993) demonstrated that in 90 newlywed couples, high-negative subjects who exhibited more negative or hostile behavior during a behaviorally coded 30-minute discussion of marital problems evidenced significantly greater down-regulated immune functioning (e.g., NK-cell lysis, poorer responses to ConA and PHA, and higher antibody titers to Epstein–Barr Virus, among other responses) over a 24-hour period relative to low-negative subjects. Also of note, blood pressure changes were more dramatic and persistent in high-negative subjects,

and women overall were more likely than men to have negative immunological alterations.

Academic Stress.   Keicolt-Glaser and her colleagues have also been
responsible for some of the most methodologically sound, large-scale human
stress studies investigating the immunological effects of the predictable acute
stressor of academic examinations on medical students (Kiecolt-Glaser,
Garner, Speicher, Penn, Holliday, & Glaser, 1984). These data have shown a
decay in NK-cell activity when compared to baseline blood samples obtained
1 month prior to the exams. Additionally, in main effects noted for stressful
life events in self-report inventories of the Holmes–Rahe Social Readjustment
Scale and the UCLA Loneliness Scale, high scorers had lower NK activity
than low scorers. The use of protein markers ruled out the possibility that the
differences in NK-cell response were due to nutritional deficiencies. Also
of note, there was no difference in received grades between students who
did and did not participate. Other data (Glaser, Kiecolt-Glaser, Bonneau,
Malarkey, Kennedy, & Hughes, 1992) have suggested that academic stress
could negatively impact the ability of hepatitis vaccines to evoke antibody
responses in a sample of medical students. Kang, Coe, and McCarthy (1996)
recently expanded this line of research when they investigated whether
differences in immune responses between healthy and asthmatic adolescents in response to academic examinations. Results revealed alterations in
immune functioning, for example, decreased NK-cytolytic activity in both
groups, without concurrent changes in lung function for the well-managing
asthmatics.

Chronic Stress.   Researchers have also investigated the effects of
chronic stressors on immune functioning. Specifically, the health of family
members who provide long-term care of loved ones with Alzheimer's disease, often considered a form of living bereavement, has been examined
over time. Results suggest that caregiving may produce more depression in
family members (Crook & Miller, 1985), in addition to impaired immune
responses compared to a matched-control sample when exposed to ConA,
PHA, and latent Epstein–Barr virus (Kiecolt-Glaser, Dura, Speicher, Trask,
& Glaser, 1991). Moreover, caregivers experienced significantly more days
ill from upper respiratory tract infections, and the poorest immune functioning was observed in caregivers who had institutionalized their spouse
within the previous year after caring for them for an average of 5 years.
Esterling, Kiecolt-Glaser, Bodnar, and Glaser (1994) expanded these findings by including a group of former Alzheimer's disease caregivers (those
whose spouse had died at least 2 years earlier) along with current caregivers and a control group. Results revealed no difference in symptoms

of depression or perceived distress between the continuing and former caregivers, and both groups were significantly more depressed than the control group. Similarly, the continuing and former caregivers did not differ in the functional responsiveness of NK-cell cytotoxicity to cytokine incubation, and both groups had a significantly poorer immune response than controls. A recent study has manipulated NK-cell composition at a cellular level to investigate the mechanisms of immune effects on caregivers (Esterling, Kiecolt-Glaser, & Glaser, 1996). Considering how the population is aging, this area of research will be increasingly valuable in the future.

HIV and AIDS. The myriad implications associated with the course of human immunodeficiency virus (HIV) and acquired immune deficiency syndrome (AIDS), first recognized in the early 1980s, provide a prototypical illness to study from a psychoneuroimmunological perspective (McCain & Zeller, 1996). Not surprisingly, HIV has been associated, albeit inconclusively due to methodological challenges and the tremendous variability of the manifestation of the virus, with depression, suicidal ideation, anxiety, and bereavement (Holland & Tross, 1987; Perry, Fishman, Jacobsberg, & Frances, 1992). For example, Kemeny and her colleagues (1995), who reported that HIV-positive men who recently lost an intimate partner to AIDS evidence decreased immune functioning, have also suggested that grief and depression may have different immunological correlates in HIV.

The hallmark of AIDS is a quantitative depletion of a subset of T-lymphocyte cells, the T-helper or CD_4 cells (CD = cluster designation) (McCain & Zeller, 1996). More recent data have reported that HIV disease is the result of a process by which CD_4 cells are continually infected, destroyed, and regenerated (Ho et al., 1995; Wei et al., 1995). The decline in CD_4 cells number is the result of the proportional rate of cell destruction exceeding cell regeneration. As the aggregate of CD_4 cells continues to decline, the signaling required for normal cellular and humoral responsivity is negatively impacted, leading to the development of opportunistic infections and various diseases that are pathognomonic of AIDS (Kemeny, 1994). The steady immunological decline noted in the beginning stages of HIV-seropositive individuals suggests that early psychosocial interventions may be particularly beneficial in helping patients to enhance their functioning (Antoni et al., 1990).

Intervention studies of individuals with HIV have generally involved exercise training and cognitive-behavioral approaches such as guided imagery and active neuromuscular relaxation (see Chapters 9, 13, and 16 for detailed discussions of these topics). Compared to a group of HIV-seropositive men who improved their aerobic capacity by riding a stationary bicycle for 45 minutes, three times per week, HIV-seropositive men who did not exercise demonstrated significant increases in anxiety and depression, and decreases in immune functioning (LaPerriere et al., 1990, 1991). More recent evidence suggests that HIV individuals who are compliant with an exercising training regimen show a significant increase in CD_4 cells, whereas those noncompliant with training (attending less than 50% of the sessions) showed a significant decrease in CD_4 cells (LaPerriere et al., 1997). Guided imagery as a therapeutic intervention gained notoriety in the area of psychoneuroimmunology when researchers claimed that cancer patients who used the technique to most likely envision their body attacking and destroying invading infections were able almost to double their mean survival time (Hall, Anderson, & O'Grady, 1994; Hall & O'Grady, 1991; Holland & Tross, 1987; Simonton, Matthews-Simonton, & Sparks, 1980). In a recent study, Eller (1996) reported that 6 weeks of training in guided imagery and progressive relaxation training (PRT) was associated with less depression and fatigue and increased CD_4 cells in a group of individuals with HIV. Recent investigators have suggested that NK cells may be a better psychoneuroimmunological marker for the effects of emotions (Sahs et al., 1994).

Humor. Norman Cousins, the noted essayist and editor of the *Saturday Review*, addressed the potential therapeutic impact of humor on the immune system when he described in detail his use of laughter during his treatment for ankylosing spondylitis, a very uncomfortable inflammation of the vertebrae. Cousins dedicated more than a decade to amassing empirical evidence for his postulate that "laughter is the best medicine," and established the Humor Research Task Force (Wooten, 1996). Controlled studies have shown that laughter lowers cortisol levels and increases lymphocytes, NK cells, and concentration of salivary IgA (Berk, 1989a,b; Dillon & Baker, 1985; McClelland & Cheriff, 1997). Therefore, through the use of what may be considered cathartic liberation, humor and laughter seem to serve a protective immune function. Some hospitals have recognized the positive emotions engendered by humor and have introduced "Laugh Mobiles" that sell humorous novelties (Erdman, 1993).

Writing. Another cathartic method that has received attention for providing a link to positive health-related outcomes, including improved immune functioning, is writing about a traumatic event (Pennebaker & Beall, 1986; Pennebaker, Kiecolt-Glaser, & Glaser, 1988). Pennebaker and his colleagues have cogently demonstrated that subjects who wrote about suppressed traumatic experiences for 20 minutes per day for 4 consecutive days had fewer doctor visits, less subjective distress, and higher overall mitogen-induced lymphocyte response. Esterling and his colleagues (1994) have more recently reported that subjects either writing or verbalizing about stressful experiences demonstrate reduced latent Epstein–Barr virus titers than control subjects. Other, more current data have shown that participants who write about traumatic events develop significantly greater antibodies to the hepatitis B vaccine compared to a control group. In an analysis of the writing style of participants from six studies, Pennebaker (1999) recently noted that the use of positive emotion words, the moderate use of negative emotion words, and an increase in both causal and insight words over the course of the writing assignment to produce a coherent story is most strongly associated with improved physical health.

Traumas.   In addition to the stressful life events described earlier, investigators have focused on acute and chronic immune system alterations following natural traumas or technological disasters. One of the first instances of this type of exploration occurred following the nuclear accident at Three Mile Island (Hatch, Wallenstein, Beyea, Nieves, & Susser, 1991). Compared to control subjects, residents near the event had greater numbers of neutrophils, and fewer B, T, and NK cells 6 years later. More recently, studies have examined immune effects following the North Ridge earthquake in Southern California and Hurricane Andrew in South Florida (Ironson et al., 1997; Solomon, Segerstrom, Grohr, Kemeny, & Fahey, 1997). In both studies, NK cell cytotoxicity (NKCC) was lower over time. In the latter study, severity of symptoms (particularly perceived loss and intrusive thoughts) was negatively related to NKCC and positively related to white blood cell counts. Of special interest for therapeutic interventions was the evidence of new-onset sleep difficulties as possibly mediating the PTSD symptom–NKCC relationship.

SUMMARY

The purpose of this chapter was to provide an overview of the extensive and evolving field of psychoneuroimmunology. We will review the main points of the chapter.

1. Generally, the immune system can be conceptually divided into innate and acquired immunity.
2. Innate immunity, also known as nonspecific immunity, includes species-specific immunity, physical barriers (e.g., skin and biochemicals such as saliva and tears), phagocytosis, natural killer (NK) cells, interferon, and inflammation.
3. Acquired immunity, also known as specific immunity, develops as part of the body's lymphatic system. Two major types of lymphocytes are T and B cells.

4. T cells, or cell-mediated immunity, specifically pursue an invading antigen and release chemical messengers (cytokines) to facilitate the immune response.

5. B cells, or humoral immunity, produce their effects indirectly by producing antibodies (known as immunoglobulins) that combine selectively with the antigen. IgG is the most common immunoglobulin.

6. The effects of circulating antibodies and cellular immunity are influenced by the body's complement system.

7. *In vitro* (removing cells from the organism) and *in vivo* tests (studying cellular function in living organisms) are commonly used to investigate the effects of mitogens such as phytohemagglutinin (PHA), pokeweed mitogen (PWM), or concanavalin A (conA) on immune functioning.

8. The link between the CNS and the immune system was investigated by examining the outcome of animal lesioning studies of the hypothalamus, limbic system, and pituitary gland.

9. Classical conditioning studies on animals and humans have also provided evidence of a functional interaction between the brain and the immune system. The area of human research most associated with classically conditioned responding is the nausea and vomiting that occurs in cancer patients undergoing chemotherapy.

10. The reciprocal link between the immune system and the CNS comes from research investigating the effects of antigens injected into animals to study CNS functioning.

11. An investigation of the neuroendocrine and endocrine axes of the stress response provides evidence of a soluble link between CNS functioning and immunity.

12. Animal studies have demonstrated the connection between biogenic and psychosocial stressors and immune function. Hans Selye's seminal work investigating the General Adaptation Syndrome (GAS) is an early example of how biogenic stressors adversely affect immune function.

13. Psychosocial stressors imposed on animals, such as lack of predictability and control, increased crowding, and isolation, have shown various immunosuppressive effects, and data suggest that animals may evidence individual coping styles to given stressors.

14. The impact of stress on immune function in humans has explored areas such as bereavement, marital conflict, and effects of taking exams, and providing long-term care to loved ones with Alzheimer's disease and AIDS. It is important to keep in mind, however, that individual variables and modifying factors need to be considered before coming to general conclusions about stress and immune function.

15. The impact of humor on immune function, most often credited to Norman Cousins, and the cathartic impact of writing about traumatic events, which is most often credited to James Pennebaker, are examples of potential therapeutic interventions that may enhance immune functioning.

16. In summary, this rather ambitious chapter has attempted to review the vast field of psychoneuroimmunology. In keeping with the mission of this volume, the emphasis has been on the impact of stress and immune function. In general, psychoneuroimmunology reinforces the widely held view that disease is a multifactorial, biopsychosocial phenomenon in terms of onset, course, and intervention.

6

Measurement of the Human Stress Response

In the final analysis, the empirical foundation of epistemology is measurement.

When an unexplained phenomenon, such as a stress-related disease, is first observed, it is common to search for possible etiological factors. This search often culminates in a phenomenological theory; in this case, perhaps a theory of stress arousal and subsequent pathogenesis. On the basis of the formulated theory, for example, of stress arousal, it is then a useful next step to design an experiment in order to test the theory and any proposed relationships critical to the theory. Inherent in the design of the experiment is the designation of key variables and some means of measuring, recording, or otherwise quantifying those relevant variables. Relevant to the present discussion, this would typically involve a means of measuring the stress response and perhaps its pathological effects.

As we review the literature concerning human stress, it is obvious that in addition to the lack of a universal definition of stress, the field has also been plagued by a plethora of inconsistencies and potential phenomenological errors in the measurement of the human stress response. If we cannot reliably and validly measure the human stress response, what degree of credibility do we place upon investigations into its phenomenology? Indeed, meta-analytic research has suggested that the measurement of independent and dependent variables may be the single most important aspect of research design—even more important than the structure of the research design itself (Cohen, 1984; Fiske, 1983; Smith, Glass, & Miller, 1980). With regard to stress research, it may be argued that the

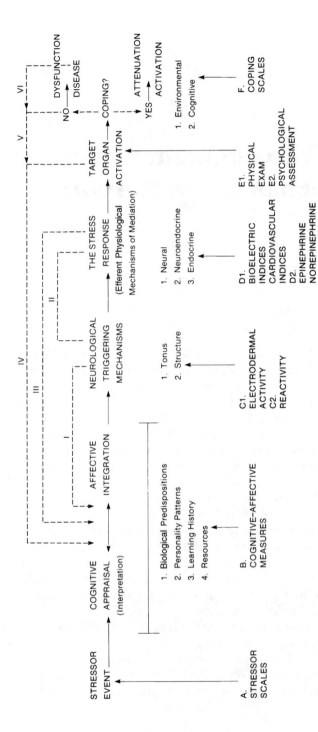

CHAPTER 6

Figure 6.1. Measurement of the human stress response.

confounded or inappropriate measurement process has the greatest ability to limit the generation of useful data regarding this important public health phenomenon (Cattell & Scheier, 1961; Everly & Sobelman, 1987). Thus, the purpose of this chapter is to discuss the measurement of the human stress response.

In Chapter 2, a systems model of the nature of the human stress response was constructed (Figure 2.6). As a means of integrating the following measurement-based discussions, that basic model is reproduced here, with key measurement technologies having been superimposed (see Figure 6.1). Let us take this opportunity to examine more closely the measurement of the human stress response.

STRESSOR SCALES

The most widely used measurement tool for the assessment of human stress, in reality, does not measure stress at all—it measures stressors. The Social Readjustment Rating Scale (SRRS), the "grandfather" of attempts at measuring stress, was developed by Thomas Holmes and Richard Rahe (1967), based upon the theory that "life change" is causally associated with subsequent illness. This notion was by no means a new idea. Adolph Meyer pioneered empirical investigations into the relationship between psychosocial events and illness with the advent of his "life chart" as a means of creating a medical history.

The SRRS contains 43 items consisting of commonly experienced "life events." Each life event is weighted with a life change unit score (LCU). Respondents are simply asked to check each of the items they have experienced within the last 12 months. The arithmetic summation of LCUs represents the total LCU score, which can then be converted to a relative health risk statement, that is, the risk of becoming ill within a stipulated time period. The association between high LCU scores and risk of subsequent illness is assumed to be a function of the fact that organisms must adapt to novel stimuli and otherwise new life events. The physiology of adaptation has long been known to be the same physiology as the stress response. Thus, stress may be seen as the linchpin between life events and illness as conceived of and measured by the SRRS.

The SRRS is not without its critics, however. Two major issues have been raised:

1. Life events scales should be modified so as to assess the perceived desirability of the life event. It has been suggested that negative life events are potentially more pathogenic than positive life events (Sarason, Johnson, & Siegel, 1978).

2. It has also been suggested that "minor hassles" are more important predictors of illness than major life events (Kanner, Coyne, Schaefer, & Lazarus, 1981).

Other noteworthy efforts in the assessment of stressor stimuli should be mentioned. In an attempt to improve the SRRS with regard to the issue of event desirability, Sarason and his colleagues (1978) created the Life Experiences Survey (LES), which not only lists a series of life events but also inquires into the desirability of each of the events. In a far more ingenious approach to the life events issue, Lazarus and his colleagues investigated the daily hassles versus major life events issue as it pertains to the prediction of subsequent illness (Kanner et al., 1981). The Hassles Scale lists a series of minor daily hassles, that is, sources of frustration that commonly recur to many individuals. The scale also includes an "uplifts" assessment that theoretically serves to mitigate the adverse impact of negative life events.

The LES and the Hassles Scale are creative and alternative approaches to the assessment of stressors, but the SRRS continues to enjoy the greatest frequency of use, both clinically and for research purposes.

A more recent entry into the genre of stressor scales is the Stressful Life Experiences Screening (SLES; Stamm, 1996). This instrument consists of 20 items that inquire as to (1) the presence of a stressful life experience, and (2) the degree of "stressfulness" of that experience. The long form (SLES-L) takes 5–10 minutes to complete.

Finally, the Life Stressor Checklist—Revised (Wolfe & Kimerling, 1998) consists of 30 "events" that satisfy the DSM-IV definition of traumatic. The self-report scale takes 15–30 minutes to complete and is designed for use with adults. The scale is not only an indicator of traumatic events, but it also serves as an assessment of the events' current impact upon the individual.

As for the genre of stressor scales, Monroe (1983) notes, "Although findings of event—illness associations appear to be consistent in that increased life events predict dysfunction in both retrospective and prospective studies, the magnitude of the association reported typically has been low" (p. 190). The recognized consistency in the life events research combined with its low-effect size leads one to believe that life events scales such as the SRRS do indeed tap some domain that has meaning in stress phenomenology; however, there appear to be other mediating variables that need to be better understood. From the view of the present model, life events scales tap the stressor domain and therefore cannot be said to assess either the stress response itself or the causal mechanisms that undergird stress arousal. Nevertheless, scales such as the SRRS can be of value, especially in stress research when the researcher wishes to obtain valid and reliable assessments of the "background noise," that is, intervening or other otherwise confounding variables in psychosocial stressor research (see Everly & Sobelman, 1987).

COGNITIVE–AFFECTIVE CORRELATE SCALES

Whereas in the preceding section we discussed the assessment of stressor stimuli, the reader will recall from Chapter 2 the agreement among most stress researchers that in order for psychosocial life events to engender a stress response and subsequent illness, they must first be processed via cognitive–affective mechanisms. It seems theoretically viable, therefore, that one might assess the cognitive–affective domain of respondents as an indirect assessment of the human stress response (Everly & Sobelman, 1987). Derogatis (1977) has argued that such a "self-report mode of psychological measurement contains much to recommend it" (p. 2). Furthermore, Everly has argued that assessment of this domain may be the most practical, efficient, and cost-effective way of measuring the human stress response (Everly & Sobelman, 1987).

There are several scales that assess the cognitive–affective correlates of the stress response. The Derogatis Stress Scale (Derogatis, 1980) is a 77-item self-report inventory derived from interactional stress theory. It purports to assess not only emotional responses and personality mediators, but also environmental events.

The World Assumption Scale (WAS; Janoff-Bulman, 1996) assesses three core assumptions, or beliefs, about life: the benevolence of the world, the inherent meaningfulness of the world, and self-worth. This self-report scale requires 5–10 minutes to complete and consists of 32 items scored according to a 6-point Likert scale.

The final inventory worthy of note within this genre is the Millon Behavioral Health Inventory (MBHI) developed by Theodore Millon and his colleagues (Millon, Green, & Meagher, 1982). The MBHI is a 150-item self-report inventory that has been normed on medical patients. "Its intent is to aid in the psychological understanding of these patients and facilitate the steps required to formulate a comprehensive treatment plan" (p. 2). The true–false inventory includes scales grouped into four categories: basic characterological coping styles, psychogenic attitudes, psychosomatic correlates, and prognostic indices. Rigorously developed yet practical in its applicability, the MBHI is the best of the broad-spectrum inventories of its kind (Everly & Sobelman, 1987). It also profits from having its theoretical foundations firmly entrenched in the personality theory of Theodore Millon.

NEUROLOGICAL TRIGGERING MECHANISMS

The assessment of the sensitivity of neurological triggering mechanisms is by no means an easy task. Aberrant evoked potentials emerging from the subcortical limbic system would be one indication of an existing hypersensitivity phenomenon within the limbic system. The accurate assessment of subcortical activity via electroencephalography (EEG) is very difficult and may be considered a gross assessment at best, however. False-negative findings are a common problem with such assessment and EEGs in general.

Electrodermal responsiveness as assessed via galvanic skin response (GSR) would be another way of assessing the reactivity of neurological triggering mechanisms (Everly & Sobelman, 1987).

Finally, the general assessment of psychophysiological reactivity is believed to be a viable process for assessing the efferent-discharge propensity of the limbic system (Everly & Sobelman, 1987). The phenomenology of this process is based upon the theories of Lacy, Malmo, and Sternbach discussed in Chapter 3.

MEASURING THE PHYSIOLOGY OF THE STRESS RESPONSE

It will be recalled from Chapter 2 that the stress response can be divided into three broad categories: (1) the neural axes, (2) the neuroendocrine axis, and (3) the endocrine axes. Let us briefly review several of the more common assessment technologies used to tap these phenomenological domains.

Assessment of the Neural Axes

Assessment of the neural axes of the human stress response is for the most part an attempt to capture a transitory state measurement phenomenon, as opposed to a more consistent trait. Technologies used for such assessment include (1) electrodermal techniques, (2) electromyographic techniques, and (3) cardiovascular measures.

Electrodermal Measures

The physiological basis of the electrodermal assessment of the stress response is the eccrine sweat gland. Located primarily in the soles of the feet and the palms of the hands, these sweat glands respond to psychological stimuli rather than heat and emerge on the terminal efferent ends of sympathetic neurons. Although the neurotransmitter at the sweat gland itself is Ach, as opposed to NE, the assessment of this activity provides useful insight into the activity of the sympathetic nervous system. Electrodermal activity may be assessed via active GSR techniques or through passive techniques such as skin potentials (SP), according to Edelberg (1972). Andreassi (1980) has stated that electrodermal techniques are useful indices of somatic arousal.

Electromyographic Measurement

The physiological basis of electromyographic measurement of the stress response is the neurological innervation of the striated skeletal muscles. Electromyography, although an indirect measure of muscle "tension," is a direct measure of the action potentials originating from the neurons that innervate the muscles.

Skeletal muscles receive their neural innervation primarily as a result of alpha motoneuron presence, on the efferent limb, and secondarily as a result of gamma motoneuron activity as well. From the afferent perspective, proprioceptive neurons arising from the muscle spindles contribute to the overall electrical activity that originates from the skeletal musculature. In a relaxed state, skeletal muscle tone serves as a very useful general index of arousal (Gellhorn, 1964; Gellhorn & Loofbourrow, 1963; Jacobson, 1929, 1970; Malmo, 1975; Weil, 1974), yet in a contracted state this utility appears to disappear. Thus, when using skeletal muscles as general indices of arousal and stress responsiveness, it becomes of critical importance to teach patients to first relax those muscles (Everly et al., 1989).

There has been considerable debate on the utility of a particular set of muscles as an index of arousal. That set of muscles is the group known as the *frontalis*.

Jacobson (1970) and Shagass and Malmo (1954) first recognized that the frontalis and related facial muscles were prime targets of the stress-arousal process. Budzynski and Stoyva (1969) and Stoyva (1979) explored and refined the clinical utility of these muscles in the treatment of stress-related disorders. Similar work was undertaken by Schwartz et al. (1978), who found the corrugator muscles of similar utility in relation to depression.

It may be argued that the frontalis muscles of the forehead provide a useful site for the assessment of stress arousal. These muscles have been termed "quasi-voluntary" muscles because of their autonomic-like properties manifest during emotional states. In support of such a view is the recent series of studies indicating that when simple facial expressions are mimicked, an alteration in heart rate and skin temperature can be observed, even when the subjects were simply asked to mimic the expression without any consideration for the cognitive or affective state that might be associated with it. Similarly, Rubin (1977) suggests that the frontalis muscles, in particular, may possess properties of dual innervation: skeletal alpha motoneuron and ANS innervation.

Although, clearly, the frontalis musculature is predominately striated in nature (thus receiving efferent innervation from the alpha motoneuron assemblies), Rubin (1977) has argued that the frontalis also possesses thin nonstriated layers of musculature. These nonstriated muscles apparently receive their innervation (directly or indirectly) from the SNS (Miehlke, 1973). Thus, assessment of the frontalis muscles through electromyographic procedures may well provide insight into alpha motoneuron activity, sympathetic neural activity, as well as neuroendocrine activity (Everly & Sobelman, 1987). Although there is not total agreement on the utility of the frontalis musculature (Alexander, 1975), Stoyva (1979) provides useful guidelines for the use of that measurement variable.

Clinical biofeedback experience shows the frontalis muscles are useful in the treatment of a wide range of stress-related disorders, including essential hypertension and disorders of the GI system. Most clinicians, over the years, have reported use of the frontalis muscle in electromyographic assessment; however, the trapezius, brachioradialis, and sternocleidomastoid muscle groups have also been utilized.

In summary, most evidence suggests that the electromyographic assessment yields insight into the activity of other major muscle groups (Freedman & Papsdorf, 1976; Glaus & Kotses, 1977, 1978) as well as the generalized activity of the SNS (Arnarson & Sheffield, 1980; Budzynski, 1979; Everly et al., 1989; Jacobson, 1970; Malmo, 1966; Rubin, 1977).

Cardiovascular Measurement

Cardiovascular measurement of the stress response entails the assessment of effects of the stress response upon the heart and vascular systems. Common cardiovascular measures include heart rate, peripheral blood flow, and blood pressure.

Heart rate activity as a function of the stress response is a result of direct neural innervation as well as neuroendocrine activity of epinephrine and norepinephrine. During psychosocially induced stress, epinephrine is preferentially released from the adrenal medullae. The ventricles of the heart are maximally responsive to circulating epinephrine and will respond with increased speed and force of ventricular contraction. Of course, direct sympathetic neural activation increases heart rate as well. The measurement of heart rate is most commonly achieved through the use of audiometric or oscillometric techniques during the normal assessment of blood pressure. Occasionally, heart rate will be measured from ECG techniques via the use of passive electrodes or even through plethysmography.

Plethysmography focuses upon the volume of blood in a selected anatomical site. The most common areas for such assessment of the stress response are the fingers, toes, calves, and forearms. During the stress response, most patients will suffer a reduction of blood flow from these areas. This vasoconstrictive effect is a result of direct sympathetic activity to the arteries and arterioles, as well as of circulating norepinephrine (Guyton, 1996). A decline of blood flow to these areas will also result in a reduction of skin temperature. Therefore, skin temperature is also sometimes utilized, although it is not as reliable as plethysmography. So we see that the assessment of peripheral blood flow can be accomplished via the use of plethysmography as well as skin temperature.

Finally, blood pressure is sometimes used as an *acute* index of the stress response. The assessment of blood pressure is generally achieved through the quantification of systolic and diastolic blood pressure, and may be considered highly state-dependent.

Systolic blood pressure is the hemodynamic pressure exerted within the arterial system during systole (the ventricular contraction phase). Diastolic blood pressure is the hemodynamic pressure exerted within the arterial system during diastole (relaxation and filling of the ventricular chambers).

Blood pressure is a function of several variables revealed in the following equation:

$$BP = CO \times TPR$$

where

BP = blood pressure
CO = cardiac output = stroke volume × heart rate
TPR = total hemodynamic peripheral resistance

Blood pressure can be measured noninvasively through auscultation, audiometry, or oscillometry. In noninvasive paradigms, a sampled artery (usually the brachial) is compressed through the use of an inflatable rubber tube or bladder. The bladder is inflated until it totally blocks the passage of blood through the artery. Air pressure, measured in millimeters of mercury (mm Hg) is slowly released from the bladder until a sound is heard or a distension sensed. This sound and distension (called a Korotkoff sound) is indicative of blood being allowed to pass through the once blocked artery. Korotkoff sounds continue until the artery is fully opened and returned back to its natural status. The first Korotkoff sound is indicative of the systolic blood pressure. The passing of the last Korotkoff sound is indicative of the diastolic blood pressure.

The technique of audiometry measures blood pressure by the use of a microphone to sense the Korotkoff sounds. Oscillometry detects the Korotkoff phenomenon via a pressure-sensitive device placed on the outside of the artery. Finally, auscultation is the sensing of the Korotkoff sound via stethoscope. Audiometric and oscillometric techniques are far more reliable than is manual auscultation.

In summary, the measurement of cardiovascular phenomena can be seen to tap both neural and neuroendocrine domains; thus there is an overlap in phenomenology. Also, when using the cardiovascular domain to measure stress arousal, the clinician is interested only in the *acute* fluctuations, as opposed to chronic levels. This is due to the fact that stress exerts its most measurable effect upon the acute status of the cardiovascular system. A multitude of other factors enter into, and otherwise confound, the measurement process when examining cardiovascular indices such as chronic blood pressure and peripheral blood flow, for example.

Assessment of the Neuroendocrine Axis

Assessment of the neuroendocrine axis of the stress response entails measurement of the adrenal medullary catecholamines: epinephrine (adrenaline) and norepinephrine (noradrenaline).

Aggregated medullary catecholamines may be sampled from blood or urine and assayed via fluorometric methods. Reference values range for random sampling up to 18 μg/100 ml urine, for a 24-hour urine sample up to 135 μg, and for timed samples, 1.4 to 7.3 μg/hour during daylight hours (Bio-Science, 1982). For aggregated catecholamines sampled from plasma, values range from 140 to 165 pg/ml via radioenzymatic procedures (Bio-Science, 1982).

Various fluorometric (Anderson et al., 1974; Euler & Lishajko, 1961; Jacobs et al., 1994), chromatographic (Jacobs et al., 1994; Lake, Ziegler, & Kopin, 1976; Mason, 1972), and radioimmunoassay (Jacobs et al., 1994; Mason, 1972) methods are available for the assessment of catecholamines. The most useful of all methods may be the high pressure liquid chromatography (HPLC) with electrochemical detection as described in Hegstrand and Eichelman (1981) and McClelland, Ross, and Patel (1985). HPLC allows multiple catecholamines to be derived from sampled plasma, urine, and saliva with superior ease and sensitivity.

Epinephrine can be sampled from urine, plasma, or saliva. When sampled from urine a typical distribution is as follows: (see Jacobs et al., 1994;

Katzung, 1992):

Unchanged epinephrine	6%
Metanephrine	40%
Vanillylmandellic acid	41%
4-Hydroxy-3-methoxy-phenylglycol	7%
3,4-Dihydroxymandelic acid	2%
Other	4%
	100%

Norepinephrine can also be sampled from urine, plasma, and saliva. Table 6.1 provides a range of epinephrine and norepinephrine values when sampled from urine.

Despite the availability of methods such as HPLC, some researchers prefer the assessment of catecholamines by indirect routes, for example, through the assessment of urinary metabolites. Metanephrines and vanillylmandellic acid (VMA) are two popular choices.

In the case of the metanephrines, one of the major deactivating substances acting upon epinephrine and norepinephrine is the enzyme catecholamine-O-methyl-transferase (COMT). Metabolites of this deactivation process are metanephrine and normetanephrine. Aggregated metanephrines range from 0.3 to 0.9 mg/day in urine. VMA levels range from 0.7 to 6.8 mg/day. VMA is the urinary metabolite of COMT and monoamine oxidase.

Assessment of the Endocrine Axes

According to Hans Selye (1976), the most direct way of measuring the stress response is via ACTH, the corticosteroids, and the catecholamines. The catecholamines have already been discussed. The most commonly used index of ACTH and corticosteroid activity is the measurement of the hormone cortisol. Cortisol is secreted by the adrenal cortices, activated by ACTH, at a rate of about 25 to 30 mg/day and accounts for about 90% of glucocorticoid activity.

**Table 6.1. Value Ranges for Urinary
Epinephrine and Norepinephrine**

	Epinephrine	Norepinephrine
Basal levels	4–5 µg/day	28–30 µg/day
Aroused	10–15 µg/day	50–70 µg/day
Significant stress	> 15 µg/day	> 70 µg/day

Cortisol may be sampled from either plasma or urine. Radio-immunoassay plasma levels for a normal adult may range from 5 to 20 μg/100 ml plasma (8 A.M. sample). The normal diurnal decline may result in a level of plasma cortisol at 4 P.M. about one half of the 8 A.M. level. Normal urinary-free cortisol may range from 20 to 90 μg/24 hours (see Bio-Science, 1982). It has been suggested that urinary-free cortisol is the most sensitive and reliable indicator of adrenal cortical hyperfunction, followed by plasma cortisol and finally 17-hydroxycorticosteroid (17-OHCS), a cortisol metabolite (Damon, 1981). Normal values for 17-OHCS measured from urine typically range from 2.5 to 10 mg/24 hours in the female to 4.5 to 12 mg/24 hours in the male adult (Porter–Silber method). Slight increases in 17-OHCS are evidenced in the first trimester of pregnancy and in severe hypertension. Moderate increases can be observed in the third trimester of pregnancy and as a result of infectious disease, burns, surgery, and stress (Bio-Science, 1982). In conditions of extreme stress, urinary 17-OHCS may exceed 15 mg/24 hours. Plasma assessments of 17-OHCS range from 10 to 14 μg% at 8 A.M. basal levels to 18 to 24 μg% under moderate stress, to an excess of 24 μg% in extremely stressful situations (Mason, 1972).

This section has discussed the assessment of the physiological constituents of the stress response. It should be noted that the assessment of this domain represents a challenging and potentially frustrating exercise. One major factor that confounds the assessment of most physiological variables is the fact that most physiological phenomena used to assess stress arousal are state-dependent variables that wax and wane throughout the course of a day as well as with acute situational demands. Normal diurnal fluctuations as well as acute situational variability can serve to yield false-positive or false-negative findings in the absence of meaningful baseline data. There has even been some question as to the predictive validity of acute physiological indices. Another issue that confounds the overall utility of many physiological measures is that such measures usually require special training, special equipment, or both. The difficulties associated with physiological assessment of the human stress response have been summarized by Everly and Sobelman (1987). Other issues, such as response specificity and organ reactivity, are also reviewed.

ASSESSMENT OF TARGET-ORGAN EFFECTS

Once the stress response has been activated to pathogenic proportions, there emerges another possible assessment strategy for measuring human stress—the assessment of the target-organ effects of the stress response.

The assessment of target-organ effects can consist of measuring physical as well as psychological variables.

Physical Diagnosis

The assessment of the physical effects of stress would involve the use of standard diagnostic techniques common to the practice of physical medicine. The goal of such assessments is to measure the integrity of the target organ's structural and functional status. An in-depth discussion of such procedures is far beyond the scope of this volume, however.

It should be mentioned that such assessments are never clearly assessments of stress. One never really knows to what degree pathogenic stress arousal has contributed to the manifestation of target-organ pathology. For this reason, the diagnosis of stress-related target-organ disease is typically a diagnosis by exclusion; that is, one systematically excludes non-stress-related etiological factors while at the same time looking for evidence of pathogenic stress arousal through the assessment of other measurement domains as well. The stress-related diagnosis then emerges from a convergence of these data sets. There are also self-report scales that have proven to be valid and reliable indices of experienced physical illness. The Seriousness of Illness Rating Scale (SIRS; Wyler, Masuda, & Holmes, 1968; see also Rosenberg, Hayes, & Peterson, 1987) is one useful self-report tool for measuring illness and weighting its impact. The Stress Audit Questionnaire (Miller & Smith, 1982) is another. It is important to keep in mind that there is still no certainty as to the extent of the role of stress arousal in the formation of the emergent illnesses/reactions.

Finally, the Family Disruption from Illness Scale (Ide, 1996) extends the assessment of physical symptoms somewhat by assessing the degree of disruption that 53 health-related symptoms impose upon daily functioning. Most items represent physical illnesses. This scale, while more recent than the SIRS, is not as comprehensive, nor have its psychometric properties been adequately assessed.

Psychological Diagnosis

The psychological diagnosis of the stress response refers to the measurement of the "psychological" effects of the stress response. There currently exist numerous and diverse methods for the measurement of psychological states and traits. To cover this topic fully would require a volume of its own. Therefore, what we shall do in this section is merely highlight the paper-and-pencil questionnaires that a clinician might find most useful in measuring the psychological effects of the stress response.

Minnesota Multiphasic Personality Inventory—2 (MMPI-2). The MMPI-2 is a revision of perhaps one of the most valid and reliable inventories for the assessment of long-term stress on the personality structure of the patient. The numerous clinical and content scales of the MMPI-2 yield a wealth of valuable information. These scales sample a wide range of "abnormal" or maladjusted personality traits (a personality trait is a rather chronic and consistent pattern of thinking and behavior).

The MMPI-2 consists of 10 basic clinical scales developed on the basis of actuarial data:

1. Hs: Hypochondriasis
2. D: Depression
3. Hy: Conversion Hysteria
4. Pd: Psychopathic Deviate
5. Mf: Masculinity–Femininity
6. Pa: Paranoia
7. Pt: Psychasthenia (trait anxiety)
8. Sc: Schizophrenia
9. Ma: Hypomania (manifest energy)
10. Si: Social Introversion (preference for being alone)

In addition to the highly researched clinical scales, the MMPI-2 has validity scales that give the clinician a general idea of how valid any given set of test scores is for the patient. This unique feature of the MMPI-2 increases its desirability to many clinicians.

The MMPI-2 offers a virtual wealth of information to the trained clinician; its only major drawback appears to be its length of over 560 items.

The Sixteen Personality Factor Questionnaire (16-PF). The 16-PF (Cattell, 1972), much the same as the MMPI, assesses a wide range of personality traits. It measures 16 "functionally independent and psychologically meaningful dimensions isolated and replicated in more than 30 years of factor-analytic research on normal and clinical groups" (p. 5).

The 16-PF consists of 187 items distributed across the following scales:

- Reserved–Outgoing
- Less Intelligent–More Intelligent
- Affected by Feelings–Emotionally Stable
- Humble–Assertive
- Sober–Happy-Go-Lucky
- Expedient–Conscientious
- Shy–Venturesome
- Tough-minded–Tender-minded
- Trusting–Suspicious
- Practical–Imaginative
- Forthright–Astute
- Self-Assured–Apprehensive

- Conservative–Experimenting
- Group-Dependent–
  Self-Sufficient
- Undisciplined Self-Conflict–
  Controlled
- Relaxed–Tense

Millon Clinical Multiaxial Inventory—II (MCMI-II). The Millon Clinical Multiaxial Inventory (MCMI) is a 175-item self-report, true–false questionnaire. The MCMI-II, although not as widely utilized as the MMPI in the diagnosis of major psychiatric disorders, is clearly the instrument of choice when the clinician is primarily interested in personologic variables and their relationship to excessive stress. Furthermore, the MCMI-II offers valuable insight into treatment planning. Another major advantage of the MCMI-II over the MMPI and 16-PF is that it consists of only 175 items. The MCMI-II includes 22 clinical scales broken down into three broad categories; 10 basic personality scales reflective of the personality theory of Theodore Millon (1981); three pathological personality syndromes; and nine major clinical psychiatric syndromes (Millon, 1983). From a psychometric perspective, the MCMI-II offers the best of both worlds: an inventory founded in a practical, clinically useful theory as well as rigorous empirical development. The scales of the MCMI-II are listed below:

- Schizoid
- Avoidant
- Antisocial
- Narcissism
- Passive–aggressive
- Compulsive
- Dependent
- Histrionic
- Schizotypal
- Borderline
- Sadistic
- Paranoid
- Anxiety
- Somatoform
- Hypomania
- Dysthymia
- Alcohol abuse
- Drug abuse
- Psychotic thinking
- Psychotic depression
- Psychotic delusions
- Self-defeating

Millon Clinical Multiaxial Inventory—III (MCMI-III). While the MCMI-II is still in use, Millon has published an even more current version of the MCMI, the MCMI-III (Millon, 1997). The MCMI-III still contains 175 items but 95 were changed or reworded from the MCMI-II. Two scales were added: Depressive Personality and Posttraumatic Stress Disorder. Item scoring was changed from a 3-point to a 2-point scale. The unique value of the Millon instruments resides in the criterion-referenced validation process that yields direct probabilistic evidence as to the clinical utility of the component scales to discriminate "cases" from "noncases" using the operating characteristics of sensitivity and specificity as the cornerstones of its clinical predictiveness. This important psychometric characteristic gives the Millon instruments greater clinical and forensic utility compared to the MMPI.

Common Grief Response Questionnaire (CGQ).   The CGQ (McNeil, 1996) consists of 86 self-report items using a 7-point Likert response scale. The purpose of the CGQ is to assess the frequency of occurrence of numerous grief reactions to the death of a loved one.

Impact of Events Scale—Revised (IES-R).   The IES-R (Weiss & Marmar, 1993) is a revision of the original IES. The IES-R consists of 22 self-report items purported to assess posttraumatic stress. Three response dimensions are tapped: intrusive ideation, avoidance and numbing, as well as hyper-arousal. The IES-R takes about 10 minutes to complete and is a widely used research tool.

Penn Inventory for Posttraumatic Stress Disorder (PENN).   Similar to the IES-R, the PENN (Hammarberg, 1992), is a measure of posttraumatic symptoms. It is, however, is a more global measure, consisting of 26 self-report items.

Stanford Acute Stress Reaction Questionnaire (SASRQ).   The SASRQ (Cardena & Spiegel, 1993; Shalev, Peri, Canetti, & Schreiber, 1996) consists of 30 self-report items that assess acute stress disorder. The scale takes 5–10 minutes to complete and appears to be useful in predicting PTSD.

Taylor Manifest Anxiety Scale (TAS).   The TAS (Taylor, 1953), unlike the inventories previously described, measures only one trait—anxiety. Its 50 items are derived from the MMPI. The TAS measures how generally anxious the patient is and has little ability to reflect situational fluctuations in anxiety.

State–Trait Anxiety Inventory (STAI).   The STAI (Spielberger, Gorsuch, & Luchene, 1970) is a highly unique inventory in that it is two scales in one. The first 20 items measure state anxiety (a psychological state is an acute, usually situationally dependent condition of psychological functioning). The second 20 items measure trait anxiety. This is the same basic phenomenon as that measured by the TAS. The STAI can be administered in full form (40 items) or be used to measure only state or trait anxiety.

Affect Adjective Checklist (AACL).   Another unusual measuring device is the AACL (Zuckerman, 1960). Like the STAI, the AACL can be used to measure a psychological state or trait by using the same items (21 adjectives) and merely changing the instructions. The client may use the checklist of adjectives to describe how he or she feels in general or under a specific set of conditions—"now" for instance. Zuckerman and Lubin (1965) later expanded the AACL by adding specific items to assess hostility and depression. The new scale is called the Multiple Affect Adjective Checklist (MAACL).

Subjective Stress Scale (SSS). The SSS (Berkun, 1962) is designed to measure situational (state) effects of stress on the individual. The scale consists of 14 descriptors that the patient can use to identify his or her subjective reactions during a stressful situation. Each of these descriptors comes with an empirically derived numerical weight, which the clinician then uses to generate a subjective stress score.

Profile of Mood States (POMS). The POMS (McNair, Lorr, & Droppleman, 1971) is a factor-analytically derived self-report inventory that measures six identifiable mood or affective states (p. 5):

- Tension–Anxiety
- Depression–Dejection
- Anger–Hostility
- Vigor–Activity
- Fatigue–Inertia
- Confusion–Bewilderment

The POMS consists of 65 adjectives, each followed by a 5-point rating scale that the patient uses to indicate the subjective presence of that condition. The instructions ask the patient to use the 65 adjectives to indicate "How you have been feeling during the past week including today." Other time states have been used, for example: "right now," "today," and for "the past three minutes."

The POMS offers a broader range of state measures for the subjective assessment of stress when compared with the STAI, the AACL-MAACL, and the SSS.

THE ASSESSMENT OF COPING

The MBHI assesses the patient's characterological coping style. The Hassles Scale measures an indirect form of coping within its "uplifts" subscale. Everly created a simple coping inventory for use in conjunction with the National Health Fair (Everly, 1979a; Girdano & Everly, 1986). This checklist can be found in Appendix H.

Finally, perhaps the most popular of the coping indices is the Ways of Coping Checklist developed by Lazarus and Folkman (1984). This 67-item checklist that assesses an individual's preference for various styles of coping patterns (e.g., defensive coping, information seeking, problem solving) enjoys a considerable empirical foundation and can be found in their 1984 textbook on stress, appraisal, and coping.

In the broadest sense, coping may be viewed as any effort to reduce or mitigate the aversive effects of stress. These efforts may be psychological or behavioral. The scales mentioned sample both domains.

LAW OF INITIAL VALUES

A final point should be made regarding the role of individual differences in the process of measurement. No two patients are exactly alike in their manifestations of the stress response. When measuring psychophysiological reactivity, or any physiological index, the clinician must understand that the patient's baseline level of functioning on any physiological variable affects any subsequent degree of activity or reactivity in that same physiological parameter. This is Wilder's Law of Initial Values (Wilder, 1950). In order to compare an individual's stress reactivity (assuming variant baselines), a statistical correction must be made in order to assure that the correlation between baseline activity and stressful reactivity is equal to zero. Such a correction must be made in order to compare groups as well. Benjamin (1963) has written a very useful paper that addresses the necessary statistical corrections that must be made. She concludes that a covariance model must be adopted in order to correct for the law of initial values, though specific calculations will differ when comparing groups or individuals.* It must be remembered that the Law of Initial Values will affect not only the measurement of stress arousal but also stress reduction.

---

*One useful formula for correcting for the Law of Initial Values when comparing individuals is the Autonomic Lability Score (ALS; Lacey & Lacey, 1962). The ALS, a form of covariance and therefore consistent with Benjamin's recommendation, is expressed as

$$\text{ALS} = 50 + 10 \left[\frac{Y_z - X_z r_{xy}}{(1 - r_{xy}^2)^{0.5}} \right]$$

where X_z = client's standardized prestressor autonomic level, Y_z = client's standardized poststressor autonomic level, and r_{xy} = correlation for sample between pre- and poststressor levels.

SUMMARY

In this chapter we have described briefly some of the most commonly used methods of measuring the effects of the stress response. The methods described have included physiological and psychological criteria.

The most important question surrounding the measurement of the stress response is "How do you select the most appropriate measurement criterion?" The answer to this question is in no way clear-cut. Generally speaking, to begin with you should consider the state versus trait measurement criterion issue. Basically, state criteria should be used to measure immediate and/or short-lived phenomena. Trait criteria should be used to measure phenomena that take a longer term to manifest themselves and/or have greater stability and duration. The psychological criteria discussed in this chapter are fairly straightforward as to their state or trait nature. The physiological criteria are somewhat less clear. Some physiological criteria possess both state and trait characteristics. Furthermore, normal values for blood and urinary stress indicators may vary somewhat from lab to lab. Therefore, the clinician should familiarize him- or herself with the lab's standard values. Before using physiological measurement criteria in the assessment of the stress response, the reader who has no background in physiology would benefit from consulting any useful physiology or psychophysiology text (see, e.g., Everly & Sobelman, 1987; Greenfield & Sternbach, 1972; Levi, 1975; Selye, 1976; Stern, Ray, & Davis, 1980). Finally, because no two patients are alike in their response to stressors, the clinician might consider measuring multiple and diverse response mechanisms (or stress axes) in order to increase the sensitivity of any given assessment procedure designed to measure the stress response (see Figure 6.1).

Having provided these closing points, let us review the major issues discussed within this chapter:

1. It has been argued that the single most important aspect of empirical investigation is the process of the *measurement* of relevant variables. This is true of investigations into the nature of human stress as well.

2. The Social Readjustment Rating Scale (Holmes & Rahe, 1967), the Life Experiences Survey (Sarason et al., 1978), and the Hassles Scale (Kanner et al., 1981) are all self-report inventories that assess the patient's exposure to critical "life events." Collectively, these scales do not measure stress; rather, they assess the patient's exposure to stressors. Stressor scales are correlated with stress arousal because the physiology of adaptation to novel or challenging stimuli is also the physiology of the stress response.

3. The Derogatis Stress Scale (Derogatis, 1980), and the Millon Behavioral Health Inventory (Millon et al., 1982) represent scales designed

to assess the patient's cognitive–affective status. The stress response is thus assessed indirectly through the measurement of cognitive–affective states known to be highly associated with stress arousal. It has been argued that such assessments may well be the most efficient, practical, and cost-effective way of assessing stress arousal. All of these scales also include symptom indices.

4. Albeit an important clinical phenomenon, the assessment of propensities for limbic efferent discharge (limbic hypersensitivity phenomenon) is extremely difficult. Subcortical electroencephalography is a crude measure at best. Electrodermal and general psychophysiological reactivity may be the best options currently available for the assessment of neurological triggering mechanisms of the human stress response.

5. Numerous measurement options exist for the assessment of the physiological stress response itself (if deemed appropriate).

5a. The neural stress axes may be assessed via electrodermal measures, electromyographic measures, as well as cardiovascular measures (heart rate, peripheral blood flow, blood pressures).

5b. The neuroendocrine stress axis can be measured via the assessment adrenal medullary catecholamines.

5c. The assessment of the endocrine stress axes is most commonly conducted via the assessment of cortisol.

6. The assessment of target-organ effects of pathogenic stress arousal can be conducted via standard physical medicine examination or the use of self-report inventories such as the Seriousness of Illness Rating Scale (Wyler et al., 1968) to measure *physical effects. Psychological effects* may be assessed via self-report scales such as the MMPI, the MCMI, the 16-PF, IES-R, PENN, SASRQ, CGO, the TAS, the STAI, the AACL, the SSS, and the POMS.

7. Coping is an important potential mediating variable. It may be assessed via the MBHI; the Hassles Scale, a coping scale developed by Everly (Everly, 1979a) for the U.S. Public Health Service; or the Ways of Coping Checklist (Lazarus & Folkman, 1984).

II

The Treatment of the
Human Stress Response

Part II, the second of three parts that constitute this volume, is dedicated to the presentation of a treatment model for excessive stress arousal, with subsequent discussions of its therapeutic components.

In Part I, Chapter 2 presented an epiphenomenological systems model of the human stress response (Figure 2.6). Each of its components was described within that chapter so as to convey the notion that the human stress response is an active, dynamic, multifaceted process. In Chapter 6, the same model was again used, but this time to demonstrate how *measurement* technologies may be superimposed on the same phenomenological process and model (Figure 6.1). We again use the phenomenological model first introduced in Chapter 2 as a means of presenting an integrated overview of the *treatment* of the human stress response.

The purpose of Chapter 7 is to briefly review the relationship between personality and human health, but more importantly, to provide a rationale for the consideration of personality factors in the cause and treatment of stress-related disorders. We construct a personologic diathesis (personality-based susceptibility to stress arousal) model so as to facilitate the integration of personality factors in treatment planning. Chapter 7 is accordingly entitled "Personologic Diathesis and Human Stress."

Chapter 8, "Control and the Human Stress Response," serves as a prologue to the chapters that cover specific technologies for therapeutic intervention. The perception of control, or self-efficacy, has been cogently argued to be the most powerful single therapeutic impetus in the treatment of excessive stress and other syndromes of dyscontrol. Chapter 8 provides extensive coverage of some of the research that serves as the basis for such an argument.

In a review of the treatment model (Figure II.1), the first technologies for therapeutic intervention to be listed are *environmental engineering* and *psychotherapy*. The term *environmental engineering*, borrowed from the work of Girdano and Everly (1986), refers to efforts to "act artfully upon" one's environment to reduce stress arousal through the alteration of one's exposure to stressors. Such strategies may be thought of as "preventive" or "reactive" problem solving through the manipulation of environmental variables. The concept of psychotherapy as used in this volume refers to any efforts that result in a more adaptive and health-promoting cognitive–affective style and expression as they pertain to the stress response. Bearing this in mind, Chapter 9, entitled "Psychotherapy: A Cognitive Perspective," briefly reviews cognitive therapy from several perspectives, while providing a framework for integrating problem solving within a cognitive therapeutic framework.

Chapter 10, "A Neurophysiological Rationale for the Use of the Relaxation Response," provides the reader with a cogent reason for employing strategies that engender the relaxation response in any treatment protocol designed to attend to pathogenic stress arousal or its target-organ effects. This chapter provides the rationale that the relaxation response may be used not only as a secondary intervention but also many cases as a primary therapeutic agent in many cases. Thus, Chapter 10 introduces the sub-sequent chapters that address specific technologies for engendering the relaxation response.

Chapters 11–14 cover the topics of meditation, respiratory control, neuromuscular relaxation, and hypnosis, respectively. As prefaced by Chapter 10, these technologies are standard methods by which the clinician can teach the patient to elicit the relaxation response, thereby reducing manifest arousal, as well as propensities for overreactivity. These chapters provide an overview of the conceptual and research foundations upon which these techniques are based. More relevant, Chapters 11–13 provide the clinician with a practical "boilerplate" protocol for employing these techniques (Chapter 14 provides a more general overview). However, these protocols are designed as a working foundation that the clinician may alter as needed.

Chapter 14, by Dr. Gravitz and Page, which addresses hypnosis, extends beyond the elicitation of the relaxation response by also covering behavior changes associated with the technique.

Chapter 15 discusses biofeedback as a therapeutic intervention. The reader will discover that biofeedback can be used to reduce pathogenic arousal and assist in engendering the relaxation response, or it can actually be used to treat the target-organ manifestations of excessive stress.

Chapter 16, "Physical Exercise and the Human Stress Response," as noted in the treatment diagram, can be used to release or ventilate the stress response once it has been engendered.

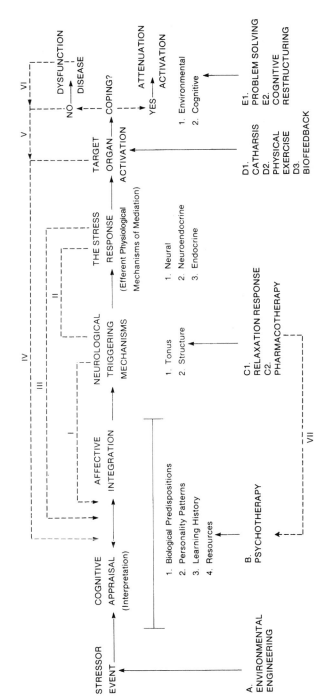

Figure II.1. A multidimensional treatment model for the human stress response.

Chapter 17, by Dr. Noel and Curtis, "The Pharmacological Management of Stress Reactions," reviews the advances in the use of psychotropic medications in the treatment of stress and stress-related disorders. This chapter covers several drug classes, how they work, their basic clinical effects, and recommended dosages.

To summarize Part II, let us return to the multidimensional treatment model contained within this introduction.

Chapters 7 and 8 introduce the topics of personality and control that serve as clinical prefaces to the treatment of excessive stress arousal.

Chapter 9, which addresses the topic of psychotherapy from a cognitive perspective, also covers the topic of environmental engineering.

Chapter 10 provides the reader with a rationale for the utilization of the relaxation response and demonstrates its central phenomenological role in any treatment paradigm for excessive arousal or its target-organ effects. Chapters 11 through 14 serve as practical guides for the use of the relaxation response in clinical practice.

Chapters 15 and 17 expand that discussion into machine-assisted and medication-assisted technologies.

Chapters 14–16 address the issues of how one can intervene at the level of the target organ once the pathogenic stress response has been initiated.

7

Personologic Diathesis and Human Stress

> Where malignant disease is concerned it may be more important to understand what kind of patient has the disease rather than what kind of disease the patient has.
>
> Sir WILLIAM OSLER, M.D.

The purpose of Part II is to review options that have proven useful in the treatment of excessive stress arousal. This chapter begins that discussion with an issue relevant to treatment planning—the role of personality in the etiology and treatment of the human stress response.

Recall from Chapter 2 that the manner in which an individual chooses to perceive and interpret his or her environment (cognitive interpretation) serves as the single most important determinant of whether the stress response will be elicited in response to a psychosocial stressor. We may then argue that the *consistent* manner in which an individual perceives and interprets the environment, in addition to the aggregation of consistent attitudes, values, and behavior patterns, serves as an operational definition of the construct of "personality." If we accept such a proposition, it becomes reasonable to assume that there may well exist individuals whose consistent personality traits, including cognitive interpretations regarding their environment, may predispose them to excessive elicitation of the stress response and, therefore, increased risk of stress-related disease. Such personality-based predispositions for stress may exist in the form of personologic diatheses, such as cognitive distortions, persistent irrational expectations, "ego" vulnerabilities, and/or consistent stress-producing overt behavior patterns.

If indeed one's personologic idiosyncrasies can predispose to excessive stress arousal, it behooves the clinician to familiarize him- or herself with the common manifestations of such personologic predispositions. Investigations into such relationships between personality factors and stress arousal have typically taken one of two perspectives.

1. Historically, investigations into the relationship between personality and stress have focused upon highly *specific* personality traits that appear to predispose individuals to highly *specific* diseases, without consideration of the global personality structure within which those traits reside (Alexander, 1950; Dunbar, 1935).

2. Investigations have pursued the proposition that there exist consistent, personality-based predispositions, that is, "vulnerabilities" unique to and inherent within each and every basic personality pattern (Millon, 1996; Millon et al., 1999). Collectively, these characterological susceptibilities serve as a form of Achilles' heel, referred to here as a *personologic diathesis*, serving, under the right set of circumstances, to predispose one to the elicitation of the stress response and a host of subsequent stress-related disorders (Everly, 1987; Frances, 1982; Millon & Everly, 1985). These characterological susceptibilities may exist in the form of "ego" vulnerabilities, consistent cognitive distortions, expectations, and repeated stress-producing behaviors. Such an approach tends not to focus on specific traits and their association with specific diseases, but rather sees each different personality style or pattern as possessing a personologic diathesis consisting of an aggregation of personality-based susceptibilities to stress. Let us pursue these notions further.

HISTORICAL FOUNDATIONS

When one first thinks of the relationship between personality and stress, the Type A coronary-prone behavior pattern invariably comes to mind (Friedman & Rosenman, 1974). Yet the search for the stress-prone personality far predates the discovery of the Type A pattern.

The work of Dunbar (1935) represents one of the earliest and most noteworthy efforts at formulating psychosomatic theory based upon personality profiles. Dunbar described various personality profiles that seemed to be predisposed to specific stress-related diseases. For example, from her perspective, the hypertensive patient could be seen as characterologically shy, reserved, rigid, yet possessing the propensity for "volcanic eruptions of feelings." The migraine patient, on the other hand, could be seen as perfectionistic and overachievement oriented.

As noted in Chapter 3, the conflict theory of French and Alexander (Alexander, 1950) argued that persons prone to repeated characterological conflicts are prone to specific stress-related disorders.

In addition to the work of Dunbar and Alexander, there were other early contributions from the analytically oriented theorists, yet early interest waned, with rather low reliability among the findings of the various theorists. Similarly, even reliable findings contributed only minimal variation to the overall disease process. Thus, research into the relationship between personality and disease significantly diminished for over a decade until interest was rekindled by cardiologists Friedman and Rosenman (1974) in their investigations into the Type A coronary-prone behavior pattern.

Friedman (1969) described the Type A pattern as a characteristic "action–emotion complex" exhibited by individuals engaged in a chronic struggle to "obtain an unlimited number of poorly defined things from their environment in the shortest period of time." Originally, the Type A pattern was believed to constitute chronic time urgency, competitiveness, polyphasic behavior, and poorly planned, often impulsive behavior (Friedman & Rosenman, 1974). The Type A pattern has also been described as consisting of primary traits of time urgency, hostility, ambition, and immoderation. Friedman and Rosenman also described secondary traits of impatience, aggression, competitiveness, and denial.

The original search for the Type A pattern was, indeed, a search for a consistent behavior pattern that predisposed to premature coronary artery disease. When diagnosed via the standardized structured interview technique, the Type A pattern has consistently shown a relationship with coronary artery disease (see Powell, 1984; Shepherd & Weiss, 1987; Williams, 1984; Williams et al., 1980). Major investigations that have failed to uncover a relationship between coronary heart disease and the Type A pattern have generally used techniques other than the structured interview to assess the pattern (Everly & Sobelman, 1987; Shepherd & Weiss, 1987). The use of diverse measurement technologies may have inadvertently added to the confusion surrounding the nature of the Type A pattern (Everly & Sobelman, 1987). Indeed, the pursuit of the Type A pattern has taken on a life of its own, so much so that individuals invariably ask if there is such a thing as a "good" Type A pattern. By definition, the answer to such a question must be "no," if one only remembers that the original quest for the Type A pattern was actually a search for a behavior pattern that predisposes to premature coronary heart disease. Considering this point, how could there be a "good" Type A?

The relationship between Type A behavior and coronary heart disease has prompted researchers to conduct various components analyses in search of the pathogenic core of the Type A pattern (Powell, 1984; Williams, 1984; Williams et al., 1980). Such endeavors have uncovered myriad Type A constituents that serve to clarify further the nature of the pattern.

Figure 7.1 represents an integration of findings reported as part of the "second generation" of Type A research designed to better understand the constituents of coronary-prone behavior (Powell, 1984; Williams, 1984, 1986; Williams et al., 1980). It portrays a deeply rooted personologic insecurity as the foundation of the Type A pattern. That characterological insecurity is thought to give rise to an extraordinary need for power and achievement, perhaps as a means of compensating for or contradicting the feelings of insecurity. Power and achievement are related to control, and it has been found that Type A individuals possess not only high achievement motives but also an extraordinary need for control. The need for control and the fear of the loss of control may then account for the observed impatience, time urgency, polyphasic behavior, competitiveness, and related traits that Type A persons exhibit. Studies by Williams and his colleagues have suggested that chronic hostility and cynicism may be an important psychological factor in the increased coronary risk that Type A individuals exhibit. Dembroski and Costa (1988) reviewed the assessment of the Type A pattern and noted that the "global" Type A pattern is not a good predictor of heart disease, but the hostility component may play a critical pathogenic role.

Research has also shown that Type A individuals exhibit extraordinary physiological reactivity when confronted with a psychosocial challenge.

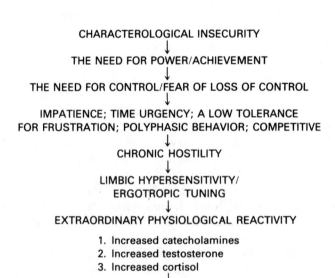

CHARACTEROLOGICAL INSECURITY
↓
THE NEED FOR POWER/ACHIEVEMENT
↓
THE NEED FOR CONTROL/FEAR OF LOSS OF CONTROL
↓
IMPATIENCE; TIME URGENCY; A LOW TOLERANCE
FOR FRUSTRATION; POLYPHASIC BEHAVIOR; COMPETITIVE
↓
CHRONIC HOSTILITY
↓
LIMBIC HYPERSENSITIVITY/
ERGOTROPIC TUNING
↓
EXTRAORDINARY PHYSIOLOGICAL REACTIVITY

1. Increased catecholamines
2. Increased testosterone
3. Increased cortisol
↓
INCREASED RISK OF CORONARY HEART DISEASE

Figure 7.1. An integrative model of Type A characteristics.

That reactivity has been shown to be manifest in increased release of cate-cholamines, testosterone, and cortisol—all well-known atherogenic agents. The physiological reactivity, according to the work of Everly (1985b), may well be based upon some form of limbic system hypersensitivity, or what Gellhorn (1967) has called the "ergotropic tuning phenomenon." Finally, the unusually high levels of circulating catecholamine, cortisol, and testoterone appear to be directly related to the increased risk of coronary artery disease manifested by Type A males. It should be noted that, at rest, the Type A indi-vidual manifests no significant differences in catecholamine, testosterone, or cortisol secretion when compared with non-Type A individuals. Only upon psychosocial challenge are the aforementioned differences seen to emerge.

The Type A pattern remains a promising area for continued research into the relationship between personality and disease, especially stress-related disease. It will be recalled that the catecholamines, testosterone, and cortisol are all key stress-responding hormones. The interested reader should refer to Shepherd and Weiss (1987) for an important review.

The next major contribution to the stress and personality phenome-non comes from Suzanne Kobasa, who investigated personality character-istics that seem to act as a buffer between individuals and the pathogenic mechanisms of excessive stress. Her research investigated the domain of "hardiness," that is, characterological factors that appear to mitigate the stress response. Kobasa (1979; Kobasa & Puccetti, 1983) defined hardiness as the aggregation of three factors:

1. Commitment, that is, the tendency to involve oneself in experi-ences in meaningful ways.
2. Control, that is, the tendency to believe and act as if one has some influence over one's life.
3. Challenge, that is, the belief that change is a positive and normal characteristic of life.

The hardiness research has shown that individuals who demonstrate a com-mitment to self, family, work, and/or other important values; a sense of control over their lives; and the ability to see life change as an opportunity will experience fewer stress-related diseases/illnesses even though they may find themselves in environments laden with stressor stimuli.

The hardiness construct is indeed a tempting concept to entertain. This formulation has received a serious challenge from Lazarus and Folkman (1984), however, who argue that there is a paucity of systematic studies that examine the relationship between antecedent variables and health. Conclusions, they suggest, are typically formulated on the basis of inference with regard to coping mechanisms. They argue that Kobasa's conclusions about hardiness are based on tenuous inferences about coping mechanisms generated through the use of questionable measurement technologies.

It seems clear that factors such as those described in the hardiness research may indeed play an important role in mitigating otherwise pathogenic circumstances. Nevertheless, it may be useful to better operationalize these factors before employing such notions in psychotherapeutic formulations.

No review of historical foundations in personality and stress research would be complete without mentioning the oldest longitudinal research investigation, specifically, the relationship between personality and disease. The Johns Hopkins Precursors Study (see Thomas & McCabe, 1980) seeks to answer the question "Do individuals have distinctive personal characteristics in youth that precede premature disease and death?" The Precursors Study cohort consisted of 1,337 graduates of the Johns Hopkins School of Medicine between the years of 1948 and 1964. Thomas and McCabe investigated, via self-report, consistent "habits of nervous tension" (HNT) and subsequent disease.

> Compared with those of the healthy group, the overall HNT patterns were significantly different for the cancer, coronary occlusion, mental illness and suicide groups. ... It therefore appears that youthful reactions to stress as self-reported in a checklist of habits of nervous tension reflect individual psychobiological differences that are linked with future health or disease. (p. 137)

Thus, in the most liberal interpretation of personality, the Precursors Study continues to reveal links between what may be argued to be characterological traits and the subsequent formation of disease.

Indeed, in a meta-analytic investigation in search of the "disease-prone personality," Friedman and Booth-Kewley (1987) reviewed a research base including *Psychological Abstracts* and *Index Medicus*. Focusing upon psychosomatic disease processes, the authors found 229 studies, of which 101 were ultimately used in the meta-analysis. They conclude: "The results point to the probable existence of a generic 'disease-prone' personality that involves depression, anger/hostility, anxiety, and possibly other aspects of personality" (p. 539).

Let us now turn to a discussion of more recent trends in personality research as it pertains to excessive stress arousal.

THE PRINCIPLE OF PERSONOLOGIC PRIMACY

Should the patient with passive–dependent traits presenting with a stress-induced chronic migraine headache syndrome be treated in the same manner as the patient with histrionic traits and a migraine syndrome of equal severity? Should the patient with avoidant traits and a panic disorder be treated in the same manner as a patient with compulsive traits and a diagnosed panic disorder of equal intensity? A growing body of evidence argues that the answer to both questions is "no" (Frances, 1982).

Theoretical (Everly, 1987; Millon, 1996; Widiger & Frances, 1985), as well as empirical evidence (Everly et al., 1987; Kayser, Robinson, Nies, & Howard, 1987; Millon et al., 1999; Strupp, 1980; Taylor & Abrams, 1975) suggests that clinical and subclinical personality patterns may be a uniquely important factor in the diagnosis and treatment of many psychiatric and stress-related disorders. More specifically, the "principle of personologic primacy" as proposed by Everly (1987) denotes that personologic style plays a uniquely important role in the following:

1. The consistent propensity to create psychosocial stressors (via some diathesis).
2. The phenomenological course of psychiatric and stress-related disorders.
3. Diagnostic refinement of major psychiatric syndromes.
4. Psychotherapeutic, as well as psychopharmacological, treatment responsiveness.
5. The long-term prognosis for many psychiatric and stress-related disorders.

The "principle of personologic primacy" further argues that basic personality patterns and their respective hosts of idiosyncratic interpretational predispositions (i.e., personologic diatheses) for stress and other clinical syndromes serve as phenomenological foundations from which major stress-related illnesses and psychiatric syndromes may emerge. Thus, such syndromes are best understood as pathological extensions of potentially malignant personologic undergirdings, for example, consistent cognitive distortions, irrational expectations, "ego" vulnerabilities, unfounded assumptions, and the like (Everly, 1987; Millon, 1996; Millon & Everly, 1985; Millon et al., 1999). Adverse environmental events, psychoactive drug reactions, and physical and/or psychological trauma may serve as sufficient impetus to cause the personologic substructure to express itself in pathological clinical manifestations such as headaches, panic attacks, and hypertensive and acute tachycardic episodes mediated through the physiological stress response (Chapter 2).

In summary, with regard to stress-related disorders, the "principle of personologic primacy" may be understood as suggesting that (1) a patient's *chronic* propensity to interpret the environment cognitively in such a manner as to engender the stress response with extraordinary frequency is more likely than not to be a function of a personality-based predisposition (diathesis); similarly, (2) a chronic and consistent pattern of elicitation of the stress response is perhaps best viewed more as a manifestation of a dysfunctional characterological predisposition, rather than merely one's exposure to a series of consistently hostile environments. This brings us to the natural corollary of the "principle of personologic primacy": personality-based psychotherapy.

PERSONOLOGIC PSYCHOTHERAPY AND STRESS-RELATED DISORDERS

If, indeed, we accept personality as playing an important role in the etiology of stress-related disease, then we might logically assume that it must play some role in the treatment of such disease as well. Everly (1987) has introduced the concept of "personologic psychotherapy" as one way of recognizing the role that personality may play in treatment formulation. According to Everly, personologic psychotherapy represents a metatherapeutic approach to the treatment of psychiatric as well as stress-related disorders. More specifically, it is the embodiment of the belief that in most chronic psychiatric and stress-related syndromes, a dysfunctional personologic style supports these syndromes and, therefore, must also become a target for therapeutic intervention, if the chronic nature of the problem is to be addressed. Similarly, the concept of "personologic psychotherapy" embodies the belief that treating only the symptoms of *chronic, recurrent* clinical syndromes may in many cases be analogous to palliatively attending to a clinical veneer while ignoring an important aspect of the etiological malignancy (see also Millon et al., 1999).

The theoretical basis for "personologic psychotherapy" is Millon's biosocial learning theory (Millon, 1988, 1996). It is referred to as a metatherapy because the specific manner in which the personologic dysfunction is treated is left to the discretion of the treating therapist.

With specific attention to stress-related disorders, personologic psychotherapy is broadly interpreted to suggest that in addition to treating the florid symptoms of *chronic* stress-related disorders, it is necessary to direct some aspect of therapeutic effort toward the personologic predispositions (diatheses) that may be serving to sustain the chronic stress-related disorder.

Let us examine one example of how these concepts may be used in treatment planning with a patient who can be said to possess a dependent characterological style while manifesting a chronic and more florid stress-related gastrointestinal (GI) dysfunction. According to the theoretical basis

(Millon, 1996; Millon & Everly, 1985), a major sustaining mechanism in a chronically dependent character structure is an extraordinary need for interpersonal affection, affiliation, and support. Such an individual is most vulnerable to chronic stress when this critical need is denied or perhaps only jeopardized. In such a scenario, alleviation of the stress-related GI symptomatology may serve to address only the immediate medical concern. If, indeed, symptom removal has been the only outcome achieved in treatment, then nothing has been done to preclude recurrent GI dysfunction. On the other hand, therapy directed with personologic considerations in mind would certainly consider the potentially self-sustaining mechanisms of extraordinary dependency needs and target the dependent pattern as an additional focus for therapy. Once again, the specific therapeutic technology employed remains at the discretion of the therapist.

The principle of personologic primacy and its therapeutic corollary by no means dictate that formal psychotherapy needs to be conducted in all stress-related disorders. Certainly, there are acute stress-related manifestations that may have little or no etiological basis in personality-related dysfunction. Similarly, "psychotherapeutic" change may well be realized on the basis of therapies not traditionally seen as being "psychotherapeutic" in nature, such as relaxation training and biofeedback therapy (Adler & Morrissey-Adler, 1983; Green & Green, 1983; Murphy & Donovan, 1984). Such therapies commonly yield outcomes such as an improved sense of self-efficacy, a more internal locus of control, improved self-esteem, and what has been called by some a state of "cultivated low arousal" (Adler & Morrissey-Adler, 1983; Green & Green, 1983; Sarnoff, 1982; Stoyva & Budzynski, 1974). In Chapter 8, however, we discuss psychotherapy in greater detail.

MILLON'S PERSONALITY THEORY AND STRESS

Preceding sections in this chapter have argued basically two points: (1) that personality type is related to disease, including stress-related disease, and (2) that treatment planning for stress-related diseases should take into consideration the undergirding personality structure if treatment is to be considered complete. It has also been argued that different personalities possess relatively unique characterological "vulnerabilities," or personologic diatheses, which serve as characterological "weak points" for the initiation of pathogenic stress mechanisms should environmental conditions support such development. Yet one factor that has served to limit the progression of the field of research related to personality and stress is the lack of a coherent superordinate theory of personality from which to extend relational investigations. This is in contrast to the traditional search for unique and specific independent personality factors, such as the Type A pattern.

The biosocial learning theory of personality is a theoretically sound but, more important, clinically useful perspective from which to examine the role that personality plays in the initiation and prolongation of the human stress response (Millon, 1996). A comprehensive review of Millon's theory is beyond the scope of this chapter. Interested readers should refer to Millon (1996). A brief description of his basic personality styles will be presented below.

Considering the realm of "normal" personologic styles, Millon (Millon & Everly, 1985) suggests that there exist eight basic and theoretically pure styles. These normal styles are fundamentally adaptive under most circumstances. Yet each one of these styles will be considered to possess, as part of its intrinsic constituency, idiosyncratic "vulnerabilities" or uniqueness that can serve to predispose to excessive stress arousal under the proper set of environmental circumstances.

A brief review of these eight normal styles seems appropriate at this point. We label each of the styles (with one exception) with the traditional diagnostic terms. The reader must keep in mind, however, that although the terms used will be those most commonly associated with personality "disorders," the present discussion refers NOT to personality disorders but to the "*normal*" personologic variants.

The individual with an *aggressive* personality has difficulty trusting others. He or she tends to usurp the rights of others and to be defensively self-centered. Action-oriented and highly independent, the behavioral style of the personality is forceful. The individual often displays intimidating interpersonal conduct and angry affective expressions, yet the self-perception is one of assertiveness. There is a significant need to control and dominate the environment. The basic, sustaining reinforcement pattern is that of negative reinforcement, in which the individual strives to avoid a loss of control, humiliation, and any position or status that is perceived as being inferior.

The individual with a *narcissistic* personality, even in its normal variation, has difficulty postponing gratification. The person is passively independent, and a poised behavioral appearance is usually manifest. Interpersonal conduct is usually seen as being unempathic, and the affective expression may be seen as serene. The self-perception of the narcissist is one of confidence. Narcissistic individuals seem preoccupied with being seen as unique or special. Such persons often resort to creating illusions of extraordinary competence or influence. They usually are so self-absorbed as to be incapable of seeing any point of view other than their own. This lack of empathy often leads to poor interpersonal communications and shallow relationships. The basic reinforcement pattern is that of positive reinforcement, wherein these individuals act to secure for themselves a position of "entitlement."

The *histrionic* personality is driven by a need for approval, affection, affiliation, and support. Histrionic individuals project an animated, sociable, sometimes dramatic, appearance. An exaggerated affective expression is often present. These individuals are often seen as superficial. However, boredom, especially interpersonal boredom, often plagues the person with histrionic traits. With a flair for the drama in life, the histrionic personality moves about searching for approval, yet it seems that this search is never-ending. Thus, these individuals tend to pursue activities that make them the center of attention. The basic sustaining reinforcement pattern is positive, in which support, approval, and affiliation are inherently reinforcing.

The *schizoid* personality style is described as a characterological pattern typified by a passive behavioral appearance and detached, unobtrusive interpersonal conduct, manifesting a rather bland affective expression. The self-perception of the character style is one of placidity. The individual with a schizoid personality style, juxtaposed to the histrionic style, expresses virtually no desire for interpersonal affiliation or support. The classic prototype of the "lone wolf," this individual appears to view interpersonal exchange as a burdensome process. The schizoid seeks isolation as a defense against excess stimulus bombardment and a sense of being overwhelmed. Thus, the reinforcement pattern of the schizoid can be said to be negative.

The *compulsive* personality is a highly respectful personologic style. Driven by the need to behave in a socially acceptable manner, and to avoid making mistakes, individuals with a compulsive personality walk the "straight and narrow." They consistently adhere to foredrawn rules and regulations, ethics and mores. They often appear as rigid and inflexible, tending to suppress emotions and any signs of distress. These people are most comfortable with the concrete things in life. The abstract and ambiguous are to be avoided as sources of distress. Their sustaining pattern of reinforcement is negative; that is, their behavior is driven by the need to avoid making mistakes and being perceived as socially inappropriate.

The *avoidant* personality desires social affiliation and support yet is so afraid of social rejection that social avoidance becomes a way of life. Shy and withdrawing, individuals with an avoidant personality remain extraordinarily sensitive and vigilant to anything that resembles interpersonal rejection. The sustaining pattern of reinforcement appears to be negative, that is, the avoidance of interpersonal rejection and/or humiliation.

The *dependent* personality is driven by the search for support. Unlike the histrionic style, which actively attracts approval and support, the dependent personality acquiesces to gain affection and support. The chronic pattern of submissiveness and passivity often prohibits the natural development of independent skills and autonomous behaviors. The sustaining pattern of reinforcement is dual, that is, both positive and negative reinforcement. The negative reinforcement is revealed as a pattern in which submissiveness "earns" the affection and support of others, thereby, through a negative reinforcement pattern, avoiding the penultimate stressor—rejection, abandonment, and interpersonal isolation.

The *passive–aggressive* personality, in its pure form, is ambivalent. In many ways it represents an adolescent, from a maturational perspective, in an adult's body. The individual with a passive–aggressive personality desires interpersonal independence but lacks the skills required to function in such a manner. This causes the individual to resort to a dependent reinforcement pattern, yet not without considerable dissonance. Such individuals tend to behave aggressively, but lacking the "adult" skills of assertiveness, cannot risk rejection, so they are aggressive in a hidden, cloaked, or "passive" manner. The sustaining reinforcement pattern for these individuals is negative. Their chronic pessimism, negativism, and interpersonal "game playing" seem to provide rewards of some kind, especially when they can see others fail, compromise, or become as negative or cynical about the world as they are. Indeed, perhaps misery does love company. More important, the passive–aggressive manipulation allows the person to avoid a sense of interpersonal impotence and dependence.

These, then, are the theoretically "pure" personologic styles as described by Millon (Millon & Everly, 1985). In reality, it should be noted that most people are combinations of two or three of these styles. Furthermore, to reiterate, each of the aforementioned personality styles can be said to be fundamentally "normal" and *not* to be considered a personality disorder, despite the descriptive labels usually used in conjunction with a personality disorder.

Returning to the issue of the human stress response, the notion of personologic psychotherapy as it pertains to the treatment of stress arousal argues that some degree of therapeutic effort needs to be directed toward the unique qualities and/or sustaining reinforcement patterns of the personality being treated, because it is felt that some idiosyncratic qualities or vulnerabilities may play a significant role in the etiology of chronic stress syndromes. Using Millon's schema, it may be argued that each of the eight basic personality styles possesses its own intrinsic personologic diathesis, that is, factors inherent in the personality that may serve to contribute to extraordinary stress arousal. These factors are listed in Table 7.1. From

Table 7.1. Personologic Diatheses and Stress

Personality style	Sustaining reinforcement pattern	Consistent personality factors that contribute to extraordinary arousal
Aggressive	R−	1. Need to exert control of, and to vigilantly monitor, the environment 2. Being placed in a position of having to rely on, or trust, other individuals 3. Fear of being taken advantage of and efforts to avoid that 4. Fear of being humiliated, and efforts to avoid that 5. Assumption that "only the strong survive" and the persistent efforts to be "strong"
Narcissistic	R+	1. Inability to postpone gratification 2. Fear of not being seen as "special" 3. Need to create illusions of extraordinary competence 4. Inability to empathize with others, leading to consistently poor communications 5. Assumption that others will recognize him/her as "special"
Histrionic	R−	1. Interpersonal instability 2. Fear of a loss of affection 3. Fear of a loss of support or actual rejection 4. Frequent changes in life events 5. Need for interpersonal approval 6. Belief that he/she must earn, or "perform" for interpersonal affection, approval, and support
Dependent	R−	1. Fear of the loss of interpersonal support 2. Fear of the loss of affection or of actual rejection 3. Chronic submissiveness and inability to be assertive when desired 4. Fear and avoidance of interpersonal confrontation
Passive–aggressive	R−	1. Desire to behave in a manner contrary to previous learning history 2. Inability to act assertively 3. Chronic tendency to compare self to others 4. Chronic negativism 5. "Successes" of peer group 6. Actual failure or rejection

(Continued)

Table 7.1. (*Continued*)

Personality style	Sustaining reinforcement pattern	Consistent personality factors that contribute to extraordinary arousal
Compulsive	R−	1. Efforts to maintain rigid self-control 2. Change 3. Coping with abstract or ambiguous situations 4. Decision making when options are not clear 5. Unclear directions 6. The "gray areas" of rules and policies 7. Fear of making a mistake 8. Need for, and excessive efforts to, earn approval 9. Fear of social disapproval 10. Belief that emotions should be suppressed 11. Assumption that others share compulsive traits and will act accordingly 12. Waste (e.g., of time, money, effort) 13. Risk taking
Avoidant	R−	1. Interpersonal intrusion 2. Fear of interpersonal rejection 3. Need to remain highly vigilant 4. Lack of interpersonal support 5. Actual rejection 6. Interpersonal hypersensitivity
Schizoid	R−	1. Interpersonal intrusion 2. Lack of interpersonal support 3. Hyperstimulation

a clinical perspective, we hope that enumeration of these factors will assist the clinician in (1) understanding how personologic factors may contribute to chronic stress arousal syndromes and (2) targeting psychotherapeutic efforts toward the personologic foundations of excessive stress, that is, the unique vulnerabilities and/or sustaining mechanisms as described in the preceding text or in Table 7.1.

SUMMARY

In this chapter, the focus has been upon the role that personality plays in the initiation, prolongation, and ultimate treatment of the human stress response. Let us review the main points:

1. There is a commonly held belief that in the case of *chronic* stress arousal and stress-related diseases, one's personality serves to play a significant role from an etiological, as well as therapeutic, perspective.

2. Historically, investigations have focused upon *specific* personality traits and *specific* disease formation (Alexander, 1950; Dunbar, 1935).

3. More contemporary perspectives have chosen to look within the global personality for characterological vulnerabilities, that is, personologic diathesis, for extraordinary stress arousal and a subsequent host of stress-related diseases (Everly, 1987; Frances, 1982; Millon, 1996).

4. The principle of personologic primacy argues that consistent characterological traits serve to undergird and therefore play a unique role in the patient's propensity to create psychosocial stressors. Such factors play a major role in treatment planning and responsiveness (Everly, 1987; Frances & Hale, 1984) as well.

5. The notion of "personologic psychotherapy" is the natural corollary of the principle of personologic primacy and basically argues that even in chronic stress-related disorders, characterological traits require therapeutic attention and therefore should be considered in treatment planning (Everly, 1987; Millon, 1996; Millon et al., 1999).

6. When attempting to better understand and concretize the role of personologic vulnerabilities as factors that predispose to extraordinary stress arousal, Millon's biosocial learning theory of personality serves as a theoretically cogent and clinically practical framework from which to operate. Table 7.1 describes common personologic factors that serve to contribute to extraordinary stress arousal within each of Millon's basic eight "normal" personality formulations. An understanding of these factors serves to foster a better understanding of *chronic* stress arousal and its subsequent disorders, and to facilitate treatment planning and intervention when one looks beyond the florid symptoms of excessive stress arousal.

7. A final point needs to be reiterated before this chapter is brought to a close. We have indeed attempted to sensitize the reader to the belief that personality traits play an important role in the nature and treatment of the human stress response. That is *not* to say, however, that formal psychotherapy needs to be an integral aspect of all stress treatment/stress management paradigms. Processes such as relaxation training, biofeedback, and even health education practices are clearly capable, in some instances, of altering dysfunctional practices. Yet there are instances where chronic, stress-related diseases are a direct function of personologic disturbances such as dysfunctional self-esteem, persistent cognitive distortions, irrational assumptions, inappropriate expectations of self and others, and so on. In such cases, some concerted psychotherapeutic effort would clearly be indicated. The most effective "mix" of therapeutic technologies (e.g., relaxation training, psychotherapy, hypnosis) remains to be determined by the therapist on a case-by-case basis. It is clearly beyond the scope of this volume to dictate such guidelines.

Consistent, then, with the belief that the treatment of excessive stress is a multidimensional enterprise, we will now proceed to address the myriad therapeutic technologies that have been found useful in the treatment of excessive human stress.

The discussion of specific therapeutic interventions begins in the next two chapters with an exploration of a "psychotherapeutic" genre that has shown special relevance to the treatment of excessive stress arousal.

8

Control and the Human Stress Response

> ...grant me the strength to change what I can, the courage to bear what
> I cannot change, and the wisdom to know the difference.
>
> REINHOLD NIEBUHR, 1934

The preceding chapter sensitized the reader to how the patient's persono-logic diathesis functions as a portentous epiphenomenological factor in the etiology, maintenance, and treatment of stress-related disorders. Lazarus (1975) stated that personality-based idiosyncracies influence an individual's appraisal and interpretation of his or her environment. He further asserted that target-organ activation and emotional arousal are derived from these personologic factors. Therefore, it may be deduced that personologic factors function as a form of "filtering mechanism" that helps to shape one's perception of reality. The present chapter addresses one specific aspect of the perceptual filtering process, namely, the construct of control and how it affects human health. Albert Bandura (1997) cogently captures the essence of this chapter with his statement: "The intensity and chronicity of human stress is governed largely by perceived control over the demands of one's life" (p. 262). More specifically, this chapter will review several theories of control and consider the function of this con-struct in linking stress with illness, recovery, aging, and the psychothera-peutic process. The relationship between controllability and immune function, addressed in Chapter 8 in the first edition of this text, is now covered separately in Chapter 5.

A DEFINITION OF CONTROL

Control is conceptualized as existing within five general domains:

- The demonstrated ability to change or manipulate an environmental transaction (Bandura, 1997, 1977; Thompson, 1981).
- The perceived ability to change or manipulate an environmental transaction (Bandura, 1997, 1977, 1982a,b; Krantz, 1980).
- The ability to predict an environmental transaction (Seligman, 1975).
- The ability to understand an environmental transaction (Averill, 1973; Krantz, 1980; Thompson, 1981).
- The ability to *accept* the environmental transaction within some meaningful cognitive framework or belief system. Some authors consider this as "relinquishing" control.

THEORIES OF CONTROL

Alfred Adler (1929) suggested 70 years ago that the desire to make decisions and affect outcomes—in other words, to enact control—is a basic tenet of human behavior. Personal control has been conceptualized in various forms (e.g., behavioral control, cognitive control, decisional control, and informational control). The construct of cognitive control, however, is typically considered to have the most impact on the stress response (Sarafino, 1998; Cohen, Evans, Stokols, & Krantz, 1980; Thompson, 1981).

Learned Helplessness

Martin Seligman and his colleagues' learned helplessness theory (Overmier & Seligman, 1967; Seligman & Maier, 1967) is often acknowledged as a progenitor of the cognitive-control focus. Employing an experimental design known as triadic, their seminal animal research typically consisted of three groups of dogs receiving different types of pretreatments. The first group (the escape group) was given a controllable event (an outcome influenced by some response); the second group (the helplessness group) was *yoked* to the first (i.e., they received the same event as the first group; however, it was now uncontrollable); and the third group (naive group) received no pretreatment. The dogs in the first two groups were then exposed to electric shock. The difference between the groups was that the dogs in the escape group were trained to turn the shock off (e.g., pressing a panel located on either side of their heads with their noses), whereas the responses of the dogs in the yoked group had no effect. The dogs in the naive group received no shock.

Twenty-four hours later, all three groups received 10 trials of signaled escape–avoidance training in a shuttle box; jumping over a shoulder-high barrier within 10 seconds of a discriminant signal (e.g., lights dimming) would prevent the shock. Failure to jump led to a shock that continued until the dog jumped, or for the duration of 60 seconds. The escape group and the naive group jumped the barrier readily; however, the yoked group initiated few escape attempts. Moreover, when they did respond successfully, they did so inconsistently. In fact, most of these dogs lay down and did not react emotionally while being shocked. Seligman and his colleagues (Overmier & Seligman, 1967; Seligman & Maier, 1967) described how these laboratory experiments produced deficits in the yoked dogs in three disinct domains: (1) motivation to respond, (2) ability to learn that responding had an impact, and (3) emotional disturbance, primarily anxiety or depression. Interestingly, Hiroto (1974) replicated these findings fairly precisely on college students. An unsignaled, loud noise served as the stimulus and moving a lever from one side of a box to the other served to eliminate the noise.

The learned helplessness model formulated by Seligman and his colleagues has had a tremendous impact in psychology on the theoretical development of the effects of uncontrollable outcomes and their impact on symptoms associated with depression and anxiety. However, as human research expanded in this area, investigators questioned why individuals exposed to uncontrollable negative events did not invariably develop a sense of helplessness and subsequent feelings of depression. They also questioned the relationship between depression and loss of self-esteem. Abramson, Seligman, and Teasdale (1978) reformulated the learned helplessness paradigm by incorporating an attributional framework to help account for the experience of human depression. They perceived noncontingency between response and outcome as leading to future expectations of no control or limited control of either internal or external situational demands. According to their theory, this perception of helplessness would lead to cognitive deficits in which the individual anticipated lack of control in subsequent challenges. Furthermore, feelings of sadness, depression, and limited motivational energy would result in the absence of coping due in part to the perceived noncontingency between previous responses and outcomes.

Abramson et al. (1978) proposed that when people perceive noncontingency between response and outcomes, they attribute their helplessness to a cause that may be stable (consistent) or unstable (inconsistent), global (broad range of situations) or specific (narrow range of situations), and internal (personal helplessness) or external (universal helplessness). Thus, depression occurs in four classes of deficits: motivational, cognitive, self-esteem, and affective. Therefore, individuals who tend to attribute failure to global, stable, and internal factors are more predisposed to feelings of depression, low self-esteem, stress, and limited control.

Although the reformulated theory of helplessness and depression had a major impact on theoretical development in social and clinical psychology, and generated a vast amount of empirical data following its inception, its emphasis was on an attributional account of human helplessness instead of a formally articulated theory of depression. Abramson, Metalsky, and Alloy (1989) later proposed the *hopelessness* theory of depression as not only a revision of their 1978 reformulation but also as a distinct clinical subtype of depression. According to this theory, hopelessness is considered a sufficient cause of depression rather than a particular symptom. Included within the hopelessness theory is the diathesis–stress component that specifies three separate vulnerability factors (cognitive diatheses) considered to interact with negative situational occurrences or stressors in leading to symptoms of depression: (1) attributional diathesis (attributing negative life events to stable and global causes), (2) cognitive diathesis about self (making negative self-statements and inferences following an inauspicious occurrence), and (3) cognitive diathesis about consequences (a sad occurrence will lead to a further, negative consequence). Several empirical studies have focused on supporting these diatheses (Alloy, Just, & Panzarella, 1997; Metalsky & Joiner, 1992) and the Hopelessness Depression Symptom Questionnaire was introduced to measure symptoms associated with the construct (Metalsky & Joiner, 1997).

According to the hopelessness theory of depression, a cognitive style typified by external, unstable, and specific attributional characteristics may reduce risk for depression when a person encounters stress (Alloy & Clements, 1992). Alloy, Kelly, Mineka, and Clements (1990) proposed that some perception of control styles associated with the hopelessness theory of depression may serve to decrease vulnerability to depression. More specifically, this proposal is partially predicated on the frequently replicated finding that mildly depressed individuals accurately judge the degree of control their responses have over outcomes (depressive realism), whereas nondepressed individuals evidence an overestimation, or illusion of control, with regard to their responses and outcomes (Ackerman & DeRubeis, 1991). Illusion of control has been suggested to operate primarily by helping to prevent increases in negative emotions following a stressful event; however, it is also suggested that positive affect may maintain or at times enhance the illusion (Alloy & Clements, 1992). Thus, the cognitive imperative of perceived control may serve as one of the principal factors mitigating the relationship between environmental events and outcomes.

Illusions of Control

The concept of the illusion of control is usually credited to Ellen Langer. In a series of cogently designed studies, she and her colleagues demonstrated that people in purely chance situations that they interpret as having skill-based components or behaviors will act as if they can control the outcome. For example, subjects who chose their own lottery tickets required more compensation to exchange their tickets than those who were not given a choice of tickets, even if the "exchange ticket" had a higher probability of winning than the original ticket (Langer, 1975). Several years after the seminal work of Langer, illusory perceptions of control were considered a key factor in understanding the effects of psychological stress on behavior. For example, Friedland, Keinan, and Regev (1992) randomly assigned Israeli flight school cadets to either a low-stress (currently involved in classroom studies) or a high-stress condition (one-half hour before a training flight). Subjects were then given four hypothetical gambling situations (e.g., a free airline ticket is inside one of six drawers; either choose a drawer or roll a die to decide which drawer to open). As expected, subjects in the high-stress condition showed a stronger preference for gambling forms that induce illusions on control. In the preceding example, this would involve choosing the drawer rather than rolling the die.

More recently, Thompson, Armstrong, and Thomas (1998) have proposed that individuals rely on a control heuristic to help account for the circumstances of illusions of control and to estimate outcomes involving control. The control heuristic considers two broad components: (1) one's intention to achieve the outcome, which includes perception of ability to enact the outcome, and desire for the outcome, and (2) the perceived connection between the action and outcome, which includes a temporal association, or frequency of action, followed by the desired outcome, a shared meaning or similarity between action and outcome, and a predictive connection of prior expectations.

Julian Rotter's (1954) social learning theory, which emphasizes behavior potential (probability that an individual will act in a certain fashion), expectancy (belief of reinforcement following a specific behavior), reinforcement value (an individual's perceived worth of an outcome), and psychological situation (how an individual views the context of behavior), offers important insights into the influences of motivation. In 1966, Rotter expanded his social learning theory to include locus of control, which is a generalized belief about the extent to which behaviors influence successes and failures. People with an *internal* locus of control perceive that outcomes are contingent on their actions, choices, or efforts, whereas individuals with an external locus of control believe their actions have minimal impact on outcomes, and that outcomes are determined by forces outside of themselves (e.g., fate, luck, powerful others). Rotter developed the I-E Scale to measure the degree of internality or externality of a person's beliefs about personal control.

SELF-EFFICACY

Comparable to Seligman, Langer, and Rotter, Albert Bandura (1977, 1982a,b, 1997), renowned for his social cognitive theory of human behavior, focuses on a cognitive locus of appraisal to help account for maladaptive stimulus–response interactions. A major construct in his more than 20 years of work is the concept of self-efficacy, which he defines as "beliefs in one's capabilities to organize and execute the courses of action required to produce given attainments" (1997, p. 3). Thus, efficacy beliefs or appraisals of competence and control influence behaviors, thoughts, feelings, and emotions. Individuals possessing a high sense of self-efficacy are often task-oriented and utilize multifaceted, integrative problem-solving skills to enhance successful outcomes when dealing with psychosocial stressors. Conversely, people with limited self-efficacy may perceive psychosocial stressors as unmanageable and are more likely to dwell on perceived deficiencies, which generates increased stress and diminishes potential problem-solving energy, lowers aspirations, and weakens commitments.

Bandura (1997) posits that people's beliefs concerning their efficacy are determined by four principal influences:

1. Enactive mastery experiences or performance accomplishments are considered the most powerful source of self-efficacy, because mastery is based on actual success.
2. Vicarious experiences (observational learning, modeling, imitation) increases confidence as people observe behaviors of others, noting contingencies of behavior, and then use this information to form expectancies of their own behavior. An observer's perception of characteristic similarity between him- or herself and the model is an important factor in vicarious experiences.
3. Verbal or social persuasion utilizes expressions of faith in one's competence. The impact of verbal persuasion is less profound than the previous two sources; however, when applied in combination with vicarious and enactive techniques, the influence of self-efficacy is more effective.
4. Finally, physiological and affective states influence self-efficacy, in that comfortable physiological sensations and positive affect are likely to enhance one's confidence in a given situation.

The preceding concepts, although unique, share a focus upon the relevance of a cognitive appraisal of control as a portentous mediator in human functioning. The following sections examine the effects of control on stress and other health-related factors.

CONTROL AND ILLNESS

The relationship between perception of control and onset of poor health is not a new phenomenon. Some of the earliest recorded work in this area is credited to Schmale and Iker (1966). In one study, 51 essentially healthy women under the age of 50 rated their perception of control after they were discovered to have suspicious, cancer-like symptoms following a routine Pap smear test. Patients with higher ratings of helplessness and hopeless were more likely to develop cancer in the future. Given the correlational nature of this study, these data could not resolve the issue of cause and effect; in other words, whether hopelessness led to cancer, or whether cancer, prior to being diagnosed, resulted in perceived helplessness. What these suggestive data did provide, however, was an important area for future exploration.

Following the work of Schmale and Iker, Engel (1968) introduced the theoretical construct of the "giving-up given-up" complex. He described a general consensus among his physician colleagues and himself that 70% to 80% of physical illness seen in their medical practices occurred after the clinical manifestation of psychological states involving the following characteristics: (1) a feeling of giving up experienced as helplessness or hopelessness; (2) a depreciated self-image; (3) a sense of loss of gratification from relationships or roles in life; (4) a feeling of disruption in the sense of continuity between past, present, and future; and (5) a reactivation of memories of earlier periods of giving up. Engel suggested that the complex is neither a coincidence nor a consequence of illness, but rather a modifier of the capacity of the person to cope with a pathogenic stressor.

Engel (1971) expanded this theoretical work when he categorized 170 examples of sudden death reported in newspapers over a 5-year period. His categories included age, gender, and eight "life settings" or circumstances representing various types of losses, threats, and even successes. In his sample, women were more often reported as suddenly dying in relationship to loss, whereas men were reported to die more suddenly in relation to perceived danger. Implicit in his interpretation of these events was the notion that persons no longer had, or believed they had, control over the situation. In turn, he concluded that people struggle to cope with the overwhelming experience and at times may give up and accept death.

Cannon (1942) is often credited with the most comprehensive study of the scientific literature on the subject of voodoo death spells in Africa, Australia, New Zealand, South America, and Haiti. He concluded that the observed sudden deaths were not due to natural causes or poisoning, and suggested that the interrelationship between debilitating intense fear, the firm belief of primitive peoples in the effects of tribal superstitions, and abandonment of the victim led to loss of control, hopelessness, and despair.

Further evidence has demonstrated the direct influence of concepts such as perceived control and self-efficacy on health, independent of health behaviors. For example, in a 7-year longitudinal study of 3,128 non-institutional persons over age 65, Mossey and Shapiro (1982) collected data on self-rated health ("For your age, would you say, in general, your health is excellent, good, fair, poor, or bad?"), as well as objective health status (reports from physicians on medical conditions and occurrence of health problems requiring hospitalization and/or surgery). The results showed that the mortality rate for those who rated their health as poor was almost three times that of persons who rated themselves as being in excellent health. More revealing, however, was the finding that subjective, self-reported health was a more accurate mortality predictor than the objective physicians' health measures. For example, "health pessimists" (those who rated their health as fair or poor despite objective measures of good or excellent health) had a greater risk of dying than "health optimists" (those who rated themselves as healthy despite negative objective reports). In a related study of 7,000 adults (Kaplan & Camacho, 1983), women with poor self-rated health were five times as likely to die compared to those who evaluated their health as excellent. For men, the difference was more than twice as great. These results remained even after controlling for health-related behaviors (e.g., drinking, smoking, and exercising), social contacts (family and friends), and mood (happiness and depression).

One of the most fascinating studies of the effects of perceived manipulated control on health was performed on patients diagnosed with panic disorder with agoraphobia (Sanderson, Rapee, & Barlow, 1989). Previous research has demonstrated that breathing carbon dioxide (CO_2)-enriched air (e.g., 5.5% CO_2-enriched) can provoke panic attacks in a majority of patients with panic disorder. While most evidence to date had focused on the biochemical effects of 5.5% CO_2, Sanderson and his colleagues, noting that "fear of losing control" was reported as the most intense symptom during a panic attack, examined the influence of instilling an illusion of control in 20 patients exposed to 5.5% CO_2-enriched air for 15 minutes.

Prior to being exposed to the enriched air, all subjects were told that a box located directly in front of them *might* light up during the exposure. They were also informed that when this box was lit, they would be able to decrease the amount of CO_2, if desired, by turning a dial attached to the chairs in which they were sitting. All were encouraged, however, to lower the CO_2 only if they felt that it was absolutely necessary. In actuality, the dial had no effect on the deliverance of CO_2. For half of the subjects, the light box was randomly illuminated periodically throughout their CO_2 exposure, whereas for the other subjects, the light never came on. Subjects who believed they could not control the quantity of CO_2 (no-light subjects) reported a greater number of symptoms and intensity of panic compared to the subjects who believed they could control the CO_2. In fact, 80% of subjects in the "no illusion of control" group reported that they experienced a panic attack compared to only 20% in the "illusion of control" group. As more recent data have shown, enhancing patients' perceived control through cognitive-behavioral interventions that provide education regarding the etiology and maintenance of panic, cognitive techniques to alter faulty appraisals, exposure exercises, and diaphragmatic breathing (see Chapter 12) has markedly alleviated the incidence of panic attacks in patients with panic disorder (Schmidt, Trakowski, & Staab, 1997).

Diagnosis with a life-threatening illness is considered one of the most profound psychological stressors that people may face in their lives, and their perceptions of control are likely to be severely challenged. According to Helgeson (1992), the maturation of chronic illness is a victimizing experience. Janoff-Bulman (1988) has written extensively on how the effects of victimization may disrupt and strongly threaten the core assumptions we have of the world. In particular, beliefs about the benevolence of the world, the meaningfulness of the world (e.g., people get what they deserve), and feelings of self-worth become considerably compromised, leading people to feel increasingly vulnerable. The process of coping involves reestablishing the basic assumptions about the world that are viable to regain a sense of control.

Bombardier, D'Amico, and Jordan (1990) examined appraisal and coping strategies to enhance controllability among 101 patients with diverse, chronic medical conditions consisting mostly of low back pain and headache. Comparable to the Mossey and Shapiro's (1982) findings, they suggested that a physician's ratings of the magnitude of structural damage was not predictive of overall dysfunction. Furthermore, their results indicated a triad of emotion-focused coping, consisting of wishful thinking, self-blame, and avoidance, predicted poorer adjustment to illness.

Patients with a chronic illness, such as debilitating coronary artery disease, rheumatoid arthritis, diabetes, or AIDS, typically lack control over certain aspects of the disease process. However, there are features of persons with chronic illness, such as persistence, self-image, and other coping skills, that remain "controllable" (Caldwell, Pearson, & Chin, 1987;

Thompson, 1981). The innovative 6-week, 12-hour program at the Stanford Arthritis Center (Lorig & Fries, 1990), which relied on self-management through illness education, relaxation, and nutrition, is an example of a successful treatment intervention. However, relevant to the topic of perceived control, the data from this program indicated that the participants who improved were not necessarily those who knew more about arthritis or most changed their behavior. Instead, interviews with participants suggested that those who improved had a positive outlook and an enhanced sense of control over their chronic illness. In other words, the best predictor of change was whether the person thought he or she would improve. Four years after the initial assessment, improved participants continued to report an increase in self-efficacy, close to a 20% reduction in subjective pain, and decreased physician visits.

Moreover, rheumatoid arthritis patients demonstrated more personal control and positive mood over symptoms that were moderate or severe, whereas personal control was not related to mood for mild symptoms. Conversely, personal control and positive mood were related if the disease process was less severe; however, a more severe disease process was associated with negative mood and poorer adjustment (Affleck, Tennen, Pfeiffer, & Fifield, 1987; Banwell & Ziebell, 1985). Helgeson (1992), in a study of 96 cardiac patients, expanded these findings to suggest additional moderators in the relationship between control and adjustment. She reported that adjustment is better if the perceptions of control are consistent and based in reality, and if the threat is more severe and perceived as contollable. For example, she found that for rehospitalized patients, the increased severity of threat coupled with appropriate perceptions of control buffered these patients from inordinate distress. She noted, however, that multiple rehospitalizations, while certainly increasing threat severity, may eventually lead to a conflict in perceptions of control and in turn to poorer coping.

Since patients with chronic illness often work closely with health care professionals, issues of vicarious control (perceptions that others have control) deserve consideration. In the Helgelson (1992) study, perceptions of vicarious control were related to better adaptedness for patients undergoing invasive, physician-based treatments such as angioplasty or bypass surgery, but not for patients treated only with medications. In other investigations, vicarious control and adjustment were associated positively among breast cancer patients who had a favorable prognosis (Taylor, Lichtman, & Wood, 1984), whereas a negative relationship was found between vicarious control and adjustment for AIDS patients (Reed, 1989).

Reed, Taylor, and Kemeny (1993) accounted for these latter findings · by suggesting that vicarious control for AIDS patients may be less adaptive given the nature and history of the response of the medical community to the illness. In a sample of 24 gay men who were generally well informed about the disease and its treatment options, Reed and colleagues reported that those with belief in personal control and responsibility over both day-to-day symptoms and the course of the illness were better adjusted than those with greater vicarious beliefs. In addition to the apparent prognostic differences between the breast cancer and AIDS groups, Reed et al. also offered the possibility that men and women may respond differently to personal and vicarious control beliefs. Clearly, circumstances such as type of illness, prognosis, and gender may be involved in the complex process of vicarious control and warrant future research consideration.

CONTROL AND AGING

Perception of control of one's immediate environment is considered an important factor in positive cognitive, psychological, and physical outcomes in older adults (Brandtstadter & Baltes-Gotz, 1990; Eizenman, Nesselroade, Featherman, & Rowe, 1997; Rowe & Kahn, 1987). Rodin and Timko (1992) hypothesized that the variety of physical, personal, and social challenges and conditions confronting elderly persons help to intensify the relationship between health and a sense of control.

Langer and Benevento (1978) reported on how subtle contextual factors surrounding activities in which one is engaged can influence control. For example, assigning a person an inferiority label such as *old* or *institutionalized* may indirectly communciate an insidious and stigmatized message of incompetence. Langer and Benevento termed the process, in which an individual erroneously infers incompetence from interpersonal situational factors, "self-induced dependence." Given the frequently false perception in American society that old age equates to deterioration combined with the actual experience of emotional losses such as retirement and bereavement, it is understandable how the elderly may be particularly susceptible to self-induced dependence. Bandura (1982b) also suggested that older people often perceive themselves as declining both intellectually and physically, since they often use younger groups rather than their peers for comparison.

Considering the negative stereotypes of aging, along with the increased perception of questionable competency on the part of elderly persons, it is not surprising that younger people interacting with older individuals may be apt to assist them in tasks that they previously performed effectively on their own. Avorn and Langer (1982) studied changes in performance on a simple puzzle task in 72 elderly residents of an intermediate-care facility, who were randomly assigned to one of three groups: (1) helped—at each of the four 20-minute sessions, an examiner sat with the subject, encouraged working on the puzzle, and actually selected pieces that solved the puzzle with the subject; (2) encouragement only—at each of the four 20-minute sessions, an examiner sat with the subject and encouraged completion of the puzzle but with minimal assistance; and (3) no contact—no participation by the examiner. There were no differences among the groups at pretesting on puzzle acumen, cooperativeness, alertness, or age; however, postexperimental puzzle testing revealed several performance differences. Subjects who were helped completed fewer puzzle pieces and performed more slowly than subjects in the encouragement-only group. Also, helped subjects performed less well on the posttest despite the practice they received, whereas, the encouragement- only and no-contact groups both improved. Moreover, on measures of confidence and autonomy gathered at the time of the posttests, helped subjects were less confident of their ability and rated the puzzles more difficult than the encouragement-only group. Taken collectively, these data suggest that assistance, although usually well intentioned, may adversely affect elderly persons' sense of control.

In addition to investigating loss of control, several studies have examined the health and emotional effects of attempting to instill control in elderly persons. Recognizing the potentially adverse stress effects of relocating to long-term-care facilities, several studies have shown that enhancing predictability and involving elderly individuals in the decision-making process to enter a home contributes to better health. For patients already in a nursing facility, Langer and colleagues conducted a series of highly regarded studies associating increased personal responsibility, choice, and control with positive health outcomes. In a study of nursing home residents, Langer and Rodin (1976) varied the type of communication residents heard from an administrator. Some subjects ($n = 47$) received a communication emphasizing responsibility and decision making, in addition to being given the choice of caring for a plant and the chance to decide on which of two nights to watch a movie. Subjects ($n = 44$) in the other group received a communication that made more explicit the policy of the nursing home (i.e., that it was the staff's responsibility to care for them). Moreover, these 44 residents were implicitly denied choice by being given a plant to care for and were assigned a night to view a movie. Questionnaires and behavioral ratings obtained 1 week prior to the communication revealed that there were no differences between the groups on measures such as perceived control or activity level. Three weeks after the communication, residents given an enhanced sense of responsibility became more active and alert, felt happier, and became more involved in a variety of activities than the comparison group.

Rodin and Langer (1977) returned to the nursing home 18 months later and found that most of these group differences endured. Residents in the responsibility group remained more active, sociable, vigorous, and self-initiating than the comparison or control groups. Moreover, during this 18-month period, the responsibility-induced group showed a significantly greater increase in general health than the comparison participants. In fact, only 15% of the responsibility-induced group died within this time compared with 30% of the comparison group.

Langer, Rodin, Beck, Weinman, and Spitzer (1979) expanded on these findings to determine whether perceptions of enhanced control could slow or reverse declines in memory and health in elderly persons. In two separate studies, the authors demonstrated that the impact of environmental variables on memory and cognitive ability many be profound. In the first study, reciprocal self-disclosure was manipulated (high vs. low) in a series of dyadic interviews with nursing home residents, and memory was assessed using pattern and probe recall tests. The results revealed that the high reciprocal self-disclosure group showed improved memory compared to the low reciprocal self-disclosure and control groups. Moreover, nurses, who were unaware of the treatment conditions, rated the high-involvement group as more aware, more active, and more self-initiating than the no-treatment controls. In the second study, researchers motivated elderly patients to practice and perform cognitive activities, including memory and information-seeking tasks, by varying whether receiving practical incentives (poker chips that could be redeemed at a later time for gifts) were contingent or noncontingent. The data revealed that the elderly subjects in the contingency condition demonstrated improved memory for recent and remote events, increased motivation, and improved social adjustment.

In another study of 73 nursing home residents, Alexander, Langer, Newman, Chandler, and Davies (1989) randomly assigned and then taught residents one of three self-control strategies: meditation, mindfulness training (a guided attention technique), or mental relaxation (a cortical deactivation technique using a familiar verse, phrase, song or poem). There was also a no-treatment control group. The three treatment groups, while seemingly similar structurally, were considered different in terms of the precise mental procedure used. Cognitive functioning, health ratings (blood pressure, nurses ratings, longevity), and personality data served as dependent variables. Results indicated that the meditation group improved most on the majority of the dependent measures, followed by the mindfulness group. For example, the survival rate for the meditation group was 100% after 3 years compared to 87.5% for the mindfulness group, and 65% for the relaxation group. Alexander and colleagues proposed that the deep state of relaxation combined with the self-referent alertness was likely responsible for the meditation's greater impact.

The mindfulness group did, however, score higher than the meditation group on perceived control, which supports Charowitz and Langer's (1981) hypothesis that mindful involvement is the most important factor in establishing a sense of control.

Given that the aforementioned results have not been universally replicated (Schulz & Hanusa, 1978), investigators have hypothesized about different mechanisms that may be involved in control-related interventions. For example, the loss of control may be perceived as more detrimental than lacking control from the outset (Rodin & Timko, 1992). In a cross-sectional analysis, Mirowsky (1995) obtained survey data on perceptions of control, physical impairment, and amount of education from more than 2,800 persons ranging in age from 18 to 90. After separating participants into age groups, his results showed comparatively high and stable levels of perceived control in the 18–50 age range, followed by successive and rapid decreases in sense of control in older groups. Respondents over age 80 had the lowest sense of control. Moreover, regression analyses showed that for the low sense of control in the elderly, low education was a more significant independent predictor than physical impairment. Interestingly, these results remained even after adjustments were made for other socioeconomic factors.

Other studies have suggested that control beliefs in elderly persons may be influenced by intellectual functioning and education. A 5-year longitudinal design by Lachman and Leff (1989) demonstrated no significant changes in intellectual functioning or internal sense of control in the 63 retested patients, whose average age was 77.5 years at the time of the second testing. However, external control beliefs in powerful others' control over intelligence increased significantly. Further analyses revealed the possible impact of education. In this sample, subjects with more education believed less in the role of powerful others; however, they also showed the greatest increase in beliefs in powerful others over the 5 years.

Other investigators, consistent with a developing trend in personality research, have suggested that the construct of variability is an important factor that warrants investigative consideration in older adults. Rakowski and Cryan (1990), using data from the National Health Interview Survey, suggested that understanding the complicated and multivaried role of health perceptions and health behavior in older adults may benefit from a focus on intraindividual consistency in addition to attempts to discover factor-type, normative interindividual data. Eizenman et al. (1997) citing "an emergent trend in personality research to identify and study personality processes as nonstatic" (p. 498), suggested that the understanding of perceived control in elderly persons could be enhanced by augmenting interindividual data with short-term, intraindividual variability data. In a study of 57 nursing home residents with a mean age of 77 years, they showed that the amount of individual standard deviation on weekly measures of locus of control and perceived competence for 7 months was a fairly stable attribute. However, using logistic regression analyses, they demonstrated that the differences in magnitude of intraindividual variability scores, not the mean scores on locus of control or competence, predicted mortality 5 years later.

CONTROL AND RECOVERY

Although similar in many respects to psychological adjustment to chronic illness, perceptions of control over the course and outcome of recovery from illness, injury, and surgery warrant separate consideration given the potential and often likely differences in outcome measures. For example, as noted by Affleck, Tennen, Croog, and Levine (1987), heart attack patients are considered well suited to study these perceived control relations for three distinct reasons. First, there are a variety of psychological responses to heart attack due to myriad accepted risk factors such as heredity, stress, and behaviors. Second, the variability in outcome following a heart attack may range from minimal to highly debilitating and chronic. Third, an increased likelihood of subsequent attacks may lead to increased fear that medical assistance may not be available at the appropriate time (Wiklund & Sanne, 1984). Certainly, there is little doubt that a myocardial infarction (MI) is a traumatic event that requires noted alterations in emotional, behavioral, and social demands involved in treatment and recovery (Ben-Sira & Eliezer, 1990). In addition to uncertainty and unpredictability, there are also likely demands to follow a medical regimen, to change dietary and smoking habits, and to alter accustomed recreational and social activities (Fowers, 1994).

While behavioral changes such as adhering to a potentially complex medical regimen and/or stopping smoking are often thought to occur with little resistance in post-MI patients, the literature is replete with data that suggest otherwise. For example, it has been estimated that for chronic illnesses with long-term treatment regimens, the rate of adherence is only around 54% (Cluss & Epstein, 1985). Moreover, Strecher et al. (1985) have reported that acknowledgment of the harmful health effects of smoking will do little to curtail the behavior unless the individual has perceived efficacy in resisting situational and emotional precipitants.

Research assessing directly how perceptions of control affect recovery from an acute MI is not a new endeavor. In fact, more than 20 years ago, Cromwell, Butterfield, Brayfield, and Curry (1977) conducted an intriguing prospective study in which 131 MI patients were randomly assigned to a factorial design investigating the effects of high versus low nursing treatment procedures termed *information, participation,* and *diversion.* High-information patients heard a recording and read literature explaining the etiology and treatment of MI. Conversely, low-information subjects received a brief recording and reassuring comments from a physician. High-participation subjects were given access to a switch that would activate cardiac monitors providing EKG tracings when they experienced concern. Low-participation subjects received typical instructions regarding bed rest and self-feeding. High-diversion treatment involved liberal visitor privileges and access to reading materials and television. Conversely, low-diversion subjects were given only limited visitor privileges and were not provided with books and television.

As expected, the three nursing care factors interacted with one another in determining length of hospital stay. The major finding was that high-information subjects were discharged quickly from coronary care and the hospital if they were also provided high levels of diversion and participation. However, high-information subjects had slower discharges if their generous information was paired with low levels of diversion and participation. Cromwell et al. (1977) termed this effect "information coupling" to describe how patients were given information about their cardiac condition. If knowledge was paired or coupled with actual opportunities to foster recovery, coronary care and hospital stays were abbreviated. However, knowledge without high-participation or diversion procedures resulted in protracted recovery and lengthier hospital stays. The construct of information coupling demonstrated the necessity of considering the balance and potential intricacies of various subtypes of control. As this study suggested, control afforded through information to MI patients was not beneficial unless accompanied by active participation in the recovery process.

Mahler and Kulik (1990) augmented this area of research in a sample of 75 male coronary bypass patients. Specifically, they assessed the way in which preoperative perceptions of personal control over recovery and desires for behavioral involvement in health care and information about health care predicted hospital recovery. Perceptions of control over recovery were assessed via a semistructured interview administered 2 days prior to surgery and rated on a 5-point scale, whereas behavioral involvement and desires for information were assessed by two subscales of a 16-item, self-report Health Opinion Survey (HOS) developed by Krantz, Baum, and Wideman (1980). A high score on the behavioral involvement scale is indicative of active self-treatment (e.g., desire for postoperative ambulation and coughing would be examples in this study), and high desire for information would be associated with acquiring health care knowledge (e.g., asking questions and reading pamphlets related to the procedures). The results indicated that patients with more perceived personal control spent less time in the hospital. Also, patients with a greater desire for information tended to experience less surgical pain and fewer negative psychological reactions defined as disoriented, agitated, anxious, or depressed. Increased desire for behavioral involvement was indeed associated with more ambulation and a shorter hospital stay, but also greater pain behavior (i.e., number of analgesics taken and number of postoperative pain complaints recorded in patient's chart by nurses and physicians). Mahler and Kulik offered an interesting interpretation of this latter finding by noting that several of the high behavioral involvement patients requested pain medication in order to keep performing the oftentimes painful recommended recovery behaviors of ambulating and coughing.

Langer, Janis, and Wolfer (1975) compared specifically the roles of information and an active cognitive coping device as mediators of psychological stress in surgical patients. A total of 60 patients about to undergo elective surgery—all with generally favorable prognoses—were administered one of four standardized interviews. The interviewer in the coping device–only condition, elaborating upon the basic premise that interpretation of events and often not the events themselves create stress, presented a strategy that encouraged reappraisal, calming self-talk, and cognitive control through selective attention to positive gains rather than negative experiences anticipated as results of the procedure. Subjects receiving the second stress-reducing strategy, preparatory information, were supplied with reassurance and factual information regarding the surgery, with the intent of producing emotional inoculation. Preparatory information did not include explicit coping suggestions. A third interactive experimental procedure combined both the preparatory information and the cognitive coping strategy. In order to control for the effect of the presence and interest of psychologists, a final group was interviewed with the focus diverted from the imminent surgery to typical hospital routines.

Dependent measures included nurses' behavioral ratings and direct behavioral measures. The admitting nurses were asked to complete a questionnaire evaluating the patient's stress level in comparison with that of most other elective preoperative patients. Ratings were obtained before and 15 minutes after the experimental interviews. Thus, positive change scores reflected improvement in coping. In addition, overt behavioral postoperative indices of stress, including the total number of pain relievers and sedatives requested, and length of hospital stay, were obtained. Physiological dependent measures—blood pressure and pulse readings recorded before and 15 minutes after the interview, and again immediately before and an hour after the surgery—were obtained.

Results from the nurses' behavioral observations of stress assessment indicated main effects for the coping and combination coping–information groups. Unlike the control and information-only communication, both coping and coping–information appeared to reduce preoperative stress. A significant main effect was also obtained for the coping device on number of pain relievers requested and percentage of patients requesting sedatives. Multivariate analysis of blood pressure and pulse rate failed to reveal any systematic variation. In general, preparatory information alone produced no significant effects on any pre- or postoperative measures.

Krantz (1980) emphasized in his controllability and predictability model that procedures facilitating recovery must be presented to the patient such that he or she perceives augmented personal control. The studies reviewed in this section support the notion that the efficacy of control may be situation-specific.

As the relevance of perceived control has assumed more prominence in health care settings, a measure designed to assess how the construct predicts recovery in a situationally specific fashion has been developed. Partridge and Johnston (1989) assessed their 9-item Recovery Locus of Control Scale (RLOC) on 20 first-time stroke victims and 20 patients who suffered a wrist fracture. Using regression analyses and controlling for initial severity level of physical disability, they demonstrated that for both groups, patients endorsing more internal beliefs on the RLOC attained better recovery as assessed by Range of Movement and Personal Care scores.

Johnston, Gilbert, Partridge, and Collins (1992), expanding on this line of research, have shown how increasing perceptions of control in rehabilitation patients prior to beginning physical therapy may facilitate recovery. In their study, 71 randomly assigned outpatients who were being treated for various diagnosed conditions were mailed a standard letter confirming their appointment; however, 39 of the patients also received additional information in the letter about how their effort and investment in the program would help them control their symptoms and facilitate recovery.

One week after the first appointment, self-report measures, including both the RLOC and expectancy and satisfaction data, were obtained. The patients in the experimental group had higher internal scores on the RLOC and tended to be more satisfied with the information they received prior to their first appointment than the subjects in the standard letter group. Johnston and colleagues (1992) suggested that increased perceived internal control might improve progress with recovery, as it did in the Partridge and Johnston study. Although rehabilitation outcome data would clearly have bolstered the strength and impact of the Johnston study, the emphasis on cognitive aspects of enhancing control and recovery through minimal input warrants further investigative consideration.

CONTROL AND PSYCHOTHERAPY

In reviewing theoretical schools of psychotherapy, the construct of control is germane to treatment paradigms and theoretical orientations. For example, both the analytic and behavioral treatment of phobias involve the phobic's confronting the avoided situation or stimulus under the direction of the therapist. The phobic individual, relying on the therapeutic alliance and responding to the therapist's recommendations and encouragement, transforms from a passive into an active, control-oriented agent.

Strupp (1970) integrated the concept of control across models of psychotherapy. According to Strupp, the basic tenet of all psychotherapies is to assist the individual in achieving greater personal control or mastery. Paradoxically, the person must initially subordinate him- or herself to someone else's control in a trusting interpersonal relationship before he or she can acquire self-control, or autonomy. This type of self-abdication may be typified in the concept of transference that develops during psychoanalysis. The patient needs to establish trust in the therapist, who then judiciously utilizes this ascendancy to enhance the patient's becoming increasingly independent.

The acquisition of control in psychotherapy is probably best conceptualized as a process. In order to test this notion, it would be advantageous to assess the construct of control throughout the course of therapy instead of selectively at termination. Peterson and Seligman (1984) blindly rated the transcripts of individual psychotherapy sessions for causal explanations for adverse events of a select group of 4 persons suffering from depression following a loss. Transcripts were available from the beginning, middle, and end of treatment. For each person, causal explanations shifted from the most internal, stable, and global in the beginning session to the least internal, stable, and global in the final session. Consistent with the formulation on depression presented earlier in this chapter, depression as a symptom of helplessness was alleviated as subjects acquired control by reinterpreting problems as transient, situation-specific, and manageable.

As reviewed earlier, Bandura has used the term *self-efficacy* as a control-relevant term. Bandura, Taylor, Williams, Mefford, and Barchas's work using enactive modeling and mastery in the alleviation of fear and autonomic arousal in 12 women with spider phobia (1985) is an example of how his social learning model utilizes enhanced perception of personal control. Through the therapist's use of individual modeling that emphasized predictability and controllability to strengthen maximally perceived self-efficacy (e.g., looking at or touching a large wolf spider in a plastic container, demonstrating to the women how to control the spider's movement as it crawled on his body, or how to catch spiders that were running loose),

11 of the subjects effectively performed coping tasks that they had judged as either weak, medium, or strong threats in the absence of catecholamine (epinephrine and norepinephrine) hyperreactivity. These data clearly suggest that the social learning model is predicated on augmenting the perception of control.

Other researchers have considered control to be more of an attribute variable that mediates the therapeutic process. For example, in a population of outpatients presenting with mild or moderate "neurotic" symptomatology, Foon (1985) matched 21 therapists' and 78 clients' locus of control scores obtained on the Rotter Scale and investigated how this match influenced therapeutic expectations and outcome. Intercorrelations between therapists' and clients' characteristics completed prior to therapy revealed that therapists had more favorable expectations of internal clients than of external clients, and clients had more positive expectations of therapy with internal than with external therapists.

Using clients' locus of control scores completed at the end of therapy, therapists evaluated internal clients more positively than external clients, and internal clients rated therapy more favorably than did external clients. As expected, Foon did not find that an initial match on locus of control produced favorable therapy outcomes. This result is reasonable given that the expectation of a dimensional shift in client locus of control from external to internal accompanied successful therapy. Foon noted that contemporaneous matching of locus of control appears to be significant at certain therapeutic stages and can thus serve as an important predictor of positive outcome.

Needless to say, the influence of control in psychotherapy is quite complex. Tracey (1991), noting the various assumptions made when operationalizing, assessing, and coding the construct of control in counseling and psychotherapy, has proposed a three-dimensional model of therapeutic control. Employing 14 therapists and 26 clients from a community mental health center, she used middle-therapy-session questionnaires and audiotapes that were rated with five different control-coding schemes. Thus, the combination of models and coding schemes yielded 15 different behavioral-control indices. Cluster analysis and complex multidimensional scaling supported her posited model of intrapersonal control (attempts at control) versus interpersonal control (type of actual control), form definitions (implied meaning of behavior exhibited) versus effect definitions, and perceived versus behavioral measures of control.

More recently, Whiteside (1998) and Shapiro and Astin (1998) have each introduced relevant texts on the importance of control in psychotherapy. Whiteside's book focuses on the transpositional approach to therapy, which encourages therapists to respect the individual differences of clients and to be flexible in their approach to therapy over the course of treatment relative to client's control issues. Shapiro and Astin's work highlights three broad, general postulates used in developing a unifying theory of control: (1) A sense of gaining and maintaining control is a major motivating life force; (2) there are higher and lower levels of control; and (3) there are important individual differences in terms of desire and gaining control. Along with these broad postulates, Shapiro and Astin offer several subpostulates, including four different modes of control that can be used for framing and interpreting therapeutic situations: (1) a positive assertive mode that is decisive and active; (2) a positive yielding mode that involves patience, trust, and acceptance, along with letting go of active control; (3) a negative assertive mode that involves too much control and is described by terms such as *manipulating, overcontrolling,* and *dogmatic;* and (4) a negative yielding mode that involves too little control and is described by terms such as *indecisive* and *manipulated.*

The prevailing influence of the concept of control on diverse psychotherapeutic schools may be most astutely conceptualized by the eminent Jerome Frank. According to Frank (1974), it may well be that all psychotherapeutic techniques, despite their seeming differences, derive their effectiveness from a collective ability to supply an "antidemoralization effect." Through the use of common factors obtained in psychotherapy, such as general information, predictability, and emotional control, patients acquire a means of alleviating demoralization that, according to Frank, serves as the basis of the majority of psychopathological conditions. Although Frank considers the common denominator in psychotherapy to be antidemoralization, this construct appears remarkably similar to the construct of control described in the present chapter. Therefore, it seems feasible that Frank's antidemoralization effect may in essence be a form of enhanced self-efficacy and control.

SUMMARY

The bulk of research reviewed in this chapter cogently presents the ubiquity of control as a mediating "filter" in psychosomatic processes. Indeed, the construct of control seems crucial in determining our perception of the world.

1. The chapter began with a review of some of the seminal and newer theories related to control. Seligman's theory of learned helplessness, along with its reformations and expansions, Langer's research on illusion of control, Thompson, Armstrong, and Thomas's control heuristic, Rotter's social

learning theory, and Bandura's social cognitive theory, which relies heavily on the concept of self-efficacy, were covered.

2. The connection between perception of control and onset of illness was then reviewed. The "giving-up given-up" complex and the concept of voodoo death are early constructs that support this proposed relationship. The quantitative study of Sanderson et al. (1989), in which perceived controllability impacted symptoms of panic and agoraphobia, serves as a classic example of control and illness. Other research examples in the areas of arthritis, cancer, and AIDS were presented, along with a brief review of the impact of vicarious control.

3. Changes in perceptions of control and its effect on the aging process have been studied for more than 20 years. Data in this chapter revealed that giving too much task assistance to elderly persons may actually be detrimental to their performance and sense of control. Other evidence suggests that enhancing perceptions of control may result in nursing home residents' increased alertness, happiness, and improved general health indices, including memory. Perceptions of control appear to decline with advancing age, and data suggest that factors such as level of education, intelligence, and measures of intraindividual variability may be important predictive components.

4. Data from enhancement of control studies following recovery from a MI or stroke suggest that numerous physical, psychological, and lifestyle behaviors need to be considered. Moreover, adherence to medical and treatment regimens are important factors in the recovery process. Partridge and Johnston (1989), who developed the 9-item Recovery Locus of Control Scale (RLOC), have demonstrated how an internal locus of control predicts better outcome in stroke victims and patients with wrist fractures. The RLOC also predicted improved recovery progress in patients beginning physical therapy.

5. The chapter concludes with a review of how the construct of control has served as a unifying theme across various theoretical schools of psychotherapy. This is the conclusion one might reach reviewing the research and theoretical offerings of Strupp (1970), Frank (1974), Whiteside (1998), and Shapiro and Astin (1998). Thus, the latent therapeutic mechanism of action in all psychotherapies might actually be instilling some aspect of enhanced control or improved self-efficacy. In the next chapter, we investigate the use of a cognitive perspective in psychotherapy as it pertains to the treatment of the human stress response.

9

Psychotherapy
A Cognitive Perspective

I'm an old man and have known a great many troubles, but most of them never happened.

MARK TWAIN

Like beauty, a stressor resides in the eye of the beholder. It should be clear by now that the patient's cognitive interpretation of the environment leads to the formation of a psychosocial stressor from an otherwise neutral stimulus. This concept has resulted in more eloquent phrasing such as "There are no things good or bad, but thinking makes them so" (Shakespeare); "It is not what happens to you that matters, but how you take it" (Hans Selye); "Men are disturbed not by things, but by the views which they take of them" (Epictetus); "No one can make you feel inferior without your consent" (Eleanor Roosevelt).

If one accepts the concept that the primary determinant of any given psychosocial stressor is the cognitive interpretation or appraisal of that stimulus (as argued in Chapter 2), then it seems reasonable to assume that a useful therapy in treating stress-related disorders might be a psychotherapeutic effort directed toward the cognitive-interpretational domain. Although clearly not the only psychotherapeutic technique of value in treating excessive stress, psychotherapy with cognitive restructuring or reinterpretation as a goal seems applicable, particularly in the treatment of pathogenic stress-response syndromes. The purpose of this chapter, therefore, is to review several cognitively based psychotherapeutic approaches that can be employed in the treatment of excessive stress arousal. This chapter also serve to integrate the first stress-management technique listed in the therapeutic model ("environmental engineering"), described in the introduction to Part II.

It is not the goal of this chapter to provide a "how-to" manual of cognitively based therapies. Excellent, practioner-oriented guides are available elsewhere (see Beck & Emery, 1985; Meichenbaum, 1985; Meichenbaum & Jaremko, 1983). Rather, it is our hope that this chapter will sensitize the reader to the critical role that cognition plays in the initiation and prolongation of human stress and to the important role of cognitively based therapies in the treatment of stress-related problems.

COGNITIVE PRIMACY

The cognitive primacy postulation is the perspective accepted within this volume. This viewpoint became apparent in Chapter 2, where we noted that the individual's interpretation of the environment is the primary determinant in the elicitation of the stress response in reaction to a psychosocial stressor. A similar yet more extensive view is summarized by Roseman (1984), who states, "A cognitive approach to the causation of emotion assumes that it is the interpretation of events rather than events per se that determine which emotion will be felt" (p. 14).

Although when discussing the stress and emotions of flight crews dealing with the threat of war, Grinker and Spiegel (1945) were two of the first researchers to refer to the notion of appraisal, Magda Arnold (1960) was the most explicit of the early theorists in support of cognitive primacy. She concluded that emotions are caused by the "appraisal" of the stimuli that one encounters. Given the perception of some environmental stimulus, subsequent emotions are a function, not of the stimulus per se but of the cognitive interpretation (appraisal) of that stimulus. Thus, Arnold was the first person to systematically state that there is a cognitive-mediational approach to the study of emotions, with appraisal as the core construct.

Lazarus first used the term *appraisal* in 1964, and by 1966 it became the essence of his theory of psychological stress (Lazarus, 1966). He and his colleagues extended Arnold's work to recognize the role of initial appraisal of a given environmental stimulus but added the notion of reappraisal, which entails the cognitive interpretation of one's perceived ability to handle, cope with, or benefit from exposure to the stimulus. This work became known as the transactional model, and as described by Coyne and Holroyd (1982),

> The Lazarus group applies the concept of appraisal to the person's continually reevaluated judgments about demands and constraints in transactions with the environment and options and resources for meeting them. A key assumption of the model is that these evaluations

determine the person's stress reaction, the emotions experienced, and adaptational outcomes. (p. 108)

Thus, the Lazarus group emphasized first a primary appraisal ("Is this situation a threat, challenge, or aversion?") and then a secondary one ("Can I cope or benefit from it?") in the origin of human adult emotions.

The basic position of the primacy of cognition in the cognitive–affective relationship is held by numerous theorists and researchers (Arnold, 1960, 1984; Chang, 1998; Dewe, 1992; Hemenover & Dienstbier, 1996; Lazarus, 1966, 1999; Levine, 1996; Peeters, Buunk, & Schaufeli, 1995; Terry, Tonge, & Callan, 1995). To reiterate, the cognitive primacy perspective argues "that cognitive activity is a 'necessary' as well as sufficient condition of emotion" (Lazarus, 1982, p. 1019). More specifically, cognitive activity here refers to "cognitive appraisal," the role of which is to mediate the relationships between people and their environments. In a recent monograph on stress and emotion, Lazarus (1999) succinctly notes that "emotions are the product of reason in that they flow from how we appraise what is happening in our lives. In effect, the way we evaluate an event determines how we react emotionally. This is what it means to speak of cognitive mediation" (p. 87). Commenting on the cognitive perspectives, Dobson and Shaw (1995) note that "they share an assumption that it is the perception of events, rather than events themselves, that mediates the response to different circumstances and ultimately determines the quality of adaptation of individuals" (p. 159).

Although the preponderance of stress researchers support the notion of cognitive primacy, not all writers have agreed. During the 1980s, Zajonc and Lazarus had vigorous literary disagreements regarding the merits of cognitive primacy. Zajonc (1984) argued that an affective reaction could occur independently or without cognitive participation under certain circumstances. While he provided specific reasons to support his contention for the independence of affect (e.g., phylogenetic and ontogenetic primacy, separation of neuroanatomical structures for affect and cognition, the periodic lack of correlation between appraisal and affect, the formation of new affective reactions established without apparent appraisal, and the consideration that affective states can be induced by noncognitive procedures), Lazarus provided effective rebuttals for each of the points. Parkinson and Manstead (1992) presented a critique of appraisal theory; however, Lazarus's (1999) response to their criticism suggests that their points of disagreement are actually quite narrow. In fact, Lazarus suggests that they generally accept most of his theory on stress and emotion. He acknowledges that a definitive empirical separation of appraisal and emotion is arduous due to the obvious methodological limitations; however, he contends that more empirical support is offered for cognitive primacy than for any other theories. Lazarus further contends that the theory of cognitive primacy should not be discarded unless one is prepared to offer a more encompassing and effective alternative explanation. Most researchers agree that a more effective alternative explanation to cognitive primacy is yet to come.

COGNITIVE-BASED PSYCHOTHERAPY

According to Bandura (1997, 1982a,b), the primary factor in the determination of a stressful event is the individual's *perceived* inefficiency in coping with or controlling a potentially aversive event. We now review several models of cognitively based psychotherapeutic interventions that may be employed to alter the patient's perception (cognitive interpretation) of an environmental transaction that might be seen as potentially aversive. We then present a brief overview of the recently defined rubric of positive psychology.

Ellis's Model

Modern cognitive therapy is considered to have emerged in 1955, when Albert Ellis developed rational-emotive therapy (RET; Arnkoff & Glass, 1992). Ellis (1971, 1973, 1984, 1991) has proposed that individuals often acquire irrational or illogical cognitive interpretations or beliefs about themselves or their environment. The extent to which these beliefs are irrational and important corresponds to the amount of emotional distress experienced by the individual. Ellis believes that the emotional disturbance experienced by the individual can be summarized using the following "A-B-C" model:

$$A \rightarrow B \rightarrow C$$

A	B	C
Activating experience	Belief	Emotional consequence

In Condition A, some environmental transaction involving the individual occurs (e.g., he or she is late for an appointment). In Condition B, the person generates some "irrational" belief about him- or herself based on the original experience (e.g., "I'm stupid, worthless, incompetent for being late"). Condition C represents the emotional consequence (e.g., guilt, depression, shame, or anxiety) that results, not from the experience itself (A) but directly from the irrational belief (B). Ellis then employs his model of RET, which consists of adding a "D" to the A-B-C paradigm, representing a conscious effort to "dispute" the irrational cognitive belief that resulted in the emotional distress. The RET therapist may use techniques such as debating, role playing, social skills training, and bibliotherapy to challenge the

Table 9.1. Disputing Irrational Beliefs

1. What irrational belief needs to be disputed?
2. Can this belief be rationally supported?
3. What evidence exists for the falseness of this belief?
4. Does any evidence exist for the truth of this belief?
5. What worse things could *actually* happen to me if my initial experience (activating experience) does not end favorably?
6. What good things can I make happen even if my initial experience does not end favorably?

individual's beliefs, often in a confrontational, forceful fashion. Therefore, regardless of the techniques use, the overall psychotherapeutic goal is to alter the individual's interpretation. Ellis has delineated a series of questions to assist in the disputation of irrational beliefs (see Table 9.1).

Beck's Cognitive Therapy Model

The cognitive therapy process of Aaron T. Beck is considered the second major cognitive restructuring therapy (Arnkoff & Glass, 1992). Similar to RET, cognitive therapy assists the client in identifying maladaptive thinking and persuades him or her to develop a more adaptive view. However, whereas RET is more philosophically driven (Ellis, 1995), Beck's cognitive therapy is more empirically based and focuses on whether thoughts and beliefs are realistic compared to whether they are rational (Meichenbaum, 1995). As Beck (1995) notes,

> Based on my clinical observations and some systematic clinical studies and experiments, I theorized that there was a thinking disorder at the core of the psychiatric syndromes such as depression and anxiety. This disorder was reflected in a systematic bias in the way the patients interpreted particular experiences. (vii)

Beck differentiates between three types of cognitions that may be involved in disrupted thinking: automatic thoughts, schemas, and cognitive distortions. Automatic thoughts are considered a "surface level" cognition that is brought to awareness quickly and readily, and leads directly to the individual's emotional and behavioral responses. Cognitive schemas are thought of as internal models of aspects of the self and the environment, and are used to process information. They often lead individuals with emotional problems to develop perceptions of threat, loss, or danger. Cognitive distortions serve in essence as a link between dysfunctional schemas and automatic thoughts. For example, when new information is processed cognitively, the material may be biased or skewed in order to make it consistent with a current schema.

Then, to challenge the patient's maladaptive thinking, Beck encourages the use of a Socratic dialogue, which relies on the ability of the treating therapist to ask questions in a probing manner that allows the patient to answer in a way to persuade *him-* or *herself* to think differently. Beck and Emery (1985) describe in elaborate detail how cognitive restructuring principles can be used in the treatment of anxiety and stress-related disorders: "Anxious patients in the simplest terms believe, 'Something bad is going to happen that I won't be able to handle.' The cognitive therapist uses three basic strategies or questions to help the patient restructure this thinking" (p. 200):

1. What is the evidence supporting the conclusion currently held by the patient?
2. What is another way of looking at the same situation but reaching some other conclusion?
3. What will happen if, indeed, the currently held conclusion/opinion is correct?

While examining each of these three strategic questions, it is important to keep in mind that individual differences may affect a patient's responses. It is also worth acknowledging that the therapist may need to employ all three strategies throughout therapy.

1. *What is the evidence?* One goal of this strategy is to analyze the patient's cognitive patterns and search for "faulty logic." Therapists may help patients to correct faulty logic and ideas through questioning techniques that may allow them better to clarify the meaning(s) and definitions of the problem. According to Beck (1993), individuals experiencing stress reactions tend to personalize events not relevant to them (egocentrism) and interpret situations in global and absolute terms. Therefore, the following are typical questions used to improve the patient's ability to process information and test reality:

- What is the evidence supporting this conclusion?
- What is the evidence against this conclusion?
- Are you oversimplifying causal relationships?
- Are you confusing habits or commonly held opinions with fact?
- Are your interpretations too far removed from your actual experiences?
- Are you thinking in "all-or-nothing" terms (i.e., black–white, either–or, on–off, or all-or-none types of decisions and outcome)?
- Are your conclusions in any way extreme or exaggerated?
- Are you taking selected examples out of context and basing you conclusion on such information?
- Is the source of information reliable?
- Is your thinking in terms of certainties rather than probabilities?

- Are you confusing low-probability with a high-probability events?
- Are you basing your conclusions on feelings or values rather than facts?
- Are you focusing on irrelevant factors in forming your conclusions?

Through the use of such questions, patterns of faulty reasoning, such as projections, exaggerations, and negative attributions, may be discovered and corrected.

2. *What is another way of looking at it?* The goal of this strategy is to help the patient generate alternative interpretations in lieu of the interpretation currently held. Strategies such as increasing both objectivity and perspective, and shifting or diverting cognitive set (Beck, 1993) may lead to reattribution, diminishing the significance of the environmental transaction, or even restructuring the transaction to find something positive in the event.

3. *So what if it happens?* The goal of this strategy is to help the patient "decatastrophize" the environmental transaction as well as to develop coping strategies and problem-solving skills. It will be recalled from the multidimensional treatment model that "environmental engineering" (Girdano, Everly, & Dusek, 1997) and "problem solving" are merely terms that describe the therapeutic processes of this third strategic phase of therapy as described by Beck and Emery (1985). These authors suggest that "therapist and patient collaboratively develop a variety of strategies that the person can use" (p. 208). Ultimately, the goal of therapy is to allow the patient to develop autonomous skills in each of the three strategic areas mentioned previously. The notions of "environmental engineering" and "problem solving" will be more formally integrated in the next model— Meichenbaum's stress inoculation training mode.

Meichenbaum's Stress Inoculation Training

Using the principles contained in his classic text, *Cognitive-Behavior Modification*, Meichenbaum (1977) developed a specialized, cognitively based therapy for the treatment of excessive stress in a therapeutic formulation called "stress inoculation training" (SIT).

Meichenbaum (1993), reflecting on 20 years of SIT, notes:

> In short, SIT helps clients acquire sufficient knowledge, self-understanding, and coping skills to facilitate better ways of handling expected stressful encounters. SIT combines elements of Socratic and didactic teaching, client self-monitoring, cognitive restructuring, problem solving, self-instructional and relaxation training, behavioral and imagined rehearsal, and environmental change. With regard to the notion of environmental change, SIT recognizes that stress is transactional in nature. (p. 381)

The SIT paradigm consists of an overlapping, three-phase intervention. The first phase, the initial conceptualization phase, includes the development of a collaborative relationship between the client and trainer through the use of Socratic exchanges. The overall objectives of this phase include data collection and education to help clients reconceptualize their stressful experiences in a more hopeful and empowered manner.

In the second phase of SIT, coping and problem-solving skills are taught and rehearsed. Table 9.2 provides examples of self-statements that may be used as coping techniques. Skills acquisition in this phase encompasses more

Table 9.2. Examples of Coping Self-Statements Rehearsed in Stress Inoculation Training

Preparing for a stressor
  What is it you have to do?
  You can develop a plan to deal with it.
  Just think about what you can do about it. That's better than getting anxious.
  No negative self-statements: Just think rationally.
  Don't worry: Worry won't help anything.
  Maybe what you think is anxiety is eagerness to confront the stressor.
Confronting and handling a stressor
  Just "psych" yourself up—you can meet this challenge.
  You can convince yourself to do it. You can reason your fear away.
  One step at a time: You can handle the situation.
  Don't think about fear; just think about what you have to do. Stay relevant.
  This anxiety is what the doctor said you would feel. It's a reminder to use your coping exercises.
  This tenseness can be an ally; a cue to cope.
  Relax; you're in control. Take a slow deep breath.
  Ah, good.
Coping with the feeling of being overwhelmed
  When fear comes, just pause.
  Keep the focus on the present; what is it you have to do?
  Label your fear from 0 to 10 and watch it change.
  You should expect your fear to rise.
  Don't try to eliminate fear totally; just keep it manageable.
Reinforcing self-statements
  It worked; you did it.
  Wait until you tell your therapist (or group) about this.
  It wasn't as bad as you expected.
  You made more out of your fear than it was worth.
  Your damn ideas—that's the problem. When you control them, you control your fear.
  It's getting better each time you use the procedures.
  You can be pleased with progress you're making.
  You did it!

Source: D. Meichenbaum (1977). *Cognitive-Behavior Modification.* Copyright by Plenum Press. Reprinted by permission.

than self-statements. Assertion training, anger control, study skills, parenting, and relaxation may be incorporated.

The third phase of SIT, application and follow-through, allows patients to apply the skills acquired in the preceding two phases across situations with increasing levels of actual stress. Therefore, techniques such as modeling, role playing, and *in vivo* exposure are used, as well as features of relapse prevention. The follow-up component allows for future extension of SIT uses.

These three phases of SIT are enumerated in greater detail in Table 9.3. (A valuable guide for practitioners on the use of SIT is also available; see Meichenbaum, 1985.)

Table 9.3. Flowchart of Stress Inoculation Training

Phase One: Conceptualization
a. Data collection–integration
- Identify determinants of problem via interview, image-based reconstruction, self-monitoring, and behavioral observance.
- Distinguish between performance failure and skill deficit.
- Formulate treatment plan—task analysis.
- Introduce integrative conceptual model.
b. Assessment skills training
- Train clients to analyze problems independently (e.g., to conduct situational analyses and to seek disconfirmatory data).

Phase Two: Skills Acquisition and Rehearsal
a. Skills training
- Training instrumental coping skills (e.g., communication, assertion, problem solving, parenting, study skills).
- Train palliative coping skills as indicated (e.g., perspective-taking, attention diversion, use of social supports, adaptive affect expression, relaxation).
- Aim to develop an extensive repertoire of coping responses to faciliate flexible responding.
b. Skills rehearsal
- Promote smooth integration and execution of coping responses via imagery and role play.
- Self-instructional training to develop mediators to regulate coping responses.

Phase Three: Application and Follow-Through
a. Induce application of skills
- Prepare for application using coping imagery, using early stress cues as signals to cope.
- Role play (a) anticipated stressful situations and (b) client coaching someone with a similar problem.
- "Role play" attitude may be adopted in real world.
- Exposure to in-session graded stressors.
- Use of graded exposure and other response induction aids to foster *in vivo* responding and build self-efficacy.

(Continued)

Table 9.3. (*Continued*)

b. Maintenance and generalization
  - Build sense of coping self-efficacy in relation to situations client sees as high risk.
  - Develop strategies for recovering from failure and relapse.
  - Arrange follow-up review.

General Guidelines for Training
  - Attend to referral and intake process.
  - Consider training peers of clients to conduct treatment. Develop collaborative relationship and project approachability.
  - Establish realistic expectations regarding course and outcome of therapy.
  - Foster optimism and confidence by structuring incremental success experiences.
  - Respond to stalled progress with problem solving versus labeling client resistant.
  - Include family members in treatment when this is indicated.

Source: "Stress Inoculation Training: Toward a Paradigm for Training Coping Skills" by D. Meichenbaum and R. Cameron in *Stress Reduction and Prevention* (p. 121) edited by D. Meichenbaum and M. E. Jaremko. Copyright 1983 by Plenum Press. Reprinted by permission.

Meichenbaum's SIT training is of special interest in this volume because it manifests the belief that stress management is most effective when it is flexible and multidimensional. Similarly, SIT allows us to integrate the concept of "environmental engineering" as delineated in the treatment model described in the introduction to Part II. The term *environmental engineering,* it will be recalled, is borrowed from the work of Girdano, Dusek, and Everly (2000) as it was first described in 1979, and refers to any conscious attempts at manipulating environmental factors to reduce one's exposure to stressor events. Both proactive, environmental change and reactive problem solving must be included under this heading. The reader will observe that there are different points within the model wherein problem solving, or any other form of environmental engineering, is obviously applicable.

As implied earlier, one of the real strengths of SIT is its inherent flexibility, structured as it is around a cognitive foundation. SIT has been demonstrated to be of value in the control of anger, test anxiety, phobias, general stress, pain, surgical anxiety, essential hypertension, and PTSD (see Meichenbaum, 1985, 1993).

Positive Psychology

The science of positive psychology is a recent designation predicated on fundamental issues such as happiness, well-being, excellence, and optimal human functioning, among others (Seligman & Csikszentmihalyi, 2000). In essence, the focus of positive psychology is on what makes life worth living for individuals, families, and communities. We recognize and appreciate that positive psychology should not be construed as a subtype of cognitive therapy (Seligman, personal communication, June 2000); however, we believe that it is important to include the topic in this current edition. The contents of this chapter seem to be the most logical and appropriate place for this brief review.

Seligman and Csikszentmihalyi (2000) acknowledge that positive psychology is not an original concept, and they give appropriate credit to many distinguished predecessors. We, of course, have made repeated references to the effects of positive human functioning within this volume. For example, in Chapter 5, we discussed the exceptional way in which Norman Cousins has demonstrated how positive thinking and humor can affect the immune system. Moreover, in Chapter 18, we discuss the association between religious faith, health, and general happiness. What Seligman and Csikszentmihalyi note, however, is that since World War II, the emphasis of psychology as a science has been on assessing and treating mental illness. At the start of a new millennium, they suggest that we have reached a time in our history when we should formalize our research efforts to understand systematically what makes individuals and communities flourish. It will be interesting to observe the empirical and theoretical impact of positive psychology over the next several years, both within and outside of the social sciences.

SUMMARY

This chapter has reviewed the first of the specific therapeutic interventions we present in this edition for the treatment of pathogenic human stress. Chapters 7 and 8 within this section have addressed issues of personality styles and personologic idiosyncrasies as they might relate to the cause and treatment of the stress response. For example, the construct of "control," which permeates all personality styles and serves as a dominant mediating factor in the etiology and treatment of excessive human stress, has been highlighted.

This chapter has focused on the role that psychotherapy can play in treating excessive stress. Reflecting the biases of the epiphenomenological model of human stress constructed in Chapter 2, we have chosen to review cognitive-based psychotherapeutic interventions. The main points in this chapter are as follows:

1. Referring back to Figure 2.6, this chapter acknowledges the primary role that cognition plays in the initiation and propagation of a psychosocially induced stress response.

2. The genesis and features of "cognitive primacy" (the notion that affect is subsequent to cognition), as well as updates and critiques of the theory, are reviewed.

3. The rational-emotive therapy of Ellis (1971, 1973, 1984, 1991) is introduced as the first of modern, cognitive-based psychotherapeutic interventions to challenge and alter dysfunctional cognitions. Its core assumption is that individuals who suffer excessive stress may have a proclivity, albeit pathogenic, to accept irrational or otherwise inappropriate beliefs about environmental transactions. This propensity can be corrected by teaching the patient to "dispute" his or her irrational beliefs as they give rise to excessive stress arousal.

4. Beck's cognitive therapy is considered the second major cognitive restructuring therapy. It is viewed as a broader spectrum cognitive intervention that not only focuses on inappropriate cognitive patterns but also assists the patient in developing other coping and problem-solving activities. Three basic therapeutic strategies are employed to assist in cognitive restructuring: (1) analyzing the nature of any evidence that affected the individual's cognitive interpretation, (2) generating alternative interpretations via cognitive reattribution and searching for positive aspects inherent in the environmental transaction ("the silver lining"), and (3) developing environmental engineering, adaptive coping strategies, and useful problem-solving techniques.

5. The broadest spectrum cognitive-based stress management intervention extends well beyond psychotherapy and is referred to as "stress inoculation training." In the paradigm developed by Meichenbaum (1977, 1985, 1993), the intervention consists of three basic stages: (1) data collection and education, (2) skills acquisition, and (3) application and follow-through to a real-world setting. The multiple components of this approach are delineated in Table 9.3.

6. Cognitive-based interventions have demonstrated their utility in the treatment of a wide array of problems, including anger, pain, phobias, anxiety, general stress arousal, headaches, and PTSD (see Meichenbaum, 1985, Table 3.1).

7. Positive psychology is a recently developed designation predicated on the fundamental issues of happiness, well-being, and optimism. It is intended to promote an empirically based systematic study of these and other positive qualities.

10

A Neurophysiological Rationale for the Use of the Relaxation Response
Neurological Desensitization

Since the original applications of behavioral technologies to the treatment of disease, it has been observed that the elicitation of what Benson (1975) has called the "relaxation response" has proved useful in the treatment of a wide variety of psychiatric and stress-related somatic diseases (Benson, 1974; Caudill et al., 1991; Domar et al., 1990; Hellman, 1990; Kutz, Borysenko, & Benson, 1985; Lavey & Taylor, 1985; Shapiro & Giber, 1978). The relaxation response is perhaps best understood as a psychophysiological state of hypoarousal engendered by a multitude of diverse technologies (e.g., meditation, neuromuscular relaxation, hypnosis). Research into the relaxation response as a therapeutic mechanism and its clinical proliferation have been hampered, however, by a lack of conceptual clarity regarding its therapeutic foundations and/or its mechanisms of action. This chapter will explore the physiological and psychological foundations of the relaxation response to set the stage for discussions in subsequent chapters of specific therapeutic technologies (e.g., meditation, neuromuscular relaxation) used to elicit the relaxation response for the treatment of stress-related diseases.

The specific aims of this chapter are (1) to explore the psychophysiological foundations of the relaxation response as a possible rationale for the use of the relaxation response as a primary therapy as well as an adjunctive therapy in the treatment of pathogenic stress arousal (while remaining aware of the fact that in some cases specific end-organ symptoms may initially require medical stabilization or amelioration); (2) to gain insight into the counterintuitive and antireductionistic observation that a single therapeutic mechanism (i.e., the relaxation response) can be of value in treating a wide and disparate variety of psychiatric and stress-related somatic disorders; and (3) to consider the relaxation response as a natural treatment for anxiety and excessive stress arousal—a treatment intrinsically antithetical to the very nature of pathogenic stress arousal.

In order to formulate such a view of the relaxation response as a therapeutic mechanism, it first becomes necessary to reformulate the common perspective on psychiatric and stress-related somatic disorders.

DISORDERS OF AROUSAL

Traditionally, science has classified diseases on the basis of their cause or their end-organ symptoms or signs. The American Psychiatric Association's *Diagnostic and Statistical Manual of Mental Disorders* (DSM-IV; American Psychiatric Association, 1994) is replete with examples of both. Regarding classification by "cause," for example, adjustment disorders are "caused" by the inability to adjust to new situations; viral disorders are caused by viruses; and bacteriological disorders are caused by bacteria. Regarding classification by symptoms, on the other hand, mood disorders are characterized by affective symptom complexes, and anxiety disorders are characterized by anxious symptomatology. The posttraumatic stress disorder is classified by both its cause (trauma) *and* its symptoms (stress). Seldom in our nosological quests, however, do we bother to consider other, less obvious, taxonomic criteria, even though these "latent taxa" might be far more utilitarian. Such a taxonomic consideration is derived from the work of Meehl (1973).

Based on an integration of the work of Selye (1976), Gellhorn (1967), Gray (1982), and Post (Post & Ballenger, 1981), it has been proposed that various anxiety and stress-related diseases be viewed in light of a new taxonomic perspective (Everly, 1985b; Everly & Benson, 1989). Evidence indicates that numerous psychiatric and somatic stress-related diseases possess a latent yet common denominator that serves nosologically as a latent taxonomic criterion—"latent taxon" for short. It has been proposed that this latent taxon is pathognomonic arousal. Thus, such disorders may be referred to collectively as "disorders of arousal." Despite a wide variety of etiological stimuli, and an even wider variety of symptom complexes, these disorders are best seen as but variations on a theme of a pathognomonic hypersensitivity for, or an overall characteristic of, arousal.

More specifically, the "disorders of arousal" concept is based on a corpus of evidence indicating that a major homogenizing phenomenological

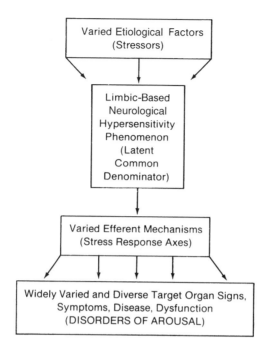

Figure 10.1. Limbic hypersensitivity phenomenon: The latent taxon in stress-related "disorders of arousal."

constituent of these disorders is a limbic-system-based neurological hypersensitivity; that is, a lowered threshold for excitation and/or a pathognomonic status of excess arousal within the limbic circuitry or its neurological, neuroendocrine, and/or endocrine efferent limbs. This neurological hypersensitivity is then capable of giving rise to a host of psychiatric and stress-related somatic disorders as noted in Chapters 3 and 4 (see Figure 10.1). These disorders are referred to collectively as "disorders of arousal."

PSYCHIATRIC DISORDERS OF AROUSAL

Over the years, clinical psychiatry anecdotes have well documented the notion that anxiety disorders and stress-related syndromes seem to be characterized by what appears to be an increased vulnerability to frustrating, challenging, or sympathomimetic stimuli. This phenomenon is best thought of as a hypersensitivity for stimulation; a sort of neurological sensitization combined with a lowered activation threshold for emotional arousal. Such reports of sensitization or hyperreactivity are consistent with the well-documented activity and function of the limbic system and its major neurological, neuroendocrine, and endocrine efferents (Cannon, 1929; Gray, 1982; MacLean, 1949; Nauta & Domesick, 1982).

In a seminal paper, Papez (1937) boldly discussed the rhinencephalon as the anatomical basis for emotional arousal. He considered the mammillary bodies, fornix, hippocampus, cingulate cortex, and anterior thalamic nuclei as key elements in a then-proposed mechanism of emotion. In a description of Papez's model, Isaacson (1982) notes:

> Neural activity representing the emotional processes originating in the cortex would be passed along into the hippocampus, the fornix, the mammillary bodies, and the anterior nuclei of the thalamus and would finally be projected onto the receptive region of the "emotional cortex" (i.e., the cingulate cortex). From the cingulate cortex, activity representing emotional processes could pass into other regions of the cerebral cortex and add emotional coloring to psychic processes occurring elsewhere. (p. 55)

The "Papez Circuit," as it came to be called, was modified as a contributor to human emotional arousal by MacLean (1949), who developed the notion of a "limbic system" (the term *limbic* is derived from limbus, which means border and refers to the fact that this system serves to undergird the cerebral neocortices). MacLean hypothesized that in addition to the basic circuitry of Papez, the amygdala, septum, and associated areas were best understood as a "system" of integrated anatomical structures that were implicated not only in emotional expression but also in the aggregation of all sensory stimulation with affect, and that ultimately provide for emotional expression, or "discharge." Such discharge would have profound potential to affect not only mental health but also physical health. According to MacLean, "This region of the brain appears to be so strategically situated as to be able to correlate every form of internal and external perception. And ... has many strong connections with the hypothalamus for discharging its impressions." (p. 351). It should be noted that the hypothalamus and hippocampus are still thought to be the prime sites of integration for visceral efferent arousal discharge (Le Doux, 1992; Reiman et al., 1986; Van Hoesen, 1982).

Finally, the work of Nauta (Nauta, 1979; Nauta & Domesick, 1982) further refined and clarified our understanding of the vital role that the limbic system plays in emotional arousal, the integration of internal and external stimulation, and the process of hypothalamically mediated "psychosomatic" processes. His work supports the conclusion that sensory input is integrated and processed via limbic structures such as the amygdala, the hippocampus, and cingulate gyrus and that such limbic structures have the potential for upward and downward efferent projections. Such projections are likely to exert influence over neocortical as well as hypothalamic, neuroendocrine, and endocrine processes.

It is important to note at this juncture that the limbic system receives efferent impulses from, as well as sending afferent impulses to, brain-stem structures—more specifically the reticular activating system and the locus ceruleus. The reticular activating system (RAS) may be thought of as a system of projections with responsibility for nonspecific arousal of the entire cerebrum. The locus ceruleus (LC) represents an aggregation of 20,000 to 30,000 cells responsible for 50% to 70% of the norepinephrine in the human brain (Redmond, 1979). Its activity is highly associated with worry, threat, and flight behavior. The reciprocal connections that the LC has with prefrontal and limbic structures suggests cognitive, affective, and LC activity are intimately interwoven (Gellhorn, 1967; Redmond, 1979) and collectively may play key etiologic roles in psychiatric and somatic disorders (Doane, 1986; Gellhorn & Loofbourrow, 1963; Gloor, 1986; Post, 1986; Post & Ballenger, 1981).

The American Psychiatric Association's own DSM-III, DSM-III-R, and DSM-IV have included references to criteria such as hyperalertness, hypersensitivity, and autonomic nervous system hyperactivity in the diagnosis of anxiety-related disorders. Considerable evidence that these symptoms arise from the limbic circuitry comes from benzodiazepine and other behavioral pharmacological research (Carr & Sheehan, 1984; Gray, 1982) as well as neurotransmitter research (Mefferd 1979). Even major reviews of the etiology, diagnosis, and treatment of anxiety disorders implicate subcortically initiated arousal and reactivity as core features of anxiety disorders (Aggleton, 1992; Barlow & Beck, 1984; Carr & Sheehan, 1984; Friedman, Charney, & Deutch, 1995; Gorman et al., 1985; Shader, 1984).

Anxiety disorders are not the only psychiatric disorders wherein arousal plays a significant role. Post and his co-workers (Post, 1985; Post & Ballenger, 1981; Post et al., 1982) have cogently argued that limbic hypersensitivity ("sensitisation") underlies various primary and secondary affective disorders. They conclude that "sensitisation models provide a conceptual approach to previously inexplicable clinical phenomena in the longitudinal course of affective illness" (p. 191). Neurological sensitization is also believed to underlie various functional psychoses, personality disorders, posttraumatic reactions, addictive disorders, and withdrawal syndromes (Aggleton, 1992; Monroe, 1970, 1982; Post, 1985; Post & Ballenger, 1981; Post, Weiss, & Smith, 1995; van der Kolk, Greenberg, Boyd, & Krystal, 1985). Similarly, Gellhorn and Loufburrow (1963) implicated propensities for excessive limbic excitation in a host of emotional disorders (see Table 10.1).

Table 10.1. Psychiatric Disorders Related to Arousal

1. Anxiety disorders (posttraumatic stress disorder, panic disorders, and diffuse generalized anxiety disorders)
2. Adjustment disorders (with anxious mood and with mixed emotional features)
3. Various primary and secondary affective disorders (especially fast-cycling bipolar disorders and secondary reactive depression)
4. Addictive disorders (cocaine, amphetamine, nicotine)
5. Temporal lobe disorders
6. Acute atypical psychotic decompensation
7. Alcohol withdrawal ($X > 6$ years alcoholism)

The sensitization phenomenon may be based upon one or more of six mechanisms (Cain, 1992; Everly, 1993; Gloor, 1992):

1. Augmentation of excitatory neurotransmitters.
2. Declination of inhibitory neurotransmitters.
3. Augmentation of micromorphological structures (especially amygdaloidal and hippocampal).
4. Changes in the biochemical bases of neuronal activation (e.g., augmentation of phosphoproteins and/or changes on the transduction mechanism *c-fos* so as to change the genetic message within the neuron's nucleus).
5. Increased neuromuscular arousal.
6. Repetitive cognitive excitation.

SOMATIC DISORDERS OF AROUSAL

The psychiatric domain is not the only arena within which pathogenic arousal may manifest itself. Many stress-related "medical" syndromes contain a core arousal constituent. A Review by Lown et al. (1976) concluded that ventricular fibrillation in the absence of coronary heart disease may be related to increased sympathetic tone or activity. Similarly, evidence indicates that increased sympathetic tone and sympathetic hyperreactivity may be key etiological factors in the development of psychophysiological essential hypertension (Eliot, 1979; Gellhorn, 1964a; Henry & Stephens, 1977; Steptoe, 1981; Suter, 1986). Other cardiovascular diseases implicated as having pathogenic arousal as a key etiological factor include nonischemic myofibrillar degeneration (Corley, 1985; Eliot, 1979), coronary artery disease (Corley, 1985; Eliot, 1979; Henry & Stephens, 1977; see Manuck & Krantz, 1984, for a more conservative interpretation), sudden death (Corley, 1985; Eliot, 1979; Steptoe, 1981), and migraine headaches and Raynaud's disease (Suter, 1986). Gellhorn (1967), Weil (1974), and Malmo

Table 10.2. Somatic Disorders Related to Arousal

1. Hypertension
2. Stress-related ventricular fibrillation
3. Nonischemic myofibrillar degeneration
4. Stress-related coronary artery disease
5. Migraine headaches
6. Raynaud's disease
7. Muscle contradiction headaches
8. Non-head-related muscle contraction dysfunctions
9. Peptic ulcer
10. Irritable bowel syndrome

(1975) have implicated excessive sympathetic tone as a major etiological factor in a host of muscle contraction syndromes and dysfunctions including muscle contraction headaches. Finally, there is some evidence that peptic ulcers (Wolf, 1985), irritable bowel syndrome (Latimer, 1985), and other gastrointestinal disorders may be related to an excessive propensity for arousal (Dotevall, 1985; Henke, 1992; see Table 10.2).

In summary, pathognomonic hypersensitivity within the limbic circuitry as a common denominator within a host of otherwise widely disparate disorders seems to warrant the proposed taxonomic reconsideration, that is, the disorders of arousal taxonomy. It may well be that research will ultimately show that disorders of arousal actually include all stress-related psychosomatic disorders (see Friedman & Schnurr, 1995; Heninger, 1995; Williams, 1995).

THE NEUROLOGICAL FOUNDATIONS OF LIMBIC HYPERSENSITIVITY AND THE DISORDERS OF AROUSAL

Ergotropic Tuning

Within this chapter, it has been argued that a limbic-system-based neurological hypersensitivity to stimulation and a propensity for sustained arousal undergirds a host of psychiatric and stress-related somatic disorders, herein called "disorders of arousal." The work of Gellhorn not only documented the existence of complex autonomic nervous system–neocortical–limbic–somatic integration (Gellhorn, 1957, 1967) but also later served as one of the most coherent and cogent explanations of the pathognomonic arousal described in this chapter. Over two decades ago, Gellhorn described a hypothalamically based "ergotropic tuning" process as the neurophysiological basis for affective lability, ANS hyperfunction, anxiety, stress arousal, and related emotional disorders (Gellhorn, 1965, 1967; Gellhorn & Loofbourrow, 1963). Gellhorn has stated:

> It is a matter of everyday experience that a person's reaction to a given situation depends very much upon his own mental, physical, and emotional state. One might be said to be "set" to respond in a given manner. In the same fashion the autonomic response to a given stimulus may at one time be predominantly sympathetic and may at another time be predominantly parasympathetic. ... The sensitization of autonomic centers has been designated "tuning" and we speak of sympathetic tuning and parasympathetic tuning ... and refers merely to the "sensitization" or "facilitation" of particular centers of the brain. (Gellhorn & Loofbourrow, 1963, pp. 90–91)

Gellhorn chose the term *ergotropic tuning* to describe a preferential pattern of SNS responsiveness. Such a neurological status could then serve as the basis for a host of psychiatric and stress-related somatic disorders.

From an etiological perspective, Gellhorn (1965) states: "In the waking state the ergotropic division of the autonomic is dominant and responds primarily to environmental stimuli. If these stimuli are very strong or follow each other at short intervals, the tone and reactivity of the sympathetic system increases" (pp. 494–495). Thus, either extremely intense, acute (traumatic) sympathetic stimulation or chronically repeated, intermittent lower level sympathetic stimulation, both of which can be environmental in origin, can lead to SNS hyperfunction. Such sympathetic activity, according to Gellhorn, creates a condition of sympathetic neurological hypersensitivity, called ergotropic tuning, which serves as the neurological predisposition, or even etiological factor, associated with the psychophysiological sequelae observed in anxiety, stress, and related disorders of arousal.

Several mechanisms may sustain the ergotropically tuned status. Gellhorn (1964) has provided cogent documentation that discharge from limbic centers sends neural impulses in two simultaneous directions: (1) to neocortical targets and (2) to the skeletal musculature via pyramidal and extrapyramidal projections (see also Gellhorn & Loofbourrow, 1963). The neocortical centers then send impulses back to the limbic areas and to the locus ceruleus by way of noradrenergic and other pathways, thus sustaining limbic activity. Simultaneously, neuromuscular proprioceptive impulses (indicative of neuromuscular status) from afferent muscle spindle projections ascend primarily via the dorsal root and reticular activating system, ultimately projecting not only to cerebellar targets but also to limbic and neocortical targets. Such proprioceptive bombardment further excites target areas and sets into motion a complex mechanism of positive neurological feedback, sustaining and potentially intensifying ergotropic tone (Gellhorn, 1964, 1965, 1967).

Thus, we see that Gellhorn has proposed a model and empirically demonstrated that intimate neocortical–hypothalamic–somatic relationships exist that use the limbic system as a central "hub" for efferent projections to the neocortex and somatic musculature as well as an afferent target for neocortical, "proprioceptive, interoceptive, and brain-stem impulses. This configuration creates a functional, potentially self-sustaining mechanism of affective and ergotropic arousal. It certainly seems reasonable that such a mechanism could play a major role in chronic anxiety and stress-related disorders of arousal.

Neurological Reverberation and Charging

Weil (1974) has developed a model somewhat similar to that of Gellhorn. In fact, Weil makes brief reference to the work of Gellhorn in his construction of a neurophysiological model of emotional behavior.

Weil notes, in agreement with Gellhorn, that the activation thresholds of the ANS (particularly hypothalamic nuclei), as well as limbic centers, can be altered. Instead of the concepts of sympathetic and parasympathetic systems, Weil uses a parallel but broader construction, that of arousal and tranquilizing systems, respectively. He calls the facilitation of activation within these systems, "charging." With regard to the concept of neurological hypersensitivity, Weil notes that two major processes can be effective in "charging the arousal system" in the human organism: (1) high-intensity stimulation and/or (2) increased rate of repeated stimulation. The processes that appear to underlie the charging of the arousal system as well as the mechanisms that could serve to sustain such a neurological status seem to be (1) the neuromuscular proprioceptive system, as described earlier, and (2) intrinsic neuronal reverberation. Regarding the latter, Weil (1974) notes:

> The reciprocal association of the hypothalamus with the midbrain and the thalamic reticular formation makes possible the establishment of intrinsic reverberating circuits. Such hypothalamic reticular circuits are in a position to be set into motion by extrinsic impulses reaching the reticular formation. They provide a neuroanatomical basis for the maintenance of a reverberating supply of impulses to reticular non-specific activation even during a momentary reduction or deficiency of extrinsic input. (p. 37)

Thus, we see that Weil's notion of charging is similar to Gellhorn's notion of tuning. Weil's formulation seems somewhat broader in the neurological mechanisms it encompasses, yet narrower in its implications for emotional and behavioral disorders. Points of agreement can be found, however, in the recognition of the fact that neurological hypersensitivity (i.e., a lowered threshold for activating limbic, autonomic, and hypothalamic effector systems) can be achieved through environmental stimulation and proprioceptive stimulation when presented in either an acute and intense (trauma-like) manner or in a lower level yet chronically repeated exposure pattern. Once achieved, such a status of lowered activation threshold could serve as a self-sustaining neurological basis for emotional and psychophysiological dysfunction.

Neuromuscular Set-Point Theory

In reviewing Gellhorn's and Weil's notions of tuning and charging theory, respectively, and the neurological mechanisms that support them, one is impressed with the central role that the striated musculature plays in sensitizing and maintaining hypersensitivity (ergotropic status). The work of Malmo seems appropriate to introduce at this juncture, for it deals directly with the role of striated muscles in psychophysiological and anxiety disorders. In a brief but cogent treatise, Malmo (1975) summarizes his classic studies on the prolonged activation of the striated musculature of anxiety patients following stressor presentation, compared with nonanxiety patients exposed to the same stressor. The work of Gellhorn clearly demonstrated that the striated muscles were target organs for limbic arousal. Malmo and his colleagues found that select groups of individuals who possessed arousal disorders, such as anxiety, seemed to demonstrate somewhat higher baseline levels of muscle tension when compared with nonpatients. More important, however, upon the presentation of a stressor stimulus, the muscle tension of the patient population reached higher levels of peak amplitude and subsequently took significantly longer to return to baseline levels once the stressor was removed. This phenomenon was interpreted by Malmo as being indicative of a defect in homeostatic mechanisms following arousal in such patients.

Malmo offered two possible mechanisms that might explain the observed homeostatic dysfunction: one neural, the other biochemical. He cites the research of Jasper (1949), who discovered that direct stimulation of the motor cortex created not only the expected electromyographic activity in the target muscle but also an "after discharge" in that muscle. The after discharge may be thought of as a residual depolarization of the neurons in the absence of direct exogenous stimulation. However, when Jasper simultaneously stimulated the thalamic–reticular system, the after discharge was eliminated. These data suggest that the thalamic–reticular system may play a role in dampening, or inhibiting, excess neuromuscular activation. Malmo then extended Jasper's work to his own and used it as a model to explain the homeostatic dysfunction observed in his own studies. Malmo saw Jasper's discovery as the homeostatic mechanism that was most likely dysfunctional in anxiety patients (i.e., a mechanism protracting neuromuscular excitation in stressful situations). More specifically, he argues that this neural inhibitory system represents a "set point" similar to that of a thermostat. This neural set point may be designed to dampen excessive muscular activity, thus preventing excessive strain. He notes that in cases where muscles are extremely tense and corresponding proprioceptive activity is sufficiently strong (i.e., exceeding the tolerances of the set point), the inhibitory neurons would be activated, thus reducing lingering peripheral muscular aftercharge activity. He further notes:

> Such a system as this would work well in providing for extra muscular exertion to meet emergencies; and by the return of the set point to normal afterwards, the motor system would have a built-in protection against excessive strain. If, however, extremely demanding life situations are prolonged ... it seems the setpoint "sticks" at the higher (above normal) level even when the individual is removed to a quiet environment.
>
> This then would be a neural mechanism that could account for the "persistence" of anxiety and the accompanying increase in muscular activity. (Malmo, 1975, pp. 152–153)

Malmo places the most emphasis on this neural mechanism in explaining the homeostatic dysfunction seen in anxiety patients, yet he does briefly mention a biochemical–neurological process that has played a central role in the formulation of current thinking on arousal disorders. Malmo notes that muscle tension leads to increased levels of lactic acid (a by-product of anerobic metabolism). Furthermore, he notes research by Pitts and McClure (1967) clearly demonstrating that lactate infusions had panicogenic properties for panic anxiety patients but had none for nonanxiety patients. It has been postulated that panic patients metabolize lactate normally, thus suggesting a neural receptor hypersensitivity existing somewhere in their CNS as the etiological site for this dysfunction. The lactate infusion data are similar to those obtained by inhalation of 5% CO_2, thus demonstrating panicogenic properties for this agent as well. The specific mechanism by which these agents induce panic attacks is unclear at this time. Interested readers should refer to Carr and Sheehan (1984), Gorman et al. (1985), and Liebowitz et al. (1985). The major point of clinical interest, however, is that Gellhorn and Weil, as well as Malmo, have shown mechanisms by which anxiety and stress may lead to chronically contracted muscles and that these muscles (while under chronic anerobic contraction) may produce a by-product (lactic acid) that may have anxiogenic properties of a biochemical nature in addition to the anxiogenic properties of excessive proprioceptive bombardment of the brain stem, limbic system, and neocortex. Thus, there appears to be remarkable agreement from researchers in diverse fields as to the probability that neurological hypersensitivity underlies anxiety and stress-related disorders of a chronic nature.

MODELS OF NEURONAL PLASTICITY

In an attempt to understand the phenomenon of neurological hypersensitivity at the most basic structural levels, this section briefly reviews popular models of neuronal plasticity.

The concept of *kindling* represents one of the most popular models of plasticity and neurological hypersensitivity in clinical literature. *Kindling* is a term originally conceived of to identify the process by which repeated stimulation of limbic structures leads to a lowered convulsive threshold (limbic ictus) and to a propensity for spontaneous activation of such structures, with resultant affective lability, ANS hyperfunction, and behavioral disturbances (Goddard, McIntyre, & Leech, 1969; Joy, 1985; Post, 1985; Post, Uhde, Putnam, Ballenger, & Berrettini, 1982). Kindling-like processes have been implicated in a host of behavioral and psychopathological conditions (Cain, 1992; Gloor, 1992; Mann, 1992; Monroe, 1970; Post & Ballenger, 1981; Reynolds, 1992).

Shader (1984) has stated, "With regard to anxiety disorders, one might speculate that kindling processes ... could increase attack-like firing from a source such as the locus ceruleus" (p. 14). Redmond and Huang (1979) support such a conclusion by suggesting that panic disorders are predicated on a lowered firing threshold at the locus ceruleus. Such discharge could then arouse limbic and cortical structures on the basis of ventral and dorsal adrenergic efferent projections arising from the locus ceruleus. Monroe (1982) has provided evidence that certain episodic behavioral disorders may be based on a kindling-like limbic ictus. He notes, "As it is known that environmental events can induce synchronized electrical activity within the limbic system, this also provides an explanation of why environmental stress might sensitize patients to acute exacerbations of an ictal illness" (p. 713). Monroe (1970, 1982) implicates explosive behavioral tirades, impulsively destructive behavior, extreme affective lability, and episodic psychotic behavior in such a neurological dysfunction. According to van der Kolk, Greenberg, Boyd, and Krystal (1985), "Long-term augmentation of LC (locus ceruleus) pathways following trauma underlies the repetitive intrusive recollections and nightmares that plague patients with PTSD (posttraumatic stress disorder)" (p. 318).

Post et al. (1982) have taken the kindling model and extrapolated from it, stating, "Kindling and related sensitization models may also be useful conceptual approaches to understanding the development of psychopathology in the absence of seizure discharges" (p. 719). They report data that demonstrate the ability of adrenergic and dopaminergic agonists to sensitize animals and humans to behavioral hyperactivity and especially affective disorders. They refer to this phenomenon as "behavioral senitisation" rather than kindling because no ictal status is obtained as an end point. Rather, the achieved end point represents a lowered depolarization threshold and an increased propensity for spontaneous activation of limbic and related circuitry (Post, Weiss, & Smith, 1995).

According to Racine, Tuff, and Zaide (1976), "Except for neural development and learning, the kindling phenomenon may be the most robust example of neural plasticity in the mammalian nervous system" (p. 19). Indeed, models of learning and memory may serve as tools for understanding the biology of kindling-like phenomena. Goddard and Douglas (1976) conducted a series of investigations designed to see if the "engram" model of memory had applicability in the understanding of the kindling phenomenon. They concluded:

> Thus it would appear that kindling is caused, in part, by a lasting potentiation of excitatory synapses. More work is needed to decide whether the changes are pre-synaptic or in the post-synaptic membrane, whether they are accompanied by alteration in synaptic morphology...
>
> Our answer to the question: does the engram of kindling model the engram of normal long term memory? is yes. (pp. 14–15)

Lynch and his colleagues at the University of California have sought to clarify this mechanism and have identified postsynaptic processes as the likely target area. Their research in long-term neuronal potentiation revealed a functional augmentation in the dendritic spines of stimulated neuronal pathways. More specifically, such changes included a 33% increase in synaptic contacts, as well as a decrease in the length and width variation of the dendritic spines (Deadwyler, Gribkoff, Cotman, & Lynch, 1976; Lee, Schottler, Oliver, & Lynch, 1980). Rosenzweig and Leiman (1982) have suggested that the number of dendritic spines as well as the postsynaptic membrane area may be increased in such neural plasticity. Delanoy, Tucci, and Gold (1983) pharmacologically stimulated the dentate granule cells in rats and found a kindling-like neurological hypersensitivity to result. Similar agonists have been shown to enhance state-dependent learning.

Joy's superb review of the nature and effects of kindling (1985) summarizes the potential alterations in biological substrata that may be involved in the kindling phenomenon. He notes that "kindling produces important changes in neuronal function and connectivity" (p. 46) and continues:

> One would expect that these changes would have morphological or neurochemical correlates. Increased connectivity could result from a morphological rearrangement of neuronal circuits, perhaps from collateral sprouting and new synapse formation. Alternatively, it could result from a modification of existing synapses, perhaps by the growth of presynaptic terminals or by an increase in the postsynaptic receptive surface or number of receptors. (p. 49)

Whatever the biological alteration underlying the neuronal plasticity associated with limbic system neurological hypersensitivity, the phenomenon (1) appears to be inducible on the basis of repeated, intermittent stimulation (Delanoy et al., 1983), with the optimal interval between stimulations to induce kindling being about 24 hours (Monroe, 1982); (2) appears to last for hours, days, and even months (Deadwyler et al., 1976; Fifkova & van Harreveld, 1977; Goddard & Douglas, 1976; Monroe, 1982); (3) appears to show at least some tendency to decay over a period of days of months in the absence of continued stimulation if the initial stimulation was insufficient to cause permanent alteration (Fifkova & van Harreveld, 1977; Joy, 1985); and (4) appears to be inducible on the basis of environmental, psychosocial, pharmacological, and/or electrical stimulation (Black et al., 1987; Doane, 1986; Monroe, 1970; Post, 1986; Post, Weiss, & Smith, 1995; Sorg & Kalivas, 1995).

In summary, the preceding sections have argued for the existence of a group of disorders that share a latent yet common denominator of limbic-based neurological hypersensitivity and arousal. The neurology of this "common thread" has been discussed in some detail. Figure 10.2 graphically depicts the hypersensitivity phenomenon.

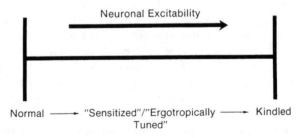

Figure 10.2. Limbic hypersensitivity phenomenon (LHP).

The etiological and/or sustaining mechanisms of the limbic-system-based neurological hypersensitivity that serves to undergird the disorders of arousal may be summarized into six basic categories:

1. Increased excitatory neurotransmitter activity within the limbic circuitry (Black et al., 1987; Post, 1985; Post & Ballinger, 1981; Post, Rubinow, & Ballenger, 1986; Post, Weiss, & Smith, 1995; Sorg & Kalivas, 1995).
2. Declination of inhibitory neurotransmitters and/or receptors (Cain, 1992; see Everly, 1993).
3. Augmentation of micromorphological structures (especially amygdaloidal and hippocampal) (Cain, 1992; Post, Weiss, & Smith, 1995; see Everly, 1993).
4. Changes in the biochemical bases of neuronal activation (e.g., augmentation of phosphoproteins and/or changes on the transduction mechanism *c-fos* so as to change the genetic message within the neuron's nucleus) (Cain, 1992; Sorg & Kalivas, 1995).
5. Increased arousal of neuromuscular efferents, with resultant increased proprioceptive bombardment of the limbic system (especially amygdaloid and hippocampal nuclei) (Gellhorn, 1964, 1968; Malmo, 1975; Weil, 1974).
6. Repetitive cognitive excitation (Gellhorn, 1964, 1968; Gellhorn & Loofbourrow, 1963; Post, Rubinow, & Ballinger, 1986).

The important point to keep in mind here is that these mechanisms appear to be inducible and responsive to environmental, psychosocial, pharmacological, and/or electrical stimulation. If, indeed, a group of psychiatric and somatic diseases exist that differ in their end-organ symptoms yet share a common pathogenic thread of neurological hypersensitivity and arousal, a therapy for the etiological and sustaining mechanisms of such disorders of arousal seems almost too obvious. If we look beyond the multitude of varied symptoms and signs that characterize these numerous disorders to the common yet latent taxonomic criterion of limbic-based neural hypersensitivity, it becomes obvious that, at least in theory, antiarousal therapies are "ideal" for achieving a neurological desensitization and amelioration of the core mechanism of pathogenesis in all of these disorders. Any such therapy, therefore, should prove of value in treating not only the *symptoms* of these varied disorders (assuming the symptoms have not become self-perpetuating) but also the *causal mechanisms* of neurological hypersensitivity and psychophysiological arousal also. Ironically, Gellhorn and Loofbourrow (1963) noted nearly 40 years ago, "If it were possible to alter the autonomic reactivity at the hypothalamic level important therapeutic results might be obtained" (p. 90).

THE RELAXATION RESPONSE

The preceding sections have argued that there exists a host of psychiatric and stress-related somatic disorders that, although diverse in their end-organ symptomatology, share a latent common thread of limbicogenic hypersensitivity (i.e., a propensity for hyperreactivity and/or sustained psychophysiological activation). These disorders have been referred to as "disorders of arousal." The available data suggest that these disorders may possess the following key etiological or sustaining constituents: (1) increased excitatory neurotransmitter activity, (2) increased neuromuscular arousal, and (3) repetitive cognitive excitation. It would seem reasonable that in order for a therapeutic intervention to work effectively to ameliorate these disorders, it should work in such a way as to neurologically desensitize and reduce overall activity within the limbic circuitry. This can be achieved by (1) reducing excitatory neurotransmitter responsivity, (2) reducing neuromuscular arousal, and (3) reducing cognitive excitation. Just such an antiarousal therapy has been uniquely captured in Benson's concept of the "relaxation response," a natural antiarousal psychophysiological phenomenon intrinsically antithetical to the mechanisms that undergird the "disorders of arousal" (Benson, 1975; Benson, Beary, & Carol, 1974; Hellman et al., 1990).

Current evidence fails to indicate reliably that there is a best way of eliciting the relaxation response; furthermore, there is no reliable evidence that only one or two specific diseases may show superior therapeutic improvement from its application (Lehrer & Woolfolk, 1993). Indeed, many technologies are available to elicit the relaxation response, such as mantra meditation, progressive relaxation, presuggestion hypnosis, and prayer (Benson, 1983, 1985), and a wide variety of diverse diseases seem amenable to its therapeutic effect (Benson, 1985; Hellman et al., 1990; Lavey & Taylor, 1985; Lehrer, 1995; Lehrer & Woolfolk, 1993; Murphy & Donovan, 1986; Shapiro & Giber, 1978).

The Physiology of the Relaxation Response

The physiology of the relaxation response is fundamentally a physiology of hypoarousal, and much of its therapeutic effect derives from this quality. According to Gellhorn, relaxation is a result of a "loss in ergotropic tone of the hypothalamus, [and] a diminution of hypothalamic-cortical discharges" (Gellhorn & Kiely, 1972, p. 404). In agreement with Gellhorn, Taylor (1978) has suggested that relaxation involves a decrease in the arousability of the central nervous system. According to Benson (1983), "The relaxation response results in physiological changes which are thought to characterize an integrated hypothalamic function. These physiological changes are consistent with generalized decreased sympathetic nervous system activity" (p. 282). A more current reinterpretation might be that the relaxation response represents a neurological "desensitization" of the limbic system and/or its sympathetic efferents.

Specific empirical investigations have traditionally shown the elicitation of the relaxation response to result in decreases in O_2 consumption and CO_2 elimination, with no change in the respiratory quotient. Other similar changes include a reduction in heart and respiratory rates with a similar reduction in arterial blood lactate (Benson, 1983, 1985). All of these alterations are consistent with a decrease in central and peripheral adrenergic excitation (Benson, 1985; Delmonte, 1984). Yet the actual mechanisms appear more complex. Research has failed to show reductions consistently in circulating adrenergic catecholamines (Michaels, Haber, & McCann, 1976). In fact, it has been observed that plasma norepinephrine may actually increase as a result of the elicitation of the relaxation response (Hoffman et al., 1982; Lang, Dehof, Meurer, & Kaufmann, 1979). Yet more recent investigations into this seeming paradox reveal that although there may be more norepinephrine available, a diminished adrenergic responsivity actually occurs at the end organ itself (Hoffman et al., 1982; Lehmann et al., 1986). In effect, the relaxation response has shown evidence of exerting effects consistent with those of an adrenergic end-organ blocking agent (Benson, 1983, 1985; Lehmann et al., 1986).

Behavioral psychophysiological studies support the notion that the relaxation response is capable of dampening a form of adrenergic responsivity. In one study, Allen (1981) used a 2,700-Hz tone at 90 dB for a duration of 0.7 sec to trigger what was assumed to be posterior hypothalamically mediated arousal in 653 subjects. He found that after training in the relaxation response for a period of approximately 10 weeks, subjects demonstrated a dampened psychophysiological responsivity to the auditory stressor. The results of Allen's study are basically in concert with those of Goleman and Schwartz (1976), who compared the stress reactivity of 30 experienced meditators with that of 30 control subjects. Results indicated that recovery from a 12-min video stressor was more rapid among the experienced meditators when compared with the control subjects. A study by English and Baker (1983) used a cold pressor to induce arousal and then measured blood pressure recovery time among 36 subjects. All subjects participated in a 4-week progressive relaxation program and then were submitted to a repetition of the cold pressor. Results indicated that relaxation training did not reduce cardiovascular response during the stressor but did facilitate a more rapid recovery within the domain of measured blood pressure.

Similar results regarding facilitated psychophysiological recovery as described in this section have been found by Praeger-Decker and Decker (1980) and by Michaels, Parra, McCann, and Vander (1979). Although not totally concordant, these studies in the aggregate still suggest that the elicitation of the relaxation response serves to reduce forms of excessive arousal (Benson & Friedman, 1985; Delmonte, 1984). Complete agreement among observers remains entangled, however, in methodological and phenomenological complexities. The interested reader is referred to Suler (1985), Delmonte (1984), Shapiro (1985), and Benson and Friedman (1985) for a useful debate of this topic.

Having addressed the notion of arousal responsivity and the relaxation response, we now consider the issue of neuromuscular arousal. Gellhorn (1964b) notes that "states of abnormal emotional tension are alleviated in various 'relaxation' therapies through reducing proprioceptive impulses which impinge on the posterior hypothalamus and maintain the cerebral cortex in an abnormal state of excitation" (p. 457). Gellhorn (1958a,b, 1964) and Weil (1974) have clearly documented the existing interconnections between the neuromuscular system and the limbic circuitry. Similarly, they have argued that reductions of neuromuscular tone achieved by the elicitation of the relaxation response would be of value in reducing abnormal states of limbic sensitivity and excitation. The primary mechanism of mediation used to achieve such a neurological desensitization, Gellhorn and Weil argue, is the reduction of proprioceptive stimulation to the limbic system.

Finally, Averill (1973), Benson (1983, 1985), Gellhorn (1958b, 1967, Gellhorn & Kiely, 1972), and Lazarus and Folkman (1984) all agree that cognitive distortion, rumination, and overall cognitive excitation can give rise to states of ergotropic and generalized psychophysiological arousal. Similarly, evidence shows that a reduction in cognitive arousal via the relaxation response contributes to a reduction in ergotropic tone and a neurological desensitization effect as well as a reduction in dysphoric psychological states (Benson, 1985; Klajner, Hartman, & Sobell, 1984; Kutz, Borysenko, & Benson, 1985; Lavey & Taylor, 1985; Shapiro & Giber, 1978).

The "psychotherapeutic effect" of the relaxation response has been hypothesized to be derived from a sense of "mental calmness" (Rachman, 1968), a sense of "control" (Klajner, Hartman, & Sobell, 1984; Stoyva & Anderson, 1982), and a reduction of cognitive–affective rumination (Gellhorn, 1964b; Gellhorn & Loofbourrow, 1963). In reviewing the evidence for the psychotherapeutic value of the relaxation response, one is struck by the recurrent theme of an increase in "self-efficacy" derived from consistent practice of the relaxation response, as well as the sense of control engendered by the physiological autoregulatory skills developed (Bandura, 1977; Romano, 1982; Sarnoff, 1982; Shapiro & Giber, 1978).

This point is especially well made by Green and Green (1977), Hamberger and Lohr (1984), and Stoyva and Anderson (1982). Bandura (1982), however, has done the most to develop this theme. He notes that the most powerful tool for combating perceptions of low self-efficacy and helplessness appears to be experience. Furthermore, he has shown that perceptions of self-efficacy can actually influence SNS activity, as well as subsequent performance. He concludes, "Treatments that eliminate emotional arousal... heighten perceived efficacy with corresponding improvements in performance" (Bandura, 1982b, p. 28). The relaxation response appears to be just such a treatment.

SELECTING A RELAXATION TECHNIQUE

As noted earlier in this chapter, many different techniques/strategies can engender the relaxation response. Such therapeutic technologies include meditation, neuromuscular relaxation, controlled breathing, imagery, and hypnosis. As Lehrer and Woolfolk (1993) point out, research has shown there to be no single, best relaxation technology; nor has any one stress-related disorder proved to be the most responsive to therapeutic amelioration by any specific relaxation technique. Not all relaxation techniques, however, are equally efficacious. The answer to this seeming paradox resides in the concept of individual differences.

"Inadequate recognition of individual differences is a methodological deficiency that has seriously slowed psychological research" (Tart, 1975, p. 140). Indeed, few outcomes in the behavioral sciences are a result of "main effects"; rather, "interaction effects" usually explain far more clinical variation.

So how does the clinician know what relaxation technology to employ? What treatment will be the most useful? Rather than ascribe main effects to therapies, perhaps the individual patient should be given primary consideration, as discussed in Chapter 7. If, then, the relaxation response can be engendered via numerous techniques, with none showing generic superiority, then the clinician should select the relaxation technique that best meets the interacting needs of patient, therapist, setting, and disorder (Paul, 1967). Unfortunately, there are no algorithmic models to guide the clinician to this end. Nevertheless, a review of Chapter 7, or texts such as that of Millon and Everly (1985), will serve to give the clinician insight into personologic differences. For example, compulsive persons may respond well to structured, directive therapy interventions (e.g., biofeedback), whereas avoidant–defensive persons may respond better to less structured technologies.

In the final analysis, it may be that the most powerful stress management/behavioral medicine programs are multicomponent programs with aspects that functionally address (1) neurological hypersensitivity via neural desensitization practices, (2) neuromuscular hypertension, and (3) pathogenic cognitive reiteration. Such a program was established by Herbert Benson (1979, 1996; Kutz et al., 1985) and evolved into a multidimensional "mind–body" behavioral medicine program through the input of Ian Kutz, Joan Borysenko, Margaret Caudill, Alice Domar, and others, and has been found to be effective in the treatment of a wide variety of "disorders of arousal" (Caudill, 1994; Caudill et al., 1991; Domar et al., 1990, 1992; Hellman, 1990a,b). Benson's formulations and clinical applications clearly represent "watershed" ideas that have evolved into the "gold standard" of clinical stress management programs.

CLINICAL PRECAUTIONS AND UNDESIRABLE SIDE EFFECTS

Until rather recently, it was assumed that the clinical use of the relaxation response was a totally harmless therapeutic intervention. Recent data have argued contrary to such a position.

Luthe (1969) was perhaps the first to point out that the relaxation response should be used with caution. A pioneer in self-regulatory therapies, Luthe has compiled an impressive list of precautions for such therapies. They include psychotic states, dissociative reactions, paranoid ideation, dysfunctional thyroid conditions, and "disagreeable cardiac and vasomotor reactions."

Stroebel (1979), another pioneer in self-regulatory therapies (especially biofeedback), has argued that fragile ego structures serve as precautions for self-regulatory interventions. Heide and Borkovec (1983) observed in 30.8% of their progressive neuromuscular relaxation patients, and in 53.8% of their meditation patients, clinical evidence of anxiety reactions during preliminary training. Edinger (1982), on the other hand, reported that undesirable side effects arose from relaxation training in 3–4% of the clinical cases surveyed.

These disparate reports led Everly, Spollen, Hackman, and Kobran (1987) to conduct a survey analysis of clinical practitioners who use relaxation training as a major component of their practice. Data were obtained from a national survey of 133 clinicians reporting on over 71,000 patients and over 700,000 patient hours. The results indicated that anxiety reactions occurred about 1.0% of the time; muscle tension headaches resulted about 0.8% of the time; a freeing of repressed ideation resulted about 0.7% of the time; and undesirable depersonalization resulted about 0.7% of the time from the elicitation of the relaxation response or some other form of self-regulatory therapy.

Based on the research of Luthe (1969), Stroebel (1979), Emmons (1978), and Everly et al. (1987), there are five major areas of concern in the elicitation of the relaxation response.

Loss of Reality Contact

The loss of reality contact during the elicitation of the relaxation response includes dissociative states, hallucinations, delusions, and perhaps parasthesias. Care should be taken when treating patients who suffer from affective or thought-disturbance psychoses or who use nonpsychotic fantasy excessively. In such conditions, the use of deep relaxation may exacerbate the problem.

Drug Reactions

Clinical evidence has clearly indicated that the induction of the relaxation response may actually intensify the effects of any medication or other chemical substance that the patient may be taking. Of special concern would be patients taking insulin, sedatives/hypnotics, or cardiovascular medications. All such patients should be carefully monitored medically (although in many cases, chronic relaxation may ultimately result in long-term reductions in required use of medications).

Panic States

Panic-state reactions are characterized by high levels of anxiety concerning the loss of control, insecurity, and, in some cases, seduction. Diffuse, free-floating worry and apprehension have also been observed. With such patients it is generally more desirable to provide a more concrete relaxation paradigm (such as neuromuscular techniques or biofeedback) rather than the abstract relaxation paradigms (such as meditation). Similarly, it is important to assure the patient that he or she is really always in control—even in the states of "passive attention," which will be discussed in the following chapter on meditation.

Premature Freeing of Repressed Ideation

It is not uncommon for deeply repressed thoughts and emotions to be released into the patient's consciousness in response to a deeply relaxed state. Although in some psychotherapeutic paradigms such reactions are considered desirable, such reactions could be perceived as destructive by the patient if unexpected and/or too intense to be dealt with constructively at that point in the therapeutic process. Before implementation of relaxation techniques, the clinician may wish to inform the patient of the possibility that such ideation may arise. Similarly, the clinician must be prepared to render support should such thoughts emerge (see Adler & Morrissey-Adler, 1983; Glueck & Stroebel, 1978).

Excessive Trophotropic States

In some instances, relaxation techniques that intended to be therapeutic may induce an excessively lowered state of psychophysiological functioning. If this occurs, several phenomena may result:

1. *Temporary Hypotensive State.* This acute state of lowered blood pressure may cause dizziness, headaches, or momentary fainting, particularly if the patient rushes to stand up following the relaxation session. The clinician should know the patient's history of resting blood pressure before employing relaxation techniques. Caution should be used if the patient's resting blood pressure is lower than 90 mm Hg systolic and 50 mm Hg diastolic. Dizziness and fainting can often be aborted if the patient is instructed to open his or her eyes and to stretch and look around the room at the first signs of uncomfortable lightheadedness. Similarly, the patient should be told to wait 1 to 3 minutes before standing up following the relaxation session.

2. *Temporary Hypoglycemic State.* This condition of low blood sugar may follow the inducement of the trophotropic state and most likely last until the patient eats. Deep relaxation, like exercise, appears to have an insulinlike action, and may induce such an action if the patient has a tendency for such conditions, or has not eaten properly that day. The acute hypoglycemic state just described may result in symptoms similar to the hypotensive condition.

3. *Fatigue.* Although relaxation techniques are known to create a refreshed feeling of vigor in many patients, a very few have reported feeling tired after relaxation practice. This is a highly unusual result and may be linked to an overstriving to relax on the part of the patient. The clinician should inform the patient that the best outcome in any attempt at relaxation is achieved when the patient *allows* relaxation to occur, rather than making it happen.

SUMMARY

Earlier in this chapter, we suggested that the disorders of arousal described earlier might be treated effectively if limbic hypersensitivity and related factors could be reduced. Operationally, this meant achieving a reduction in (1) adrenergic catecholamine activity and responsiveness, (2) neuromuscular arousal, and (3) pathogenic cognitive processes, such as rumination and perceptions of powerlessness and a lack of control. We have reviewed the concept of the relaxation response as described by Benson and found it to be capable of achieving all three of the aforementioned therapeutic goals necessary for the successful treatment of the stress-related psychiatric and somatic disorders of arousal. Thus, it would appear that a cogent rationale for the use of techniques that engender the relaxation response in the treatment of the human stress response has emerged. To briefly review, this chapter has suggested the following:

1. Neuronal hypersensitivity for excitation residing within the limbic system may be a latent common denominator serving to undergird a host of stress-related psychiatric and somatic disorders.

2. These disorders, in the aggregate, have been referred to as "disorders of arousal" by Everly and Benson (Everly, 1985b; Everly & Benson, 1989).

3. The relaxation response, as described by Benson, represents a broad-spectrum psychophysiological phenomenon antithetical to the stress-related disorders of arousal.

4. As such, the relaxation response may be a valuable tool in the treatment of all of the disorders of arousal, despite their wide varieties of etiological mechanisms and their diverse target organ symptom complexes.

5. There is no best relaxation technology. Clinicians should consider the interaction of the needs of the patient, therapist, setting, and disorder in the selection of the technology for the elicitation of the relaxation response.

6. Contrary to popular opinion, the elicitation of the relaxation response is not without its precautions and undesirable side effects. Precautions include patients with psychotic disorders, major affective disorders, patients on pharmacotherapy, and those with dysfunctional thyroid conditions, fragile ego structure, and delusion conditions. Undesirable side effects appear to occur between 3% and 4% of the time (Edinger, 1982; Everly et al., 1987) and include depersonalization, excessive trophotropic states, anxiety reactions, freeing of repressed ideation, and headaches.

In summary, this chapter has reviewed in detail the neurophysiology of the limbic system and the relaxation response. The notion of the disorders of arousal has also been introduced. In effect, we see the emergence of a rationale for using the relaxation response in the treatment of a multitude of diseases spanning a wide spectrum of traditional diagnostic boundaries—something counterintuitive to traditional, linear, Pasteurian conceptualization.

Thus, we hope that this chapter has given new credibility and importance to therapeutic technologies such as meditation, controlled respiration, and, especially, progressive neuromuscular relaxation exercises (given the important role of proprioception in the prolongation of stress-related disorders). With these points in mind, let us now move to a discussion of techniques that engender the relaxation response and see how they can be used in the treatment of all stress-related disorders of arousal described in this chapter and in Chapter 4.

11

Meditation

Chapter 10 provided a rationale for the use of the relaxation response in the treatment of stress-related disorders. We now explore several techniques used to create the relaxation response. The purpose of this chapter is to provide a clinically relevant introduction to meditation.

In our culture, *meditation* refers to the act of thinking, planning, pondering, or reflecting. Our Western definitions are, however, not representative of the essence of the Eastern notion of meditation, in whose tradition, meditation is a process by which one attains "enlightenment." It is a growth-producing experience along intellectual, philosophical, and existential dimensions. Given the focus of our text, we use the term *meditation* to mean, quite simply, the autogenic practice of a genre of techniques that have the potential for inducing the relaxation response in the participant through the use of a repetitive focal device. Inherent in the success of using these procedures is achieving a mental state characterized by a non-ego-centered and nonintrusive mode of thought processing. According to Sethi (1989), meditation provides an "attempt to achieve a blissful state where stress has lost all its negative psychophysiological impacts" (p. 10).

HISTORY OF MEDITATION

It is difficult to trace the history of meditation without considering it within the context of religion. The origins of religion date back to prehistoric times, and data suggest that it was common practice for older civilizations to use repetitive, rhythmic chants and sacrificial offerings (e.g., gold, food, animals, or sometimes humans) in attempts to appease the gods (Joseph, 1998). Therefore, a legacy of strong religious beliefs is used to instill a calming, relaxing effect on the mind, often at the expense of imposing fear on the worshipers.

Some of the earliest written records on the subject of meditation come from the Hindu traditions of Vedantism around 1500 B.C.E. These records consist of scriptures called Vedas, which discuss the meditative traditions of ancient India. Around 500 to 600 B.C.E., other forms of meditation developed, such as the Taoist in China and the Buddhist in India. From 1000 C.E. to 1100 C.E., the Zen form of meditation, called "zazen," gained popularity in Japan.

In Christianity, the use of repetitive prayers to effect a calming response spread by word of mouth. One of these earliest prayers, recorded in the 14th century on Mount Athos in Greece (Benson, 1993), required participants to concentrate on their breathing and to repeat to themselves on each exhalation, "Lord Jesus Christ, have mercy on me." Like other meditative practices, participants were instructed to discard intrusive thoughts passively and return to the repetitive prayer (Benson, 1993). Until the 18th century in the Western Hemisphere, medicine was the domain of the church, and monks treated the majority of physical and emotional symptoms. Thus, chanting and repetitious prayers may be considered the beginnings of formal meditative practices specifically designed to mitigate stress and anxiety (Joseph, 1998).

In the 1960s, a form of "westernized" style in the Hindu tradition was started in the United States. Called "transcendental meditation" (TM), it was brought to this country by Maharishi Mahensh Yogi. TM gained immense popularity in America during a time of political and social unrest and activism. Part of TM's appeal was its secular emphasis, its elimination of unnecessary elements of traditional yoga practices, and its relative simplicity of initiation. It is worth noting that although the preponderance of the literature on meditation attests to its relaxing effects, some recent literature suggests that meditation may have widely differing effects on consciousness and the body, including the potential, under some circumstances, for physiological arousal (Cortright, 1997).

TYPES OF MEDITATION

As mentioned earlier, and for the purpose of our text, we refer to the practice of meditation as a group of techniques or procedures that have the potential of inducing the relaxation response. Although many different kinds of meditation are used to manage stress (concentration meditation, insight meditation, mindfulness practices, and strategic meditation; see Sethi, 1989, for a review), one element common to all forms of meditative practice is a stimulus, or thing, on which the meditator focuses his or her awareness. According to Naranjo and Ornstein (1971), this stimulus is something to "dwell upon," in effect, a focal device.

Therefore, meditative techniques may be categorized by the nature of their focal devices. Using this criterion, there are four general forms of meditative techniques:

1. *Mental Repetition.* This form of focal device involves dwelling on some mental event. The classic example of a mentally repetitive focal device is the "mantra," a word or phrase that is repeated over and over, usually silently to oneself. We include chanting in this category as well. TM uses a mantra format, with the mantra chosen from a list of Sanskrit words. Benson (1975, 1993) employs neutral words such as *one, peace,* or *love* to evoke the relaxation response. One Tibetan Buddhist mantra in verse form is "Om mani padme hum." In Sikh meditation, the word *Vahiguru,* which literally means "wonderful light," is repeated for 10–20 minutes daily.

2. *Physical Repetition.* This form of focal device involves focusing one's awareness on some physical act. An ancient Yogic (Hindu) style of repetitive meditation focuses on the physically repetitive act of breathing. There are many different approaches to Yoga (which means "union"), and one of them, Hatha Yoga, uses various forms of breath control and breath counting (called *pranayama*). Hatha Yoga focuses on physical education, and the aspect most recognized by the public involves the practice of postures (called *asanas*). The Moslem Sufis are known for their practice of continuous, circular dancing or whirling. The name "whirling dervishes" was given to the ancient practioners of this style. Finally, the popularity of jogging in the United States has given rise to the study of the effects of such activity. One effect reported by some joggers, either on the open road or on a treadmill, is a meditative-like experience, which could be caused by repetitive breathing or the repetitive sounds of feet pounding on the ground or treadmill.

3. *Problem Contemplation.* This focal device involves attempting to solve a problem with paradoxical components. The Zen *koan* is the classic example. In this case, a seemingly paradoxical problem is presented for contemplation. "What is the sound of one hand clapping?" is a commonly used *koan.*

4. *Visual Concentration.* This focal device involves visually focusing on an image—a picture, a candle flame, a leaf, a relaxing scene, or anything else. The *mandala,* a geometric design that features a square within a circle, representing the union of humanity within the universe, is often used in Eastern cultures for visual concentration.

MECHANISMS OF ACTION

Even after more than 60 years of scientific study, the exact mechanisms at work in meditation remain unclear. However, the focal device or stimulus to "dwell upon," considered the common and essential link between various forms of meditation, appears to be a potential source of applied exploration (Benson, 1975, 1993; Glueck & Strobel, 1975, 1978; Naranjo & Ornstein, 1971; Ornstein, 1972).

It appears that the role of the focal device is to allow the intuitive, non-ego-centered mode of thought processing (considered to be activity of the brain's right neocortical hemisphere) to dominate consciousness in place of the normally dominant, analytic, ego-centered mode of thought processing (thought to be left-hemisphere activity). The focal device appears to prepare the cortex for this shift by sufficiently engaging the left hemisphere's neural circuitry to allow the right hemisphere to become dominant (see Davidson, 1976; Naranjo & Ornstein, 1971; Ornstein, 1972). The focal device may occupy the left hemisphere by engaging it in some monotonous task, such as attending to a mantra, focused breathing, or a set of postures. Also, it may overwhelm and frustrate the left hemisphere. This would occur when the meditator dwells on seemingly paradoxical problems, as in Zen, or engages in intense physical activity, as practiced by the Sufis (whirling dervishes), the Tantrics, or perhaps even the American jogger.

When the focal device is successfully employed, the brain's order of processing appears to be altered. "When the rational (analytic) mind is silenced, the intuitive mode produces extraordinary awareness" (Capra, 1975, p. 26). This awareness, or heightened attention, is the goal of all meditative techniques.

Although the thought of meditation as a "right-hemisphere experience" is compelling, other researchers, using EEG and test performance data, have suggested that the left to right hemispheric shift considered to occur in the beginning stages of learning meditation is not as pronounced or simply does not occur, particularly in experienced, well-trained meditators (Earle, 1981; Pagano, 1981). However, because most people using meditation to induce relaxation as described in this text are likely classified as novices, the idea of a basic shift away from the left, verbal hemisphere to the right, intuitive hemisphere appears to remain a viable neurophysiological explanation (see Carrington, 1993).

Other EEG data suggest that meditation produces a burst in theta wave activity (often associated with a daydreaming-like state) (Herbert & Lehmann, 1977), along with increased frontal lobe alpha wave activity and coherence (associated with being awake and in a resting state) (Wallace, Benson, & Wilson, 1971). Jevning, Wallace, and Beideback (1992), in their review of the physiology of meditation, acknowledge these brain wave occurrences and suggest that increased EEG coherence "may be most significant in that this phenomenon correlates with subjective experience of pure consciousness and may be a predictor of other behavioral and physiological concomitants of meditation" (p. 419).

Austin (1998), in his summary of EEG data, acknowledges that episodes of "microawakening" and "microsleep" (going directly from sleeping to waking back to sleep again, without the usual stepwise progression of surface EEG findings) are common during meditation. He further suggests that this implies that the brain may pass suddenly through its brain wave activity, and that "during meditation, some unstable fragments of physiological mechanisms seem to be briefly 'loosened' and are then available to recombine in new, unexpected ways" (p. 93).

Part of this recombining may lead to the state of "extraordinary awareness" alluded to earlier. This state has been called many things. In the East, it is called *nirvana* or *satori*. A liberal translation of these words means "enlightenment." Similar translations for this state include "truth consciousness" or "being-cognition." In the early Western World, those few individuals who understood it used the term *supraconsciousness* or the "cosmic consciousness." Benson (1975, 1993) has called this state the "relaxation response," as described in the preceding chapter.

Although modern research investigations continue to attempt to qualify the neurophysiology of this supraconscious state, results remain inconclusive. Part of the difficulty in gathering more conclusive results is subject selection. Most participants in meditation studies are considered beginners by traditional standards. Current data suggest, however, that possible neurophysiological explanations include simultaneous EEG amplitude increases and decreases in various parts of the brain, particularly in alpha waves, and primarily in subjects with many years of meditative experience (Jevning et al., 1992; Walsh, 1996).

It is important at this juncture to emphasize that meditation and the achievement of the supraconscious state are not always the same! It should be made abundantly clear to the patient that meditation is the process, or series of techniques, that the meditator employs to achieve the goal of attaining the relaxation response and its associated supraconsciousness.

THERAPEUTIC HALLMARKS

As just mentioned, the "extraordinary awareness" of the relaxation response, or supraconsciousness state, is the desired goal of the devoted practitioners of all meditative styles. However, it is important for the clinician *and* the patient alike to understand that achievement of this state is never assured, and that this state may not be achieved every time, even by very experienced meditators. Given this fact, the question must then arise,

"Is the time spent in the meditative session wasted if the meditator is unable to achieve the supraconscious state?" The answer to this question is a resounding No! Positive therapeutic growth can be achieved without reaching the supraconscious state. The rationale for this statement lies in the fact there exist several "therapeutic hallmarks" inherent in the process of meditation as one approaches the supraconscious state. While Shapiro (1978), in his seminal work, discusses five steps in the meditative process: (1) difficulty in breathing, (2) wandering mind, (3) relaxation, (4) detached observation, and (5) higher state of consciousness, we have chosen to describe and expand upon the hallmarks we see in the meditative process.

The first and most fundamental of these hallmarks resides in practice itself. Even the ancient Hindu and Zen scriptures on meditation acknowledge that the attempt to achieve the supraconscious state is far more important than actually reaching it. By simply taking time to meditate, the patient is making a conscious effort to improve his or her health and reduce the effects of excessive stress. Similarly, by emphasizing to the patient the importance of simply meditating, rather than achieving the supraconscious state, the clinician removes much of the competitive, or success-versus-failure, component in this process. As summarized nicely by Kabat-Zinn (1993), "Practice simply means inviting yourself to embody calmness, mindfulness, and equanimity right here, right now, in this moment, as best you can" (p. 267).

The second hallmark is a noticeable increase in somatic relaxation: a decline in oxygen consumption (by as much as 40%) and a lowering of respiratory rate (by as much as 50%) (Farrow & Herbert, 1982), reduced sensitivity to CO_2 (Kesterson & Clinch, 1989), acute decline of adrenocortical activity (Bevan, 1980), an increase in galvanic stein response (GSR) activity (which is inversely related to stress) (Farrow & Herbert, 1982; O'Halloran et al., 1985), and decreases in heart rate and blood pressure (Murphy & Donovan, 1988; Shapiro & Walsh, 1984). The combination of these and other physiological factors leads to an autogenically induced state of somatic relaxation. This awakened state of hypometabolic functioning referred to in the literature is therapeutic in that (1) the body is placed into a mode equal or superior to sleep with regard to the restorative functions performed (Jevning et al., 1992; Orme-Johnson & Farrow, 1978) and (2) ergotropic stimulation of afferent proprioceptive impulses is reduced, and trophotropic responses are enhanced (Davidson, 1976; Gellhorn & Kiely, 1972).

The third hallmark is that of detached observation (see Shapiro, 1978). In the Indian scriptures, this is described as a state in which the meditators remain "a spectator resting in him- or herself" as he observes his environment. In this state egoless, passive state of observation, the meditator simply "coexists" with the environment rather than confronting or attempting to master it. It is a nonanalytic, intuitive state. One similar experience that many individuals have had is that of "highway hypnosis," a state often experienced by individuals driving on monotonous expressways. At one point they may notice that they are at Exit 6; in what seems a mere moment later, they may notice they are at Exit 16 yet have no immediate recollection of the 10 intervening exits. Many refer to this as a "daydreaming state." It is important to note that the driver of the car is fully capable of driving; this is not a sleep state. Had an emergency arisen, the driver would have been able to react appropriately. Therefore, the clinician should explain that this state is not one of lethargy or total passivity, which happens to be a concern for many patients.

The final step in the meditative experience is the "supraconscious state" or *nirvana*. This appears to be a summation of all the previous states except that it is more intense. Davidson (1976) and Sethi (1989) have characterized its nature:

1. A positive mood (tranquillity, peace of mind)
2. A dissolving of worry and anxiety
3. An experience of unity, or oneness, with the environment; what the ancients called the joining of microcosm (human) with macrocosm (universe)
4. A sense of ineffability (being inexpressible or transcendent)
5. A feeling of active peace
6. An alteration in time–space relationships
7. An enhanced sense of reality and meanings
8. A development of new creative energy
9. Paradoxicality, that is, acceptance of things that seem paradoxical in ordinary consciousness

Given that most clinicians receive myriad questions concerning the active nature of meditation, we have placed some common experiences on a continuum (see Figure 11.1). This continuum of meditative experiences is not completely progressive from one discrete state to the next. A meditator may progress from any one state to another and then back again. Also, varying degrees of depth may be experienced within each state. Note, specifically, that boredom and distracting thoughts often precede more

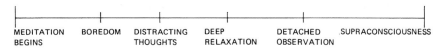

MEDITATION   BOREDOM   DISTRACTING   DEEP   DETACHED   SUPRACONSCIOUSNESS
BEGINS   THOUGHTS   RELAXATION   OBSERVATION

Figure 11.1. A meditative continuum.

positive effects. The clinician should explain to the patient that this is a natural occurrence, and that he or she should be tolerant when this happens
and simply return his or her concentration to the focal device.

As mentioned earlier, the meditator should be discouraged from evaluating the meditative sessions in a success–failure paradigm. Simple, descriptive reports to the clinician are useful to monitor the course of the activity for
a period of 2–3 weeks. A daily log might be kept by the patient, as long as it
is descriptive and not evaluative.

RESEARCH ON THE CLINICAL APPLICATIONS AND EFFECTS OF MEDITATION

Well-controlled research studies on the clinical effectiveness of meditation are increasingly abundant (see Austin, 1998; Lehrer & Woolfolk,
1984; Scotton, Chinen, & Battista, 1993; for discussions and reviews). These
studies recognize a potentially wide range of stress-related therapeutic
applications for meditation. One general area of benefit entails strategies
for refocusing or retraining attention. As noted by Sethi (1989),

> The importance of strategic meditation (SM), in enabling cognitive
> shift, becomes a crucial tool in allocation of attention as a resource for
> stress management. This proposition is based on the conceptualization
> that consciousness is a cybernetic system that can be managed through
> attention via strategic choice (meditation). (p. 86)

Other, specific meditative techniques have been found useful for the
following:

1. In the treatment of generalized autonomic arousal and excessive
   ergotrophic tone (Astin, 1997; Benson, 1985; Shapiro, Schwartz, &
   Bonner, 1998)
2. In the treatment of anxiety disorders (Kabat-Zinn et al., 1992;
   Lehrer & Woolfolk, 1984; Miller, Fletcher, & Kabat-Zinn, 1995)
3. For increasing "self-actualization," "positive mental health," and
   "happiness enhancement" (Benson, 1985; Kutz et al., 1985; Smith,
   Compton, & West, 1995)
4. In the treatment of psoriasis (Gaston, Crombez, & Dupuis, 1989;
   Kabat-Zinn et al., 1998)
5. For treatment of binge eating (Kristeller & Hallett, 1999)
6. As an adjunct in the treatment of cancer (Brennan & Stevens, 1998;
   Gawler, 1998)
7. To reduce the impact of patients with fibromyalgia (Kaplan,
   Goldenberg, & Galvin-Nadeau, 1993)

8. In the regulation of chronic pain (Kabat-Zinn, Lipworth, & Burney, 1985)
9. As an intervention for patients with myocardial infarction (MI) or coronary artery disease (CAD) (Buselli & Stuart, 1999; Zamarra, Schneider, Besseghini, Robinson, & Salerno, 1996)
10. As an adjunct in the treatment of essential hypertension (Barnes, Schneider, Alexander, & Staggers, 1997; Benson et al., 1974; Sothers & Anchor, 1989)
11. As an adjunct in the treatment of drug and alcohol abuse (Benson, 1969; Brooks, 1994; Gelderloos, Walton, Orme-Johnson, & Alexander, 1991; Lazar, 1975)

Having provided a rationale for the clinical use of meditation, we now examine its implementation.

HOW TO IMPLEMENT MEDITATION

The following discussion is provided as a guide to the clinical use of meditation.

Preparation

In addition to the general precautions for relaxation mentioned in an earlier chapter, the following preparations are important for the implementation of meditation:

1. Determine whether the patient has any specific contraindications for the use of meditation. For example, affective or thought disorders may possibly be exacerbated by meditation. Similarly, the clinician should use care with patients who demonstrate a tendency to employ nonpsychotic fantasy, as in the schizoid personality. There are also possible instances of muscle or gastrointestinal spasms. It should also be noted that some compulsive or action-oriented individuals appear to have greater difficulty in learning to meditate effectively than do less compulsive individuals. Boredom and distracting thoughts appear to compete with meditation.

2. Inquire into the patient's previous knowledge or experience in meditation. Pay particular attention to any mention of cultic or religious aspects. These are the most common misconceptions that patients find troublesome. Some may feel that by meditating, they will be performing a sacrilegious act.

3. Provide the patient with a basic explanation of meditation.

4. Describe to the patient the proper environment for the practice of meditation (see next section).

Components

In his original book, *The Relaxation Response*, and in later reviews and updates of his work, Benson (1975, 1993, 1996) describes the following basic components in successful meditation:

1. A quiet environment
2. A mental device
3. A passive attitude
4. A comfortable position

In elaborating and expanding Benson's paradigm to some extent, the first condition we recommend is a *quiet environment*, absent of external stimuli that would compete with the meditative process. Many patients state that it is impossible to find such a place. If this is so, then some creativity may be needed. The patient may wish to use music or environmental recordings to "mask" distractions. For example, the steady hum of a fan or an air conditioner may effectively drown out noise. If this is not possible, the patient may choose to cover his or her eyes and/or use earplugs to reduce external stimulation.

The second condition (for physically passive meditation) is a *comfortable position*. Muscle tension can be disruptive to the meditative process. When first learning, the patient should have most of his or her weight supported. The notable exceptions would be the head and neck. By keeping the spine straight, and the head and neck unsupported, there will be sufficient muscle tension to keep the patient from falling asleep. If the patient does continually falls asleep during meditation, then he or she should use a posture that requires greater muscle tension.

The third condition, a *focal device*, is the link between all forms of meditation, even the physically active forms, as discussed earlier. The focal device appears to act by allowing the brain to alter it normal mode of processing.

The fourth condition, a *passive attitude*, has been called "passive volition" or "passive attention" by some. Benson (1975) states that this "passive attitude is perhaps the most important element" (p. 113). With this attitude, the patient "allows" the meditative act to occur rather than striving to control the meditative process. As Benson (1993) has noted, "Don't worry about how well you're doing. When other thoughts come to mind, simply say to yourself, 'Oh, well,' and gently return to the repetition [focal device]" (p. 240).

If the patient is unable to adopt this attitude, he or she will ask questions:

"Am I doing this correctly?"—usually indicative of concern regarding performance.

"How long does this take?"—usually indicative of concern for time.
"What is a *good* level of proficiency?"—usually indicative of concern for
performance outcome rather than process.
"Should I try to remember everything I feel?"—usually indicative of
overanalysis.

The more the patient dwells on such thoughts, the less successful he or she
will be. Distracting thoughts are completely normal during the meditative
process and are to be expected. However, adoption of a passive attitude
allows the patient to recognize distracting thoughts and simply return
concentration to the focal device.

The fifth and final condition that we would recognize is a *receptive
psychophysiological environment.* By this we mean a set of internal psychophysiological conditions that will allow the patient to meditate. It has
been noted, for example, that psychophysiologically aroused patients have
a very low success rate when they attempt to meditate. Therefore, it may be
necessary to teach the patients to put themselves in a more "receptive condition" for meditating (this applies to biofeedback, hypnosis, and guided
imagery as well). To achieve this receptive condition, the patient may wish
to use a few neuromuscular relaxation techniques before the meditation,
in order to reduce excessive muscle tension. We have recommended in
some circumstances that the patient take a hot bath before meditating. In
fact, some patients have reported high levels of success when they meditate
while sitting in a hot tub. We have found this infrequently mentioned
concept of psychophysiological receptivity to be a critical variable in many
clinical experiences. Therefore, the meditative continuum is expanded
(Figure 11.1) to include this variable (see Figure 11.2).

Example Protocol

This section provides an example of a protocol for a physically passive,
mantra-like form of meditation. Use it as a guideline and make necessary
revisions in the margins in order to tailor the protocol to your specific
needs.

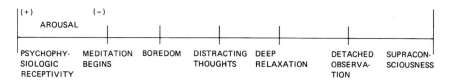

Figure 11.2. Arousal and the meditative continuum.

Background Information.   The purpose is to familiarize you with the use of meditation as a way of reducing the stress in your life. These instructions consist of background information and specific directions for the use of four techniques from which you may choose in order to meditate. Follow all the instructions closely. Later you may wish to modify a part of the technique to fit a personal preference or situation, but in the initial learning phase, you should do all the exercises exactly as instructed. Once you have chosen one of the meditative techniques, employ that technique as instructed for 15 to 20 minutes of uninterrupted meditation once or twice a day.

Some people, not familiar with the nature and origins of meditation, confuse its pure form with its possible uses. There are important differences. The techniques of meditation presented here are derived from ancient Eastern philosophies that have then been blended with modern relaxation and stress-reduction techniques. Although some of the techniques were used in the practice of specific religions, to say that meditation is a religious practice is like saying wine is a religious instrument simply because in many religions wine is used in the ceremonies. Meditation is a technique of quieting the mind, which, of course, is a necessary prerequisite for reducing anxiety and tension.

As taught here, a quiet mind is an end in itself. What you do with this valuable skill is, of course, up to you.

The fundamentals of meditation are often misunderstood, as meditation itself is difficult to define. It is not a physiological state. Nor is it any specific psychological feeling or a religion. Rather, as used here, meditation is a technique so basic that it has transcended time, cultures, races, religions, and ideologies. The physiological, psychological, and philosophical goals of meditation cannot be achieved without training, and mastery of technique cannot be achieved except through continued practice.

Although there are many types of meditation, the most popular meditative techniques in Western society are derived from specific practices of ancient Yoga and Zen. Each type of meditation represents a variation of purpose and technique. Those presented here are thought to be the best suited for stress reduction. The technique is the easiest to learn and the one most devoid of cultic, religious, and spiritual overtones. It is complete and can be all the meditation one will ever need; or, it may serve as an introduction to more specific types.

There are several essential steps you should follow when learning to meditate.

A first essential step is to find a quiet environment, both external and internal. A quiet room away from others who are not meditating is essential, especially while learning. Take the phone off the hook, or at least go into a room without one. Generally, do whatever can be done to reduce external noise. If you cannot completely eliminate the noise, which is often the case in busy households or in college dorms, and so forth, use ear plugs. Play a record or tape of some soft instrumental sounds, or use any of the numerous environmental sound recordings that are commercially available. Even the steady hum of a fan or an air conditioner can effectively block out, or mask, external noise. You may also wish to turn down, or completely off, any lights in the room. Now that you have quieted your external environment, the next essential step is to work on quieting your internal environment. One way is to reduce muscle tension, which represents one of the biggest obstacles to successful meditation. Spend some time relaxing your muscles. One way is to reduce muscle tension is to sit comfortably, You may not feel like a real meditator unless you are sitting in the Eastern, cross-legged lotus position, but that takes a great deal of flexibility and training. For now, sit comfortably on the floor, or, better yet, sit in a straight-backed, comfortable chair, feet on the floor, legs not crossed, hands resting on the thighs, with fingers slightly opened, not interlocked. You should sit still, but remember, meditation is not a trance. If you are uncomfortable or feel too much pressure on any one spot, move. If you have an itch, scratch. Do not assume a tight inflexible position or attitude. Relax. It is best not to lie down or support your head, or you will tend to fall asleep. Keep the head, neck, and spine in a straight vertical line. A small but significant amount of muscle tension is needed to maintain this posture, and this effort helps prevent sleep from occurring, while at the same time creating an optimal position for learning to meditate.

There are many types of meditation. Some focus on inner forces, inner power, or self-identity. Others focus on external things, such as words, lights, or sounds. Meditation is simply a natural process. And though techniques may differ, the core experience is essentially the same. The basic meditative experience involves concentrating passively on some stimulus, whether it be a word, an image, your breath, or nothing at all. The stimulus acts as a vehicle to keep distracting thoughts out of your mind. And yet, the harder you concentrate on the stimulus, the harder it is to meditate. Although this sounds confusing, it is true, simply because meditation is a "passive" activity. You must allow the stimulus, whatever it is, to interact passively with you. You must learn to concentrate passively on your stimulus. The skill of passive concentration takes time to develop—so don't be discouraged if it seems difficult for the first few weeks. Just continue to practice.

Actual Instruction.   You are now ready to begin the actual instruction. To begin with, close your eyes. Notice the quietness. Much of our sensory input comes in through our eyes. Just by closing your eyes, you can do much to quiet the mind.

The Use of Breath Concentration.   What we are going to do now is clear our minds. Not of all thoughts, but of ongoing thoughts that use the imagination to increase stress arousal. Focus on your breathing. Shift your awareness from the hectic external world to the quiet and relaxing internal world.

As you breathe in, think in. Let the air out. Think out. In and out. Concentrate on your breathing. Think in. Think out. Breath in through your nose and let the air out through the mouth very effortlessly. Just open your mouth and let the air flow out. Do not force it. Become involved with the breathing process. Concentrate on your breathing. In and out. Now, each time you breathe in, I want you to feel how cold the air is, and each time you breathe out, feel how warm and moist the air is. Do that now. (*Pause 30 seconds.*)

The Use of One.   Now we would like to replace the concentration on breathing with the use of a mantra. A mantra is a vehicle that is often a word or phrase to help keep your mind from wandering back to day-dreams. An example of a mantra, suggested by Herbert Benson in his book *The Relaxation Response,* is simply the word *one* (o-n-e). This is a soft, non-cultic word that has little meaning as a number. Every time you breathe out, say the word *one* to yourself. Say *one.* *One.* Say it softly. *One.* Say the word *one* without moving your lips. Say it yet more softly, until it becomes just a mental thought. (*Pause 75 seconds here.*)

The Use of *Om*.   The word *one* is an example of a mantra: a vehicle to help clear your mind. By concentrating on a word without emotion or significance, your mind's order of processing begins to change. The mind begins to wander, with a quieter, more subtle state of consciousness. Many people like to use words from the ancient Sanskrit language, feeling that they represent soft sounds with spiritual significances that can also be used as a focus for contemplation. The universal mantra is the word *om;* spelled o-m, it also means one. Each time you breathe out say the word *om. Om. Om.* Breathe softly and normally, but now do not concentrate on your breathing. Repeat the mantra in your mind. Just think of saying it. Do not actually move your lips. Just think of it. Do not concentrate on your breathing. Let the mantra repeat itself in your mind. Do not force it. Just let it flow. Gradually the mantra will fade. The mind will be quiet. Occasionally, the quiet will be broken by sporadic thoughts. Let them come. Experience them, then let them leave your mind as quickly as they entered, by simply going stronger to your mantra. Let us now use *om* as a mantra. Say the word *om, om.* (*Pause here 75 seconds.*) Remember, the mantra is a vehicle to help clear the mind when you cannot do so without it. Also remember, keep your movements to a minimum, but if you are uncomfortable, move. If you are worried about time, look at a clock. Discomfort or anxiety will prevent full attainment of the relaxed state.

The Use of Counting.   A final mantra that you may select if you find your mind wandering too much requires a little more concentration than the three previous meditation techniques.

As you breathe out, begin to count backward from 10 to 1. Say a single number to yourself each time you exhale. As you say the number, try to picture that number in your "mind's eye." When you reach 1, go back to 10 and start over. Let us do that now. (*Pause here 3 minutes.*)

Reawaken.   Now I want to bring attention back to yourself and the world around you. I will count from 1 to 10. With each number you will feel your mind become more and more awake and your body more and more refreshed. When I reach 10, open your eyes, and you will feel the best you've felt all day—you will feel alert, refreshed, full of energy, and eager to resume your activities. Let us begin: 1–2 you are beginning to feel more alert, 3–4–5 you are more and more awake, 6–7 now begin to stretch your hands and feet, 8 now begin to stretch your arms and legs, 9–10 open your eyes *now!* You feel alert, awake; your mind is clear and your body refreshed.

Having read the preceding example, please note the following points:

1. In the example, the patient was given four different mantras from which to choose. Such "freedom of choice" may increase clinical effectiveness. It is important to ask the patient which mantra was best for him or her, and why. Such questions foster introspection and self-understanding.
2. The meditation example contains a *reawaken* step, as does the neuromuscular relaxation example in Chapter 12.
3. The clinician should indicate, at some point, when the patient should meditate. We have found once or twice a day to be sufficient, 15 to 20 minutes in duration for each session. As with neuromuscular relaxation, before lunch or before dinner is generally the best time to meditate, although practice in the morning may provide a relaxing start for the entire day.

SUMMARY

In this chapter we discussed the first of several techniques that can be used to engender the relaxation response, specifically, the technique of meditation. Let us review several of the focal points:

1. The history of meditation is rich, vast, and provides the rationale for its clinical applications.
2. The practice of meditation is one way to engender a relaxation response. We will review other techniques in later chapters (e.g., neuromuscular relaxation, controlled respiration).
3. The "supraconscious state," as described in this chapter, may be considered one of the end points along a meditative continuum within the relaxation response.
4. Research has now clearly shown that the relaxation response, as engendered by the practice of meditation via a focal device, can be useful in the treatment of a wide variety of stress-related disorders.
5. Within this chapter, a typical protocol for teaching meditation has been provided. The clinician should tailor it to the personal needs of each patient when practical.
6. Finally, always practice meditation, or any other relaxation technique, in an office setting before assigning it as homework. This gives you the opportunity to (1) observe whether the technique is done properly, and (2) talk with the patient about his or her experiences.

12

Voluntary Control of Respiration Patterns

Controlled respiration is one of the oldest and certainly the single, most efficient acute intervention for the mitigation and treatment of excessive stress. Any clinician treating patients who manifest excessive stress syndromes should consider controlled respiration as an potentially suitable intervention for virtually all patients. The purpose of this chapter is to discuss the uses of voluntary control of *respiration patterns* in the treatment of excessive stress. As used in this text, this term refers to the process by which the patient exerts voluntary control over his or her breathing pattern—in effect, breath control. There are hundreds of diverse patterns of controlled respiration; we examine several that we feel have particular introductory utility for the clinician concerned with the treatment of the stress response. The exercises presented in this chapter are by no means inclusive. We have simply chosen several patterns that are simple to learn and effective. Again, the goal of voluntary, controlled respiration in the treatment of excessive stress is to have the patient voluntarily alter his or her rhythmic pattern of breathing to create a more relaxed state.

HISTORY

As mentioned earlier, voluntary control of respiration patterns (breath control) is perhaps the oldest stress-reduction technique known. It has been used for thousands of years to reduce anxiety and to promote a generalized state of relaxation. The history of voluntary breath control dates back centuries before Christ. References to voluntary breath control for obtaining a relaxation state can be found in the Hindu tradition of Hatha Yoga. In fact, "the word *hatha* itself comes from the Sanskrit root *ha*, meaning sun, and *tha*, meaning moon, and refers to the incoming and outgoing breaths in breathing" (Sethi, 1989, p. 69). Thus, Hatha Yoga (the yoga of postures) is built on various patterns of breathing known as *pranayama*. The term *prana* literally means "life force," and more than 3000 years ago, yogis proclaimed that "life is in the breath." Therefore, we can see that *pranayama* loosely translates into breath control or breath restraint (Fried, 1993).

While in ancient India breath control was developing in the Hindu tradition, the Chinese were practicing it as well. The development of the movement arts of T'ai Chi and Kung Fu both included controlled breathing as an essential component. These "martial arts" continue to enjoy popularity in the United States.

Perhaps the most widely used form of breath control today is the procedure for "natural" childbirth, in which various types of controlled breathing are used to reduce pain for the mother during delivery and to facilitate the descent of the child through the birth canal.

In this chapter, we focus on the voluntary, controlled breathing patterns that seem most useful as general aids to relaxation, without any specific goal other than common stress reduction.

BASIC PATTERNS OF BREATHING

In this section, we describe briefly the fundamentals involved in the breathing process by examining the four phases of the respiratory cycle and describing three basic types of breathing.

According to Hewitt (1977), and elaborated upon by Austin (1998) and Fried (1993), four distinct phase of the breathing cycle are relevant in learning voluntary control of respiration patterns (the clinician may find this cursory phasic division useful in teaching any form of deep-breathing technique):

1. *Inhalation or inspiration.* Incidently, it is no coincidence that the word *inspiration* is used to recognize the connective link between breathing and vital energy (i.e., we all have at times felt "inspired" by a creative idea or an influential other). Inhalation occurs as air is taken into the nose or mouth, descends via the trachea, the bronchi, and bronchioles, and finally inflates the alveoli, which are the air sacs constituting major portions of the lobes of the lungs. As the lungs expand, their stretch receptors tighten, which in turn sends inhibitory signals from the vagus nerve to the brain stem, signaling inhalation to stop.

2. *The pause that follows inhalation.* During this pause, the lungs remain inflated.

3. *Exhalation or expiration.* Again, note the connection between breathing and life force in the term *expiration.* For example, when someone passes away, we say that they have expired, or that they have breathed their last breath: in essence, that their life energy is now gone. Exhalation occurs as the lungs are deflated, emptying the waste gases from the alveoli.

4. *The pause that follows the exhalation phase.* During this phase, the lungs are at rest in a deflated state.

Ballentine (1976) describes three basic types of breathing that differ primarily according to the nature of the inhalation initiating the breathing cycle: clavicular, thoracic, and diaphragmatic.

The clavicular breath, the shortest and shallowest of the three, can be observed as a slight vertical elevation of the clavicles, combined with a slight expansion of the thoracic cage upon inhalation.

The thoracic breath represents (in varying degrees) a deeper breath—deeper in the sense that a greater amount of air is inhaled, more alveoli are inflated, and the lobes of the lungs are expanded to a greater degree. It is initiated by activation of the intercostal muscles, which expand the thoracic cage up and outward. The thoracic breath can be observed as a greater expansion of the thoracic cage, followed by an elevation of the clavicles on inhalation. Thoracic breathing is the most common breathing pattern.

Finally, the diaphragmatic breath represents the deepest of all the breaths, with the most air inhaled and the greatest number of alveoli inflated. In addition, for the first time, the lowest levels of the lungs are inflated. The lower third of the lungs contains the greater part of the blood when the individual stands vertically; therefore, the diaphragmatic breath oxygenates a greater quantity of blood per breathing cycle than the other types of breathing. During the diaphragmatic breath, the diaphragm (a thin, dome-shaped sheet of muscle that separates the chest cavity and the abdomen) flattens downward during inhalation. This causes the abdominal muscles to relax and rise, and pushes the organs in the abdominal cavity forward, which creates a partial vacuum and allows air to descend into the lungs. Thus, the movement of the diaphragm becomes the major cause of the deep inhalation. The full diaphragmatic breath may be observed as the abdominal cavity expands outward, followed by expansion of the thoracic cage, and, finally, elevation of the clavicles.

Variations of the diaphragmatic breath are considered by many to be the simplest and most effective form of controlled respiration in the reduction of excessive stress. Therefore, we limit our discussion to the role of diaphragmatic patterns in reducing excessive stress. It would, however, be helpful to the clinician to learn to identify all three basic patterns of breathing.

MECHANISMS OF ACTION

Although the specific mechanisms involved in stress reduction via breath control may differ from technique to technique, a general therapeutic factor is thought to be the ability of the diaphragmatic breath to induce a temporary trophotropic state. Hymes (1980) notes that the tone of the sympathetic and parasympathetic nervous systems is greatly affected by the process of respiration. Harvey (1978) recognizes that "diaphragmatic breathing stimulates both the solar plexus and the right vagus nerve in a manner that enervates the parasympathetic nervous system, thus facilitating full relaxation" (p. 14).

Expiration is also thought to affect the relaxation response. In fact, the mere act of breathing out may increase parasympathetic tone (Ballentine, 1976) and serve to slightly decrease neural firing in the amygdala and hippocampus (Frysinger & Harper, 1989). Moreover, prolonged expiration, along with quieter breathing, may further reduce neural firing in the amygdala that could lead to physiological calming (Zhang, Harper, & Ni, 1986). It is notable that during most types of diaphragmatic breathing, expiration is protracted. Interestingly, the normal person spends less time breathing in (about 43%) than breathing out; however, monks practicing the meditative art of zazen have been known to increase the exhalation phase of their respiratory cycle to around 75% (Austin, 1998). Austin also notes that breathing techniques that prolong exhalation may increase the inhibitory tone of the vagus nerve and reduce respiratory drive in the brain stem. In summary, Hymes (1980) states, "Autonomic functioning may be voluntarily shifted back to calm by exercising conscious breath control (with an associated reduction of anxiety and pain)" (p. 10).

Independent of the predominately physiological mechanisms, voluntary breath control may prove therapeutic from a cognitive perspective as well. The rationale for this statement comes from the supposition that concentration on respiration patterns may serve to enhance a perception of internal control, along with ways to compete with obsessive thought patterns, and maybe even compulsive behaviors.

CLINICAL RESEARCH

1. In a frequently cited study of 105 male participants awaiting imminent electric shocks to the hand, those who were instructed to regulate their breathing to only eight breaths per minute evidenced lower subjective arousal, and less change in skin resistance and finger pulse volume than control participants not taught respiratory control (McCaul, Solomon, & Holmes, 1979).

2. Controlled breathing has been used effectively as part of the treatment of patients with hyperventilation (Han, Stegen, de Valck, & Clement, 1996; Hegel et al., 1989; Holloway, 1994).

3. The benefits of controlled breathing have been observed in 76 post-MI patients (van Dixhoorn, 1998) and also patients experiencing noncardiac chest pain (Van Peski-Oosterbaan, Spinhoven, van Rood, Van der Does, & Bruschke, 1997).

4. Cognitive-behavioral interventions for panic disorder, which rely on deep, controlled respiration, have been associated with decreased frequency and intensity of attacks (DiFilippo & Overholser, 1999). After receiving an automatic implantable cardioverter defibrillator (AICD), a 36-year-old woman with panic and agoraphobia underwent breathing retraining as part of an effective treatment strategy to decrease anxiety and depression scores.

HOW TO IMPLEMENT

Voluntary breath control appears to be the most flexible of the interventions for the reduction of excessive stress. It can be used under a wide variety of environmental and behavioral conditions.

Despite its versatility, voluntary breath control should not be used without precautions. When breathing is used as a meditative device, the precautions discussed in the chapter on meditation are relevant. The primary precaution, relatively unique to voluntary breath control, is that regarding hyperventilation. Simply defined, hyperventilation is a condition in which the patient "overbreathes," which can quickly create the condition of hypocapnia, a decreased production and availability of CO_2. Hypocapnia results in decreased blood flow to the extremities and to the brain (Fried, 1993). The symptoms of hyperventilation, which include dizziness, panic, fatigue, feelings of suffocation, chest pain, stomach cramps, racing heart, trembling, loss of consciousness, tenseness, hot flashes, and nausea, overlap considerably with symptoms of stress and anxiety. Many of these symptoms could appear after several minutes of prolonged hyperventilation. According to Grossman and DeSwart (1984), dizziness, tiredness, and feelings of suffocation and panic are the most commonly reported hyperventilation symptoms.

Fried (1993) offers the following insights, recommendations, and additional precautions in the use of diaphragmatic breathing:

1. Some individuals with a high stress profile may unknowingly hold their diaphragm in a partially contracted position; therefore, diaphragmatic breathing may initially produce cramps.

2. If pain or discomfort is experienced due to muscle or tissue injury, then the diaphragmatic breathing exercise should be stopped.
3. In cases where metabolic acidosis may occur, such as severe hypoglycemia, kidney disease, heart disease, or diabetes, approval from a physician should be acquired before beginning diaphragmatic breathing.
4. Since diaphragmatic breathing may significantly lower blood pressure, individuals with normally low blood pressure or syncope should use the technique cautiously.

It is interesting to note that some clinicians (Barlow & Craske, 1989; Hardonk & Beumer, 1979; Lum, 1975) use a procedure known as a "hyperventilation challenge," which involves having the patient breath rapidly and deeply for about 2 minutes in an attempt to induce, and then modify, hyperventilation-like symptoms by breathing more diaphragmatically. However, not all clinicians support the use of this technique (Fried, 1993).

Listed below are three diaphragmatic breathing exercises reported to be useful in promoting a more relaxed state. In teaching any form of diaphragmatic breathing, the clinician must monitor the activities of the patient to assure proper techniques. Hewitt (1977) offers the following guidelines, which we believe are appropriate for all forms of diaphragmatic breathing:

> You fill the lungs to a point of fullness without strain or discomfort (p. 90). If after retention [of the inhalation] the air bursts out noisily, the suspension has been overprolonged; the air should be released in a steady smooth stream. ... Similarly, following the empty pause, the air should unhurriedly and quietly begin its ascent of the nostrils [as the new inhalation begins]. (p. 73)

We consider these general guidelines useful to avoid patients' overbreathing, as well as other inappropriate breathing practices. These guidelines should be followed when instructing a patient in each of the following three breathing exercises.

Breathing Exercise 1

This breathing technique may be thought of as a "complete breath." In fact, variations of this breath appear with similar names in the Yogic literature. The technique is extremely simple to complete. In order to assist the clinician in teaching the exercise to patients, we present the four phases of breath described by Hewitt (1977).

Inhalation. The inhalation should begin through the nose if possible. The nose is preferred to the mouth because of its ability to filter and warm the incoming air. On inhalation, the abdomen should begin to move outward, followed by expansion of the chest. The length of the inhalation should be 2 to 3 seconds (or to some point less than that in which the lungs and chest expand without discomfort).

Pause after Inhalation. There should be no pause. Inhalation should transfer smoothly into the beginning of exhalation.

Exhalation. Here, the air is expired (through the mouth or the nose, whichever is more comfortable). The length of this exhalation should be 2 to 3 seconds.

Pause after Exhalation. This pause should last only 1 second, then inhalation should begin again in a smooth manner. We have found that this exercise can be repeated by many patients for several minutes without the initiation of hyperventilation. However, patients should usually be instructed to stop when light-headedness occurs.

Breathing Exercise 2

This breathing exercise may be thought of as a form of "counting breath," of which variations appear in the Yogic literature. The term *counting* is applied to this exercise because the patient is asked literally to count to him- or herself the number of seconds each of the four phases of the exercise will last. In order to assist the clinician in teaching this exercise, we present the four phases of breathing described by Hewitt (1977).

Inhalation. The inhalation should begin through the nose if possible. The abdomen should begin to move outward, followed by expansion of the chest. The length of the inhalation should be 2 seconds (or to some point less than that in which the lungs and chest expand without discomfort). The length of the inhalation should be counted silently, as one thousand, two thousand.

Pause after Inhalation. There should be a pause here, following the 2-second inhalation. The counted pause here should be 1 second in duration.

Exhalation. Here, the air is expelled. The counted exhalation should be 3 seconds in duration.

Pause after Exhalation. This counted pause should last 1 second. The next inhalation should follow smoothly. We have found that this exercise can be repeated by many patients for several minutes without the occurrence of hyperventilation. However, patients should usually be instructed to stop when light-headedness occurs.

Breathing Exercise 3

This technique, developed by G. S. Everly, is designed to rapidly induce (within 30 to 60 seconds) a state of relaxation. Research has shown it to be effective in reducing muscle tension and subjective reports of anxiety, as well as having some potential for reducing heart rate (see Everly, 1979b,c; Vanderhoof, 1980). The following description is presented as if instructing a patient:

> During the course of an average day, many of us find ourselves in anxiety-producing situations. Our heart rates increase, our stomachs may become upset, and our thoughts may race uncontrollably through our minds. It is during such episodes that we require fast-acting relief from our stressful reactions. The brief exercise described below has been found effective in reducing most of the stress reaction that we suffer from during acute exposures to stressors—it is, in effect, a quick way to "calm down" in the face of a stressful situation.
>
> The basic mechanism for stress reduction in this exercise involves deep breathing. The procedure is as follows:
>
> *Step 1.* Assume a comfortable position. Rest your left hand (palm down) on top of your abdomen, over your navel. Now place your right hand so that it rests comfortably on your left. Your eyes can remain open. However, it is usually easier to complete Step 2 with your eyes closed (see Figure 12.1).
>
> *Step 2.* Imagine a hollow bottle, or pouch, lying internally beneath the point at which your hands are resting. Begin to inhale. As you inhale imagine that the air is entering through your nose and descending to fill that internal pouch. Your hands will rise as you fill the pouch with air. As you continue to inhale, imagine the pouch being filled to the top. Your rib cage and upper chest will continue the wavelike rise that was begun at your navel. The total length of your inhalation should be two seconds for the first week or two, then possibly lengthening to two and a half or three seconds as you progress in skill development (see Figure 12.2).
>
> *Step 3.* Hold your breath. Keep the air inside the pouch. Repeat to yourself the phrase, "My body is calm." This step should last no more than two seconds.
>
> *Step 4.* Slowly begin to exhale—to empty the pouch. As you do, repeat to yourself the phrase, "My body is quiet." As you exhale, you will feel your raised abdomen and chest recede. This step should last as long as the two preceding steps, or may last one second longer, after a

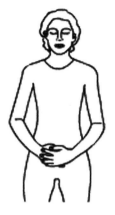 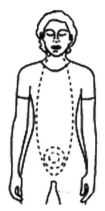

Figure 12.1. Step 1.   **Figure 12.2.** Step 2.

week or two of practice. (*Note:* Step 1 need only be used during the first week or so, as you learn to breathe deeply. Once you master that skill, you may omit that step.) Only repeat this four-step exercise three to five times in succession. Should you begin to feel light-headed, stop at that point. If light-headedness recurs with continued practice, simply shorten the length of the inhalation and/or decrease the number of times you repeat the exercise in succession.

Practice this exercise 10 to 20 times a day. Make it a ritual in the morning, afternoon, and evening, as well as during stressful situations. Because this form of relaxation is a skill, it is important to practice at least 10 to 20 times a day. At first you may not notice any on-the-spot relaxation. However, after a week or two of regular practice, you will increase your capabilities to relax temporarily. Remember, you must *practice regularly* if you are to master this skill. Regular, consistent practice of these daily exercises will ultimately lead to the development of a more calm and relaxed attitude—a sort of antistress attitude—and when you do have stressful moments, they will be far less severe.

SUMMARY

This chapter has presented a discussion of voluntary, controlled patterns of respiration for use in reducing excessive stress. As mentioned earlier, the goal of voluntary respiration in the treatment of excessive stress is to have the patient voluntarily alter his or her rhythmic pattern of breathing to create a more relaxed state.

1. Dating back to centuries before Christ, there is a rich and lengthy history of using breath control as a means to enhance relaxation.

2. There are three basic types of breathing patterns—clavicular, thoracic, and diaphragmatic. The first two are associated with (and may stimulate) a sympathetic response. The latter is associated with (and may stimulate) a parasympathetic response (see Ballentine, 1976). It has been found useful for the clinician to learn to recognize these patterns in patients and to teach them how to recognize these patterns in themselves.

3. Although the literature (especially that of Yoga) presents myriad diverse respiratory techniques for relaxation, we have focused in this chapter on diaphragmatic breathing. This emphasis is based on the conclusion that variations of diaphragmatic breathing are the simplest to teach and among the most effective for achieving a relaxed psychophysiological state. For these reasons, the clinician may find the variations of the diaphragmatic pattern most useful.

4. In the final analysis, the clinician needs to assess the suitability of using voluntary, controlled respiration with each patient on a case-by-case basis. The clinician may attempt to teach the three different exercises presented in this chapter in order to assess which may be of most utility. These variations of diaphragmatic breathing are not provided as a prescription, but as a sample of breath control techniques that have been beneficial in reducing excessive stress. Many other useful variations exist (see Fried, 1993; Hewitt, 1977; Jencks, 1977).

5. The primary precaution in the use of breath control in stress reduction regards the hyperventilation reaction. This is usually not a problem when the patient uses breathing exercises (such as those described in this chapter) for short time durations and ceases if light-headedness ensues. The Yogic literature reports that no more than 15 minutes of any hour should be spent in *pranayama* practice. Again, this topic should be addressed with patients individually.

6. In conclusion, Patel (1993) states that "if breath influences both the body and the mind, not only physical, mental, and emotional states are reflected in the pattern of breath, but through breathing we can also influence our physical, psychological, and spiritual well-being" (p. 119). This analysis certainly seems accurate. Additionally, teaching breath control may serve to enhance an overall perception of enhanced personal control.

13

Neuromuscular Relaxation

Chapter 10 presented a neurophysiological rationale for the use of the relaxation response in the treatment of stress-related disorders. In developing that rationale, we reviewed the research efforts of Gellhorn (1958a,b, 1964b, 1967), Weil (1974), and Malmo (1975). A reader of these respective literatures is likely impressed by the convergence these independent authors reached regarding the critically central role that the neuromuscular system plays in the determination of emotional and stress-related manifestations. Yet it was Gellhorn (1958a,b, 1964b) who, through a series of well-designed experiments, demonstrated that the nuclear origin of the SNS, the posterior hypothalamus, is dramatically affected by neuromuscular proprioceptive feedback from the skeletal musculature. Such findings led him (1964b) to conclude "that states of abnormal emotional tension are alleviated in various 'relaxation' therapies which impinge on the posterior hypothalamus" (p. 457). This chapter explores the clinical corollary of this notion.

The purpose of this chapter is to provide a clinically useful introduction to a genre of interventions termed *neuromuscular relaxation* (NMR). As used here, this term refers to a process by which an individual can perform a series of exercises to reduce the neural activity (*neuro*) and contractile tension in striate skeletal muscles (*muscular*). This process usually consists of isotonic and/or isometric muscular contractions performed by the patient with initial instruction from the clinician. The proper practice of NMR ultimately leads to the elicitation of the relaxation response.

HISTORY

The NMR procedure presented in this chapter comes from four primary sources: (1) the "progressive relaxation" procedures developed by Edmund Jacobson (1970), (2) the research of Bernstein and Borkovec (1973), (3) research protocols developed by this text's senior author, and (4) the clinical work of Vinod Bhalla (1980) applying neuromuscular interventions to the field of physical medicine and stress.

Edmund Jacobson is often considered the originator of relaxation techniques. His distinguished career took him from undergraduate studies at Northwestern to Harvard, where he worked with William James, among others, and received his Ph.D. in 1910, to a fellowship with Edward Titchner at Cornell, and finally to Rush Medical School (part of the University of Chicago). After receiving his M.D., Jacobson did psychophysiological research until his death in 1983 (see Gessel, 1989, for a biographic article of Jacobson). According to Gessel, Jacobson's "contributions, taken in their totality, create the basis for a comprehensive discipline of neuromuscular psychophysiology" (p. 5).

Early research by Jacobson and his colleague Carlson on the knee-jerk reflex led to the observation that in participants who appeared most deeply relaxed, the knee-jerk reflex was absent or noticeably diminished (Gessel, 1989). This type of work led Jacobson (1938) to conclude that striated muscle tension plays a major role in anxiety states. By teaching individuals to reduce striated muscle tension, Jacobson reported success in reducing subjective reports of anxiety. Later work in the area of mind–body functioning led Jacobson to hypothesize that all thought occurs with collateral skeletal muscle activity of varying, and often extremely low, response amplitudes. As Jacobson stated, "It might be naive to say that we think with our muscles, but it would be inaccurate to say that we think without them" (cited in McGuigan, 1993, p. 18).

Gellhorn (1958b, 1964b), who was particularly impressed with Jacobson's research, offered a neurophysiological rationale for the use of progressive relaxation in the treatment of stress-related disorders. After the 1940s, Charles Atlas developed a program of muscular "dynamic tension" for general health, but the model developed by Jacobson gained greater popularity among practicing clinicians.

Jacobson called his system "progressive relaxation." It consists of a series of exercises in which the subject tenses (contracts) and then relaxes selected muscles and muscle groups so as to achieve the desired state of deep relaxation. Jacobson considered his procedure "progressive" for the following reasons:

1. The subject learns progressively to relax the neuromuscular activity (tension) in the selected muscle. This process may require several minutes to achieve maximal NMR in any selected muscle.

2. The subject tenses and then relaxes selected muscles in the body in such a manner as to progress through the principal muscle groups, until the entire body, or selected body area, is relaxed.
3. With continued daily practice, the subject tends progressively to develop a "habit of repose" (1978, p. 161)—a less stressful, less excitable attitude.

Progressive relaxation gained considerable popularity when Wolpe (1958) used the same basic relaxation system in his phobia treatment called "systematic desensitization." This treatment paradigm, which has become a classic behavioral therapeutic intervention, consists of relaxing the subject before and during exposure to a hierarchy of anxiety-evoking stimuli. Wolpe has successfully employed the principle that an individual cannot concurrently be relaxed and anxious; that is, relaxation acts to inhibit a stress response. An excellent review of Jacobson's work is that of McGuigan (1993).

MECHANISMS OF ACTION

Jacobson (1978) argues that the main therapeutic actions of the NMR system reside in having the patient *learn* the difference between tension and relaxation. This learning is based on having the patient enhance his or her awareness of proprioceptive neuromuscular impulses that originate at the peripheral muscular levels and increase with striated muscle tension. These afferent proprioceptive impulses are major determiners of chronic diffuse anxiety and overall stressful sympathetic arousal, according to Jacobson. This conclusion is supported by the research of Gellhorn, who demonstrated the critical role played by afferent proprioceptive impulses from the muscle spindles in the determination of generalized ergotropic tone (Gellhorn, 1958a,b, 1964b, 1967). The neuromuscular mechanisms of action were discussed in detail in Chapter 10. Please refer back to the work of Gellhorn, Malmo, and Weil discussed in that chapter.

Once the patient learns adequate neuromuscular awareness, he or she may then effectively learn to reduce excessive muscle tension by consciously and progressively "letting go," or reducing the degree of contraction in the selected muscles. It has been argued that it is difficult for "unpracticed" individuals to achieve a similar degree of conscious relaxation, because they are not educated in the sensations of tension versus conscious deep relaxation—as a result, measurable "residual tension" remains during conscious efforts to relax.

Other studies on progressive relaxation have suggested that there are two principal therapeutic components at work. Although it is generally accepted that the traditional Jacobsonian concept of *learned awareness* of the differences between the tension of contraction and relaxation experienced on the release of contraction is an important therapeutic component, there may be more. It has been suggested that the actual procedure of *contracting* a muscle before attempting to relax it may add impetus to the total amount of relaxation achieved in that muscle, over and above the process of learned awareness (Borkovec, Grayson, & Cooper, 1978).

RESEARCH ON CLINICAL APPLICATIONS AND EFFECTS

A review of research and clinical literature on the genre of techniques considered part of NMR (including Jacobson's procedures) reveals myriad stress-related therapeutic applications. Specifically, neuromuscular relaxation has been suggested to be effective for the following:

1. Non-insulin-dependent diabetes mellitus (Henry, Wilson, Bruce, Chisholm, & Rawling, 1997)
2. Peptic ulcers (Thankachan & Mishra, 1996)
3. Vascular and muscle tension headaches (Blanchard et al., 1988, 1991)
4. Essential hypertension (Argas, Taylor, Kraemer, Southam, & Schneider, 1987; Shoemaker & Tasto, 1975)
5. Tinnitus (Jakes, Hallam, Rachman, & Hinchcliffe, 1986)
6. General arousal and development of a calmer attitude (Jacobson, 1978; McGuigan, 1991; Stoyva, 1977)
7. Assistance in the treatment of cancer chemotherapy (Carey & Burish, 1987)
8. Assistance in the treatment of HIV infection and AIDS (Kocsis, 1996)

Given these research findings, it seems that NMR strategies may be an effective component in a variety of treatment programs designed to mitigate the impact of both chronic stress and stress that exacerbates a disease process. We now present a structure for clinical implementation.

HOW TO IMPLEMENT A PHYSICALLY ACTIVE FORM OF NEUROMUSCULAR RELAXATION: PREPARATION

To review, NMR represents a series of exercises during which the participant tenses (contracts) and then releases (relaxes) selected muscles in a predetermined and orderly manner. Some preliminary activities that the clinician should perform before implementing the procedure are as follows:

1. In addition to the general precautions for relaxation mentioned in an earlier chapter, determine whether the patient has any muscular or neuromuscular contraindications: for example, nerve problems, weak or damaged muscles, or skeletal problems that would be enhanced through the neuromuscular exercises. When in doubt, avoid that specific muscle group until a qualified opinion can be obtained.

2. Ask about the patient's previous knowledge or experience of NMR techniques. Because the clinician must consider whether such knowledge or experience will facilitate or be detrimental to the current treatment situation, it is usually helpful to discuss in relative detail any previous exposure that the patient may have had with NMR techniques.

3. Provide the patient with background and rationale for use of NMR techniques.

4. Discuss with the patient the proper environment for the practice of NMR techniques: (a) quiet, comfortable surroundings; darkened, if possible, in order to enhance concentration on bodily sensations; (b) loose clothing; remove contact lenses, glasses, and shoes if desired; (c) body supported as much as possible (with exception of neck and head, if patient falls asleep inadvertently).

5. Educate the patient about the difference between the desired muscle "tension" and undesirable muscle "strain." Tension is indicated by a tightened, somewhat uncomfortable sensation in the muscles being tensed. Strain is indicated by any pain in the muscle, joints, and tendons, as well as any uncontrolled trembling in the muscles. Strain is actually excessive muscle tension.

6. Instruct the patient in proper breathing: Do not hold the breath while tensing muscles. Instead, breathe normally, or inhale on tensing and exhale on relaxing the muscles.

7. Before beginning the actual protocol with the patient, informally demonstrate all the exercises you will be employing. Take this opportunity to answer any questions that the patient may have.

8. Finally, explain to the patient exactly "how" you will provide the instructions. For example: "In the case of each muscle group that we focus upon, I will always carefully describe the relaxation exercise to you first, before you actually do the exercise. Therefore, don't begin the exercise until I say, 'Ready? Begin.'"

The order of these steps may vary. In order to facilitate awareness of some of this preliminary information, the clinician may present a handout to patients.

HOW TO IMPLEMENT NEUROMUSCULAR RELAXATION: PROCEDURE

Whenever possible, begin the total protocol with the lowest areas of the body to be relaxed and end with the face, because once a muscle has been tensed and then relaxed, we attempt to ensure that it is not inadvertently retensed. The quasi-voluntary muscles of the face are the most susceptible to retensing; therefore, we relax them last to eliminate the opportunity.

The Sequential Steps to Follow for Each Muscle Being Relaxed

Once the clinician is ready to initiate the actual protocol, he or she should be sure to follow a fundamental sequence of steps for *each* muscle group.

Step 1. Describe to the patient the specific muscle(s) to be tensed and how it/they will be contracted. "We are now going to tense the muscles in the calf. To begin, I'd like you to leave your toes flat on the floor and raise both of your heels as high as you can."

Step 2. Have the patient initiate the response with some predetermined cue: "Ready? Begin."

Step 3. Have the patient hold the contraction for 3 to 5 seconds. During this time, you may wish to encourage the patient to exert an even greater effort: "Raise your toes higher, higher, even higher."

Step 4. Signal the patient to relax the concentration: "And now relax."

Step 5. Facilitate the patient's awareness of the muscles just relaxed by having him or her search for feelings of relaxation: "Now sense how the backs of your legs feel. Are they warm, tingling? Do they feel heavy? Search for the feelings."

Step 6. The clinician may wish to encourage further relaxation: "Now let the muscles relax even more. They are heavier and heavier and heavier."

Step 7. Pause at least 5 to 10 seconds after each exercise to allow the patient to experience relaxation. Pause 15 to 20 seconds after each major muscle group.

Step 8. When possible, go directly to the opposing set of muscles. In this case, it would involve leaving the heels flat on the floor and raising the toes as high as possible.

Example Protocol

The following brief protocol includes previously discussed components. See whether you can identify the major preliminary activities (only a few can be included in this example) and the sequenced steps (some sample muscle groups have only six or seven of the steps to avoid monotony).

As you read the example, make notes in the margins provided as to what changes you might make in order to make the protocol more effective for your needs in teaching a general NMR protocol.

Background Information. As early as 1908, researchers at Harvard University discovered that stress and anxiety are related to muscle tension. Muscle tension is created by a shortening or contraction of muscle fibers. The relationship between stress and anxiety on one hand, and muscle tension on the other, is such that if you are able to reduce muscle tension, stress and anxiety will be reduced as well.

Progressive NMR is a tool that you can use to reduce muscle tension and, therefore, stress and anxiety. It is a progressive system by which you can systematically tense and then relax major muscle groups in your body, in an orderly manner, so as to achieve a state of total relaxation. This total relaxation is made possible by two important processes.

First, by tensing a muscle and then relaxing it, you will actually receive a sort of running start, in order to achieve a greater degree of muscular relaxation than would normally be obtainable. And second, by tensing a muscle and then relaxing it, you are able to compare and contrast muscular tension and muscular relaxation. Therefore, we see that the basic premises underlying your muscular relaxation are as follows:

1. Stress and anxiety are related to muscular tension.
2. When you reduce muscular tension, a significant reduction in stress and anxiety will be achieved as well.
3. NMR provides you with the unique opportunity to compare and contrast tension with relaxation.
4. NMR has been proven to be a powerful tool that can be used to achieve relaxation and peace of mind. However, relaxation is an active skill and, like any skill, it must be practiced. The mistake that most individuals make is to rush through this relaxation procedure. NMR works, but it takes practice and patience to succeed. But, after all, isn't your health and well-being worth at least 15 minutes a day?

Preliminary Instructions. Before beginning the progressive NMR procedure, let us review some basic considerations.

First, find a quiet place without interruptions or glaring lights. You should find a comfortable chair to relax in, though you will also find progressive relaxation useful when performed lying in bed, in order to help you fall asleep at night. Loosen tight articles of clothing. Glasses, jewelry, and contact lenses should be removed.

Second, the progressive NMR system requires you to tense each set of muscles for two periods, lasting about 5 seconds each. However, it is possible to tense each set of muscles up to several times if you continue to feel residual tension. Muscular tension is not equal to muscular strain. They are not the same. You will know that you have strained a muscle if you feel pain in the muscle or any of the joints around it, or if it begins to shiver or to tremble uncontrollably. In either case, these should be signs to you to employ a lesser degree of tension, or simply avoid that exercise. The entire NMR procedure lasts about 20 to 30 minutes, should you wish to relax your entire body. The time may be less if you choose to relax only a few muscles groups.

Last, don't hold your breath during contractions. Breathe normally, or inhale as you tense and exhale as you release the tension.

Actual Instructions.   You are now ready to relax progressively the major muscle groups in your body, in order to achieve a state of total relaxation. I would like you to settle back and get very, very comfortable. You may loosen or remove any tight articles of clothing, such as shoes or coats, ties, or glasses. You should also remove contact lenses. Try to get very, very comfortable. I would like you to close your eyes. Just sit back and close your eyes. Begin by directing your attention to your breathing. The breath is the body's metronome. So let us become aware of the metronome. As you inhale, become aware of how the air comes in through your nostrils and down into your lungs, and how your stomach and chest expand, and how they recede as you exhale. Concentrate on your breathing. (*Provide 30 second pause here.*)

In the case of each muscle group that we focus on, I shall always carefully describe the relaxation exercise to you first, before you are actually to do the exercise. Therefore, do not begin the exercise described until I say, "Ready? Begin."

Chest.   Let us begin with the chest. At my request, and not before, I would like you to take a very, very deep breath. Breathe in all the air around you. Let's do that now. Ready? Begin. Take a very deep breath. A very deep breath; hold it... and relax. Just exhale all the air from your lungs and resume your normal breathing. Did you notice tension in your chest as you inhaled? Did you notice relaxation as you exhaled? If you had to, could you describe the difference between tension and relaxation? Let us keep that in mind as we repeat this exercise. Ready? Begin. Inhale very deeply, very deeply. Hold it, and relax. Just exhale and resume your normal breathing. Could you feel the tension that time? Could you feel the relaxation? Try to concentrate on that difference in all the muscle groups that we shall be attending to. (*Always pause 5–10 seconds between exercises.*)

Lower Legs. Let us go now to the lower legs and the muscles in the calf. Before we begin, place both your feet flat on the floor. Now, to engage in this exercise, I should like you simply to leave your toes flat on the floor, and raise both your heels at the same time as high as they will go. Ready? Begin. Raise your heels. Raise them both very high (see Figure 13.1). Hold it, and relax. Just let them fall gently back to the floor. You should have felt some contraction in the back of your calves. Let us repeat this exercise. Ready? Begin. Raise the heels high. Hold it, and relax. As you relax, you may feel some tingling, some warmth. Perhaps some heaviness as the muscle becomes loose and relaxed. To work the opposite set of muscles, leave both your heels flat on the floor, point both sets of your toes very high. Point them as high as you can toward the ceiling. This is the same motion that you would make if you lifted your foot off the accelerator pedal in your car (see Figure 13.2). Except that we shall do both feet at the same time. Let us do that now. Ready? Begin. Raise the toes very high. Hold it, and relax. Now let us repeat this exercise. Ready? Begin. Raise the toes high. Hold it, and relax. You should feel some tingling or heaviness in your lower legs. That feeling is there. You must simply search for it. So take a moment and try to feel that tingling, warmth, or perhaps that heaviness that tells you that your muscles are now relaxed. Let those muscles become looser and heavier, and even heavier. (*Pause for 20 seconds.*)

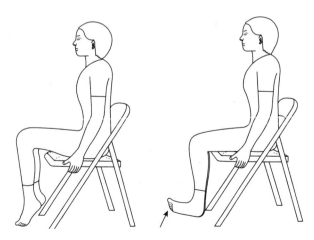

Figure 13.1.   **Figure 13.2.**

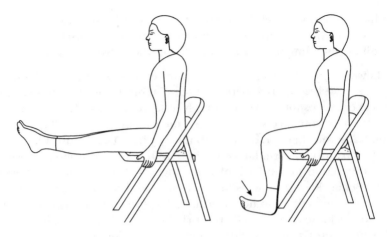

Figure 13.3.   Figure 13.4.

Thighs and Stomach.   The next set of muscles that we shall concentrate on are those of the thigh. This exercise is a simple one. At my request, I should like you simply to extend both your legs out in front of you as straight as you can (see Figure 13.3). (*If this is uncomfortable for the patient, let him or her exercise one leg at a time.*) Remember to leave your calves loose. Do not tense them. Let us do that now. Ready? Begin. Straighten both your legs out in front of you. Very straight. Hold it, and relax. Just let the feet fall gently to the floor. Did you feel tension in the top of your thighs? Let us repeat this exercise. Ready? Begin. Straighten both your legs out. Hold it, and relax. To work the opposite set of muscles, I should like you to imagine that you are at the beach and are digging your heels down into the sand (see Figure 13.4). Ready? Begin. Dig your feet down into the floor. Harder. And relax. Now let us repeat this exercise. Ready? Begin. Dig your heels down into the floor and relax. Now the top of your legs should feel relaxed. Let them become more and more relaxed—more and more relaxed. Concentrate on that feeling now. (*Pause here 20 seconds.*)

Hands and Arms.   Let us move now to the hands. The first thing that I should like you to do, with both your hands at the same time, is make very tight fists (See Figure 13.5). Tighten your fists and arms together. Ready? Begin. Clench your fists very tightly. Tighter. Hold it, and relax. This exercise is excellent if you type or do a lot of writing during the day. Now let us repeat. Ready? Begin. Clench both your fists very tightly. Hold it, and relax. To work the opposing muscles, simply spread your fingers as wide as you can (see Figure 13.6). Ready? Begin. Spread your fingers very wide. Wider.

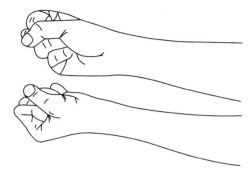

Figure 13.5.

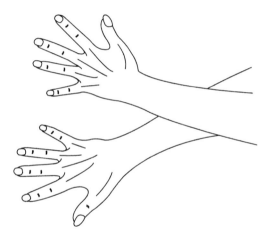

Figure 13.6.

Hold it, and relax. Now let us repeat this exercise. Ready? Begin. Spread the fingers wide. Wider. Widest of all. Hold it, and relax. Concentrate on the warmth or tingling in your hands and forearms. (*Pause here 20 seconds.*)

Shoulders.   Now let us work on the shoulders. We tend to store a lot of our tension and stress in our shoulders. This exercise simply consists of shrugging your shoulders vertically up toward your ears. Imagine trying to touch your ear lobes with the tops of your shoulders (see Figure 13.7). Let us do that now. Ready? Begin. Shrug your shoulders up high. Higher than that. Hold it, and relax. Now let us repeat. Ready? Begin. Shrug the shoulders. Higher. Hold it, and relax. Let us repeat this exercise one more time. Ready? Begin. Shrug the shoulders as high as you can. Hold it, and relax.

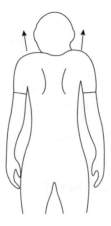

Figure 13.7.

Very good. Now just concentrate on the heaviness in your shoulders. Let your shoulders go, let them completely relax—heavier and heavier. (*Pause here 20 seconds.*)

    Face.   Let us move now into the facial region. We shall start with the mouth. The first thing I should like you to do is smile as widely as you possibly can (see Figure 13.8). An ear-to-ear grin. Ready? Begin. Hold it, and relax. Now let us repeat this exercise. Ready? Begin. Grin very wide. Wider. Hold it, and relax. The opposite set of muscles will be activated when you pucker or purse your lips together, as if you were trying to give someone a kiss (see Figure 13.9). Ready? Begin. Pucker the lips together. Purse them together very tightly. Hold it, and relax. Now let us repeat that exercise. Ready? Begin. Purse the lips together. Hold it, and relax. Let your mouth relax. Let the muscles go—let them relax, more and more; even more.

    Now let us move up to the eyes. (Be sure to remove contact lenses.) I should like you to keep your eyes closed, but to clench them even tighter. Imagine that you are trying to keep shampoo suds out of your eyes (see Figure 13.10). Ready? Begin. Clench the eyes tightly, and relax.

    Let us repeat this exercise. Ready? Begin. Clench the eyes, tighter. Hold it, and relax.

    The last exercise consists simply of raising your eyebrows as high as you can. Now, remember to keep your eyes closed, but raise your eyebrows as high as you can (see Figure 13.11). Ready? Begin. Raise the eyebrows high. Hold it, and relax. Now let us repeat this exercise. Ready? Begin. Raise the eyebrows higher. Highest of all. Hold it, and relax. Let us pause for

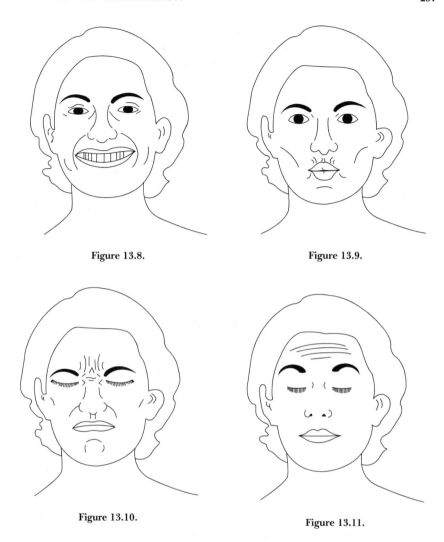

Figure 13.8.

Figure 13.9.

Figure 13.10.

Figure 13.11.

a few moments to allow you to feel the relaxation in your face. (*Pause 15 seconds.*)

Closure. You have now relaxed most of the major muscles in your body. To make sure that they are all relaxed, I shall go back and name the muscles that we have just activated and just relaxed. And, as I name them, let them go even further into relaxation. You will feel a sense of relaxation descend over your entire body in a warm wave. You will feel the muscular relaxation now in your forehead, and as it goes down into your eyes, down into your cheeks, you can feel the heaviness of relaxation descend into your jaws, into your neck, down through your shoulders, to the chest and arms, to the stomach, into your hands. Relaxation is descending into your legs, into the thighs and calves, and down to the feet. Your body now feels very heavy. Very relaxed. This is a good feeling. So take a moment and enjoy this feeling of relaxation. (*Pause here 2 minutes.*)

Reawaken. Now I want you to bring your attention back to yourself and the world around you. I shall count from 1 to 10. With each count, you will feel your mind become more and more awake, and your body more and more refreshed and responsive. When I reach 10, open your eyes, and you will feel the *best* you've felt all day—you will feel alert, refreshed, full of energy, and eager to resume your activities. Let us begin: 1–2 you are beginning to feel more alert, 3–4–5 you are more and more awake, 6–7 now begin to stretch your hands and feet, 8 now begin to stretch your arms and legs, 9–10 open your eyes *now!* You feel alert, awake, your mind is clear and your body refreshed.

SUMMARY

This chapter has presented an introduction to a series of techniques known as *neuromuscular relaxation,* which has been employed in the mitigation of the human stress response. The chapter highlighted the work of Edmund Jacobson, considered by many to be the originator of relaxation training.

The mechanisms of therapeutic action include learning the difference between feelings of tension and relaxation, which is predicated on enhanced awareness of proprioceptive neuromuscular impulses. It has also been suggested that the actual process of contracting a muscle before attempting to relax it may increase the relaxation response beyond learned awareness.

We then reviewed the preparation and actual procedures involved in implementing a series of exercises that are part of a brief NMR protocol. It is not a prescription for use with patients so much as an example of how such a protocol may be created. Usually, greater specificity is included for muscle groups, and even individual muscles, depending on the requirements of the patient. It is worth noting that Jacobson emphasizes the utility of relaxing the facial muscles, particularly the throat, mouth, and eyes, to obtain maximal relaxation. Therefore, far more specialization directed toward those muscle groups may be considered in developing a protocol:

1. The clinician may encourage the patient to develop his or her own personalized protocol. He or she may further encourage or provide the patient with a home practice audiotape.

Table 13.1. Summary Checklist of NMR Components

Preparation for implementation:
—— 1. Identify contraindications and precautions.
—— 2. Inquire as to previous knowledge/experience in techniques.
—— 3. Provide patient with background/rationale for use of technique.
—— 4. Describe proper environment for practice of technique.
—— 5. Instruct patient in the difference between muscle "tension" and muscle "strain."
—— 6. Instruct patient in proper breathing.
—— 7. Informally demonstrate all specific muscular contractions to be used.
—— 8. Describe "how" you will provide instruction and cues.

Implementation of sequential steps for *each* muscle being relaxed.
—— 1. Describe the specific muscle and "how" it will be contracted.
—— 2. Signal the patient to begin contraction.
—— 3. Hold contraction and encourage greater contraction.
—— 4. Signal the patient to release tension, that is, relax.
—— 5. Facilitate patient awareness of muscles just relaxed through verbal and intonational cues.
—— 6. Encourage further relaxation.
—— 7. Pause and allow patient to become aware of sensations.
—— 8. Proceed with opposing muscle group, if applicable.

2. Jacobson's text, *You Must Relax* (1978), and Davis, Eshelman, and McKay's *Relaxation and Stress Reduction Workbook* (1988) are excellent resources for additional, far more specific exercises. However, in the final analysis, it is the clinician's discretion to assess the suitability of any form of NMR on an individual basis.

3. Table 13.1 may be used as a checklist of important procedural information that should be addressed when teaching NMR to patients. As each step is completed, simply check it off. This same table may be used to evaluate clinical student's mastery of these procedures. As in the first edition, it is designed to be reprinted from this text and used clinically or in educational settings.

4. Finally, Appendix B contains a different version of NMR, consisting of a physically passive form that uses focused sensory awareness and directed concentration for the reduction of striated muscle tension. The clinician may consider this a potential clinical alternative to the form of NMR just described.

14

Hypnosis in the Management of Stress Reactions

Melvin A. Gravitz and Roger A. Page

The modality known in modern times as hypnosis has been a useful and recognized remedial method for more than 200 years. Originally conceptualized by Franz Anton Mesmer (1734–1815) as a physical fluid (animal magnetism) that could be transferred from one person to another, that theory has since been discredited; but even today the fundamental principles and mechanisms underlying hypnosis have not yet been definitively established. Even so, there are useful applications of hypnosis in numerous areas, including stress management.

HISTORICAL PERSPECTIVES

Originating as a medical dissertation submitted to the University of Vienna in the late 1700s, Mesmer's techniques soon became controversial, even though they were undeniably effective with many of his patients. That was understandable, because the medical establishment was threatened by his thesis that there was only one sickness (so-called magnetic illness) and only one treatment (*animal magnetism*, or *mesmerism*, as it was soon

Melvin A. Gravitz • Clinical Professor of Psychiatry and Behavioral Sciences, George Washington University Medical Center, Washington, D.C. 20036.   **Roger A. Page** • Professor of Psychology, Ohio State University at Lima, Lima, Ohio 45804.

termed). Consequently, he was compelled to relocate to Paris, where, once again, his practice flourished and his techniques proved to be ameliorative for many. Controversy again dogged his steps, however, and his opponents prevailed on the king to initiate an investigation. Two commissions comprised of prominent figures in science and medicine conducted a series of generally well-designed studies, although, curiously, they never interviewed Mesmer himself. Their finding, published in 1784, was that no fluid existed. They also concluded that the effectiveness of mesmerism was due to collusion and to deception of naive patients and, above all, to the force of imagination. Since the imagination at that time had no scientific status, Mesmer was labeled a charlatan, and he soon left France in disgrace. To his credit, one of the investigators, Laurent de Jussieu, an eminent botanist, dissented from the majority view and proposed that the imagination could have a therapeutic benefit. Mesmer's method survived him, however, and in France, elsewhere in Europe, and in the newly established United States, a number of followers modified his work and managed to keep mesmerism going for a number of years. During the first decade of the 1800s, several French investigators began using the nomenclature of *hypnotisme*, because they believed that it was a state of sleep, and Hypnos was the name of the ancient Greek god of sleep (Gravitz, 1997). By 1820, however, the modality was dormant.

In the mid-1800s, practitioners in England and elsewhere revived hypnotism (later to be termed *hypnosis*), principally as a form of pain management, but that use also faded as the more acceptable ether and chloroform were developed as surgical anesthetics. News of animal magnetism had earlier been brought to the United States in 1784 by the Marquis de Lafayette, a dedicated disciple of Mesmer. Influential opponents, notably Benjamin Franklin, who had chaired one of the French investigative commissions while serving as the first American diplomatic representive to Paris, intervened, with the result that hypnosis did not flourish in the United States until decades later.

In the late 1800s, influenced by the earlier work of the British, notably James Braid, hypnotism was revived in France, and important French scientific figures became involved in practice and research. Within the same time frame, an Austrian physician studying hypnosis in Paris helped launch the new psychotherapy called *psychoanalysis*: this was Sigmund Freud, whose contributions to hypnosis, however, were minimal. By the turn of the century, mainly because of the rise of psychoanalysis, the modality had once again faded in significance, although a number of prominent workers in the field continued their efforts. Among others, these included Pierre Janet and Alfred Binet in France, Morton Prince and Boris Sidis in the United States, Ivan Pavlov in Russia, Albert Moll in Germany, and Charles Baudouin in Switzerland.

There was a brief revival of hypnosis during World War I, when it was employed on both sides as surgical anesthesia and front-line psychotherapy for so-called shell shock and soldier's heart. These latter reactions to the effects of overwhelming stress became known in later times as combat fatigue and, in more recent years, posttraumatic stress disorder. During the 1920s, Clark L. Hull and Milton H. Erickson helped revive research and clinical interest in the method through their teaching and research. During World War II, clinical hypnosis became an important means of treating stress in the military services, where psychological problems comprised a large percentage of overall causalities. The current wave of professional and scientific interest in hypnosis had its origins in the demonstrated value of the modality during those years. The fact that hypnosis has always returned to the stage of history can be attributed to its undoubted effectiveness in assisting with the management of a wide variety of disorders, including those resulting from inordinate stress.

HYPNOSIS, STRESS, AND MIND–BODY INTERACTION

Stress can be either physical or psychological, or, as is usually the case, both. Stress of whatever kind can impact negatively on bodily chemistry and function, as Hans Selye (e.g., 1976) demonstrated many years ago, and there is truly no demarcation between the mind and body—however one may define those constructs. There are two ways of viewing the implication of these truisms. One is the recognition that psychological forces can result in physical problems. The other is that psychological forces can positively impact the healing process. The demonstrated effectiveness of psychological means, including hypnosis, in treating psychosomatic disorders is a prime example of what is involved here. These considerations have evolved into the current interest in the so-called mind–body interaction, which in turn has generated important and at times admittedly speculative thinking about the underlying mechanisms involved. Ernest Rossi (1986), in particular, may be cited as a reference for further reading. Throughout these hypotheses, hypnosis has played significant historical and modern roles.

THEORIES OF HYPNOSIS

A number of theories, at times conflicting, have been proposed (Gravitz, 1991) to explain the process of hypnosis. These have been broadly grouped into state versus nonstate positions, and each view has presented scientific findings in support of its stance. A related approach has been the advocacy of either neurophysiological or sociocognitive perspectives, again, with evidence submitted for both positions. Recently, Gruzelier (2000) has proposed an overarching integration of these various viewpoints: His theory is that hypnosis is an altered state of brain function involving interrelations of, and between, certain brain regions initiated through the intervention of the hypnotist and the situation in which the process is undertaken. He has also emphasized the central role of cognitive and neuropsychological dissociation. Thus, Gruzelier has integrated social and interpersonal contexts, as well as psychological and neurobiological findings, into a comprehensive and coherent system that merits further study.

Despite the absence so far of a generally accepted understanding of the hypnotic process, the modality has proven effective in managing a broad array of problem areas, including stress management. The basis for such applications has been the observation that hypnosis can in many instances facilitate the enhancement of human behaviors and then apply them more effectively on behalf of the individual subject or client, as the case may be. The mechanisms for these applications have included the long-known, hypnotically induced phenomena of enhanced suggestibility, hypermnesia, distortion of the time sense, regression and revivification, response to posthypnotic instructions, dissociation, ideomotor communication, tolerance for distortion of reality, modified physiological processes, and suspension of critical thinking. These phenomena are a function of individuals' unique talents as hypnotic subjects and the source of individual differences.

HYPNOSIS AND STRESS

In its definition of hypnosis and hypnotherapy, the *Policy and Procedures Manual of Division 30* (*Psychological Hypnosis*) of the American Psychological Association states, "Hypnotherapy is not a type of therapy, like psychoanalysis or behavior therapy. Instead, hypnotherapy is the use of hypnosis to facilitate psychotherapy" (p. 5). These statements emphasize a major point: Hypnosis is not a therapy, but a technique to be used as an adjunct to therapy. For example, hypnosis has been used with Albert Ellis's (1962) rational-emotive therapy (RET) by Stanton (1989) to reduce stress in high school teachers. Ellis (1984) had previously suggested the use of hypnosis with RET to reduce the number of sessions necessary to achieve positive results. Hypnosis has also been used with an extension of RET developed by Tosi (1974) called rational stage directed hypnotherapy (RSDH) to treat pathological nonassertiveness (Gwynne, Tosi, & Howard, 1978) and anxiety neurosis (Tosi, Howard, & Gwynne, 1982). RSDH combines cognitive restructuring, imagery, and hypnosis. A variation of RSDH was also used by Der and Lewington (1990) in the treatment of panic attacks to reduce panic symptoms in stressful situations.

The use of hypnosis with cognitive-behavioral therapies such as Wolpe's (1958) systematic desensitization is far from new; Wolpe and Lazarus (1966) reported using it with a number of their patients. Since then, a few examples of hypnosis used in conjunction with systematic desensitization include both Frankel (1976) and Seif (1982) in treating phobic behavior, Taylor (1985) in treating an obsession, Moore (1965) in treating bronchial asthma, and Barabasz and Spiegel (1989) in treating obesity. The literature is replete with such examples of hypnosis used with various therapies over several decades, including the more traditional insight-oriented therapies (e.g., Brenman & Gill, 1947; Crasilneck & Hall, 1975).

In recent years, support for the use of hypnosis as an adjunct to therapy has been mounting. An earlier argument by Holroyd (1987) that hypnosis serves to potentiate psychotherapy has recently been confirmed by Kirsch and his associates. In an initial meta-analysis of 18 studies, Kirsch, Montgomery, and Sapirstein (1995) found a substantial effect size (mean effect size = .87 standard deviations) when hypnosis was used as an adjunct to cognitive-behavioral psychotherapy (in the treatment of various presenting problems, including obesity) compared to the same therapy without hypnosis. This effect size is in the order of magnitude found by Smith et al. (1980) for psychotherapy compared to no treatment! Furthermore, long-term follow-ups of the obesity studies (ranging from 2 months to 2 years) indicated that participants who had received hypnosis continued to lose weight *after* treatment had ended. These findings were confirmed by a second meta-analysis conducted by Kirsch (1996) that included additional data obtained from two of the original studies, corrected for computational inaccuracies, excluded results from a questionable study, and employed conservative calculation methods. The mean effect size for the hypnosis compared to therapy without hypnosis for obesity studies was .66 standard deviations for the initial assessment and .98 standard deviations for the final assessment, leading Kirsch to conclude, "The addition of hypnosis appears to have a significant and substantial effect on the outcome of cognitive-behavioral treatment for weight reduction and this effect increases over time" (p. 519).

Given the well-established usefulness of hypnosis as a technique, a brief description of a "prototypical" hypnotic induction and suggestions as used in the treatment of stress is appropriate. The typical induction begins with the client sitting comfortably while focusing on some target. Suggestions for progressive muscle relaxation are given, usually accompanied by counting as a deepening technique, while the client is instructed to visualize a pleasant scene (e.g., lying on a beach on a warm, sunny day). A word of caution is in order here. Suggestions are most effective when tailored to fit the individual. For example, visualizing a beach may work perfectly well for a given client, whereas being asked to visualize lying in front of a cozy fire on a cold winter day may produce an adverse reaction if the client is pyrophobic. This sort of reaction can be easily avoided by administering a checklist of fears, likes and dislikes, and so on, prior to the induction.

Following the induction, the stress-specific suggestions will vary depending upon the client and particular treatment regimen employed. For example, one may have a client recall a pleasant memory while associating this with a cue (e.g., a simple motor act), then instruct the client to self-present the cue (or perform the motor act) when faced with a stressful situation. Or one may use a desensitization strategy in which the relaxation achieved through hypnosis is first paired with low stress-producing situations and eventually with high stress-producing situations. For examples of specific suggestions that have a variety of applications not only in psychology but also in medicine and dentistry, the reader is directed to the *Handbook of Hypnotic Suggestions and Metaphors* (1990) edited by Hammond, or *A Syllabus on Hypnosis and a Handbook of Therapeutic Suggestions* (1973) published by the American Society of Clinical Hypnosis Education and Research Foundation.

As we return to the primary focus of this chapter, the use of hypnosis with stress, our review of this body of work indicates that it can somewhat arbitrarily be divided into two broad types, with an admittedly gray area, without a sharp, clear-cut distinction between them. The first type would be studies that have involved reducing stress associated with a variety of *specific* situations (or external stressors). The second would be those studies dealing with stress in general and/or learning techniques to cope with it (stress management). We begin with the former.

In noting that both physical and psychological stressors have the *perception of threat* as a final common pathway for the stress response, Bowers and Kelly (1979) list created a four of "generic stressors" that

> the relevant literature deems threatening and hence stressful: (a) a perceived lack or loss of control (together with related factors such as event uncertainty and unpredictability), (b) the anticipation and occurrence of physical or psychological pain, (c) the loss of close emotional and social supports, and (d) effortful "trying" to avoid aversive stimuli or conditions. (p. 491)

In the following examples, hypnosis was employed and often compared to other techniques in treating individuals exposed to various stressors, ranging from surgeries to college exams.

Enqvist, von Konow, and Bystedt (1995) utilized preoperative hypnosis to reduce stress during maxillofacial surgery, including suggestions to reduce bleeding and edema, and to improve recovery. Compared to control patients, hypnosis patients displayed reduced swelling, fever, and postoperative consumption of anxiolytics.

In a similar vein, Faymonville et al. (1997) conducted a randomized study comparing the effectiveness of hypnosis to stress-reducing strategies (including emotional support, deep breathing/relaxation, and positive emotion induction) in decreasing discomfort during plastic surgery under local anesthesia and intravenous sedation (midazolam and alfentanil) upon request. Patient anxiety, pain, and perceived control before, during, and after surgery, along with postsurgical nausea and vomiting, were recorded. Results showed that the hypnosis patients (during and following surgery) had significantly less anxiety, pain, nausea, and vomiting than controls. They also reported experiencing more intraoperative control. The authors noted that the reduction in anxiety and pain were achieved in spite of the fact that the hypnosis group required significantly less midazolam and alfentanil during surgery! Furthermore, no direct suggestions for analgesia were given.

Another example of hypnosis used to control anxiety in a surgical setting is when oral surgical procedures are necessary in hemophiliacs. These procedures can be extremely stressful to the patient for obvious reasons. Lucas (1975) makes a case for the use of hypnosis, since anxiety can trigger (or complicate an ongoing) hemorrhagic episode, and this tendency (during and following surgery) is decreased considerably if the patient is relaxed and tranquil. An additional benefit is a reduction in pain and capillary bleeding through suggestion.

In a unique intervention for a psychosomatic condition, Gravitz (1995) successfully used a hypnosis-based paradigm to relieve functional infertility in several patients. Verbal suggestions coupled with mental imagery to relax fallopian tube musculature were provided to two patients. Since hypnosis is known to relax muscle tension, it was theorized that the consequent dilation of the tubular lumen would enable an ovum to travel successfully down the fallopian tube and achieve uterine implantation. In both cases, pregnancy resulted within several months.

Two final examples deal with what is commonly called test anxiety, admittedly a less dramatic stressor than surgery, but certainly far from mundane for those experiencing the stress. Boutin and Tosi (1983) employed the previously mentioned technique RSDH in the modification of irrational ideation and test anxiety in female nursing students. Participants were randomly assigned to one of four treatment conditions: RSDH, hypnosis-only treatment, placebo condition, or no-treatment control. Primary treatment was 1 hour per week for 6 weeks. Dependent measures included the State–Trait Anxiety Inventory (STAI; Spielberger, 1983) and the Test Anxiety Scale (Sarason, 1957), among others. Results showed a significant advantage for the RSDH and hypnosis-only groups at both posttest and at 2-month follow-up, with RSDH being more effective than hypnosis-only at both test times.

The last example involving test anxiety is a study by Palan and Chandwani (1989) that compared hypnotic suggestions, waking suggestions, and passive relaxation in medical school students. In addition to suggestions for reduced test anxiety, suggestions were also calculated to enhance self-image and improve study habits (e.g., suggestions that concentration and memory of material would improve). Although results showed that all treatment conditions produced a significant increase in motivation to study, only the hypnosis group reported significant increases in variables such as self-confidence, general health, sleep, and so forth.

The final type of study to be examined deals with reducing stress in general and/or stress management; that is, techniques to cope with stress. This type of treatment falls into what Bowers and Kelly (1979), in describing attempts to treat psychosomatic disorders psychologically, called an "intermediate level of specificity... that focuses on the reduction of stress by altering the threatening character of the environment" (p. 494). One way this is typically accomplished is that "patients' resources to deal with threats are increased through some combination of enhancing their ability to relax, to cope with a threat, and to defend themselves more adequately against its stress-producing characteristics". (p. 494)

A list of some stress management techniques *other than hypnosis* includes the following: progressive muscle relaxation (Jacobson, 1970), deep abdominal breathing (Fried, 1987), meditation (including TM), listening to music, frontalis electromyographic feedback (EMG-FB; Budzynsky, Stoyva, & Adler, 1976), distraction (and focused) imagery, and emotional support. Several studies have examined the effectiveness of these techniques compared to controls (usually sitting quietly with eyes closed), hypnosis, or other stress management techniques. For example, Avants, Margolin, and Salovey (1990) compared a brief (20 minute) treatment of 4 different techniques (progressive muscle relaxation, distraction, focused imagery, and listening to music) to sitting quietly and found that only distraction imagery and listening to music reduced anxiety to a greater extent than sitting quietly.

Raskin, Bali, and Peeke (1980) compared the effectiveness of EMG-FB, TM, and progressive relaxation in reducing general anxiety. Although 40% of their participants showed marked anxiety relief, they found no differences between the treatments with respect to efficacy.

In an effort to reduce stress in high school teachers, Stanton (1989) compared hypnosis combined with Ellis's RET to controls who spent an equal amount of time discussing stress management, with emphasis on cognitive restructuring to promote more rational thinking. Although both groups showed reductions on measures of irrational thinking and stress following treatment, the experimental group showed significantly more improvement than controls. Furthermore, they showed continued improvement at a 1-year follow-up, whereas control group scores were comparable to those immediately following treatment.

Elton (1993) compared the efficacy of hypnosis and hypnosis combined with EMG-FB in the treatment of stress-related conditions, including emotional problems such as frustration, anxiety, and low self-esteem, as well as conditions such as migraines and tension headaches. Although no control group was included, participants' scores on several variables (e.g., state and trait anxiety, self-esteem, and body stress) were compared to their baseline scores following treatment at 12- and again at 24 weeks. Both groups showed significant improvement over baseline on all variables. At week 12, the hypnosis/EMG-FB group showed a significantly greater reduction on trait anxiety (as measured by Spielberger's STAI) than the hypnosis-only group; at week 24, the former group showed a significantly greater reduction in trait and state anxiety, and a greater increase in self-esteem. No significant differences were found between groups on other variables at either 12 or 24 weeks.

In a similar combinatory vein, Sapp (1992) employed relaxation therapy combined with hypnosis in treating anxiety and stress in adults with neurogenic impairment. Several measures of anxiety and stress were significantly reduced both posttest and at 4-week follow-up.

The next three studies explored the use of *self-hypnosis* for stress management, a skill that, once learned, can be practiced outside of the therapist's office, accounting in part for its growing popularity. Soskis, Orne, Orne, and Dinges (1989) taught executives either self-hypnosis or meditation as part of "an organization stress-management program aimed at promoting health through the use of effective coping strategies" (p. 286). Depending upon their group assignment, participants were encouraged to practice self-hypnosis (or meditation) twice daily, 5 days per week for 2 weeks, then as needed. Telephone follow-ups occurred 1 month and 6 months after the training session. The rate of use dropped equally for both groups over the 6-month follow-up interval (from 90% to 42% for all participants). In addition, the frequently described uses of self-hypnosis or meditation were similar for both groups (e.g., to relax, to aid in sleep onset, to reduce effects of external stressors, etc.), as were problems encountered (e.g., scheduling difficulties, obtaining the necessary privacy, etc.).

Whitehouse et al. (1996) trained first-year medical school students in the use of self-hypnosis as a means of coping with stress and potentially reducing the impact of stress on immune function. Although the self-hypnosis group did not differ from controls with respect to immune function at four measurement times, they did report lower anxiety and stress ratings at exam time, and less variability in ratings of sleep quality throughout the measurement period.

Finally, Benson et al. (1978) compared self-hypnosis to meditation/relaxation in the treatment of anxious patients in an 8-week follow-up assessment. Both treatments showed moderate (and comparable) success in reducing anxiety at follow-up, with 37.5% of the self-hypnosis group and 31.3% of the meditation/relaxation group showing improvement.

This study, one of only a few thus far reviewed that assessed a key variable that can potentially moderate treatment outcome—hypnotic ability or hypnotizability—is worthy of further attention. To illustrate, Bowers and Kelly (1979) noted that when participants in the Benson et al. (1978) study were divided into low, moderate, and high hypnotic ability based on a pretest assessment, 47.6% (10 out of 21) of the moderate to high hypnotizable subjects showed significant reductions in anxiety, while only 9.1% (1 out of 11) of low hypnotizable participants showed a comparable reduction. Bowers and Kelly concluded,

> Clearly, differences in hypnotic ability were far more important to treatment outcome than the ritualistic differences of the two therapeutic regimens being compared.... In sum, self-hypnosis and relaxation were equally effective in reducing psychological and physiological manifestations of anxiety in moderate to high hypnotizables, and equally ineffective for low susceptibles. (p. 499)

To reiterate, despite the importance of hypnotizability, few studies have formally assessed it. Although the aforementioned Elton (1993) study did assess hypnotizability, there was no analysis of how it may have affected treatment outcome. Although the Barber Suggestibility Scale (Barber, 1969) was used in the Sapp (1992) study, it was administered without a prior hypnotic induction and was therefore a measure of *waking* suggestibility, which correlates only moderately with hypnotic susceptibility. In addition, only a single item was administered in hypnosis. Thus, it is not surprising that hypnotic susceptibility was not related to treatment gains. Finally, Whitehouse et al. (1996) obtained a pretest measure of hypnotizability and found that it was not related to treatment outcome, but their measure of self-hypnosis correlated only a modest .42 with a standard susceptibility scale, suggesting that "self-hypnosis and heterohypnosis involve

distinctive processes that may render standard heterohypnosis scales...
poor predictors of self-hypnosis skill when used on their own". (p. 251)

A series of studies by Pekala and his associates (Pekala & Forbes, 1988,
1990; Pekala, Forbes, & Contrisciani, 1988) is relevant to the importance of
hypnotizability as a moderating variable. These studies, based on 300 nursing
students who experienced progressive relaxation, deep abdominal breathing,
and hypnosis, respectively, all following a baseline condition of sitting quietly
with eyes closed, revealed not only that techniques such as progressive relaxation and hypnosis are *not* experienced as phenomenologically equivalent,
but also that the experience is moderated by an individual's hypnotic susceptibility. Specifically, high susceptible participants reported not only more hypnoidal effects than low susceptible across all conditions but also essentially
equivalent hypnoidal effects for both progressive relaxation and hypnosis.
(This suggests the possibility that high susceptible participants may be experiencing hypnosis, or something akin to it, when engaged in techniques such
as progressive relaxation.) The low susceptible participants, however, experienced more hypnoidal effects during progressive relaxation than hypnosis,
suggesting that for lows, progressive relaxation may be functioning as an
indirect hypnotic technique (i.e., a technique not defined as hypnosis to the
subjects, but possibly being hypnotic in nature; Barber, 1977).

SUMMARY

In this chapter, we have discussed the potentially valuable role of
hypnosis in the treatment of excessive stress. The information presented
can be summarized as follows:

1. Hypnosis has been used for more than 200 years in the treatment of
human ailments. It was first introduced by Franz Anton Mesmer; however,
his controversial conceptualization of animal magnetism was discredited.

2. Hypnotism was later revived in France and Austria; however, with
the rise and popularity of psychoanalysis, hypnosis faded in significance by
the end of the 20th century.

3. Interest in hypnosis was revived following the clinical applications
that occurred during World Wars I and II primarily for stress-related disorders. The current interest in hypnosis is credited in part to the successes
that occurred during those years.

4. There are a number of theories to explain the hypnotic process.
Gruzelier (2000) has recently proposed a viewpoint that comprehensively
integrates the social, interpersonal, psychological, and neurobiological
contexts.

5. There are also several proposed mechanisms of action responsible for the hypnotic effect, including but not limited to enhanced suggestibilty, hypermnesia, distortion of time, regression, and response to posthypnotic instructions.

6. It is important to emphasize that hypnosis is not therapy but a technique used as an adjunct to therapy. Hypnosis has been used with cognitive-behavioral therapies, insight-oriented therapies, rational-emotive therapy (RET), and rational stage directed hypnotherapy (RSDH), which is an extension of RET.

7. The use of hypnosis relative to stress can generally be divided into studies that address two broad categories. The first is the use of hypnosis to reduce stress associated with specific stressors that may fall with the generic categories of (a) loss of control, (b) anticipation of physical or psychological pain, (c) loss of emotional and social support, and (d) attempts to avoid aversive stimuli. Studies examining specific stressors such as surgeries, and college exams are examples of this first category. The second category includes studies examining how hypnosis compares to other stress management techniques such as biofeedback, progressive muscle relaxation, deep breathing, and meditation.

8. In summary, more research is needed that assesses relevant variables such as hypnotizability and expectancies, especially when comparing hypnosis to other stress management techniques. To date, the data suggest that hypnosis is at least as effective, if not more so, than other techniques for reducing stress and helping the individual learn to cope with stress. In addition, the efficacy of hypnosis seems to be enhanced when combined with other techniques such as biofeedback.

15

Biofeedback in the Treatment of the Stress Response

The purpose of this chapter is to provide a basic introduction to biofeedback in general and to discuss how it relates to the treatment of excessive stress. Biofeedback may still be considered "high-technology" therapy that may be used to (1) engender a relaxation response, thus treating the stress response itself, or (2) alter target-organ activity, thus treating the symptoms of excessive stress arousal.

Biofeedback may be conceptualized as a procedure in which data regarding an individual's biological activity are collected, processed, and conveyed back to the person so that he or she can modifying that activity. In essence, biofeedback allows for the construction of a "feedback loop," which is illustrated in Figure 15.1.

Feedback loops exist in almost all functions of the human body, from the rate-modifying feedback loops concerned with the most elementary biochemical reactions to the most complex human endeavors. Information regarding the result of any event is necessary at some level if it is to be modified.

Thus, the concept underlying biofeedback is fundamental in biology, and is becoming more widely employed in the therapeutic sciences. In the traditional medical model, the patient presents a physiological disturbance, and data regarding his or her physiological functioning are collected by the clinician, who draws conclusions and institutes appropriate interventions. The patient in this model has a basically passive role. This interaction, as visualized in Figure 15.2, represents an indirect closed loop of information, starting and ending with the patient and including information-gathering devices, the clinician, and therapeutic devices.

As can be seen in a comparison of Figures 15.1 and 15.2, the principle on which biofeedback is based involves the active participation of the

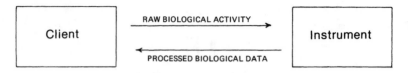

Figure 15.1.

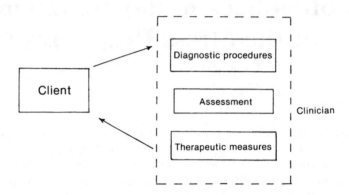

Figure 15.2.

patient in the modification of his or her condition. Consider the case of a function such as breathing, which is unique in the sense that we can control it voluntarily but, fortunately, occurs without conscious awareness. It is as if there are priorities for the human brain, with many functions occurring at subcortical levels—especially those that must be maintained in an ongoing fashion, such as heartbeat and biochemical reactions. Although this may be the most efficient way to function, it keeps the organism from being able to monitor many of its autonomic functions consciously and thus actively change them. This is what biofeedback provides for the individual—the potential to exert some control over autonomic biological activity.

Given the information provided with biofeedback, we have repeatedly found that we can learn to alter bodily functions that were once thought to be inaccessible, including greater finite control over the activities of both the voluntary and the autonomic nervous systems.

The purpose of this chapter is to expand the principles on which biofeedback is based and describe how it may be beneficial in the treatment of the stress response. We also review some of the historical trends that have led to the present state of the art and then discuss some of the biofeedback modalities in current use. Finally, we examine the role of the therapist in the biofeedback paradigm.

HISTORY

The term *biofeedback* was reportedly coined at the first annual meeting of the Biofeedback Research Society in 1969, as a shortened version of "biological feedback." Although the term itself may have been new, its foundations are not.

The historical development of biofeedback can be traced back to the early 1900s and the work of Pavlov and Watson on the one hand and Thorndike on the other. Pavlov and Watson's research on classical conditioning of the autonomic nervous system (ANS) was thought to be discretely separate from the work of Thorndike on operant conditioning of the musculoskeletal system. Early researchers were convinced that conditioning that affected the ANS had to be accomplished through a classical conditioning paradigm (an S(stimulus) → R(response) model involving conditioning on the basis of association rather than as a function of behavioral consequence as in an operant model). In fact, Kimble (1961), in his edited textbook *Conditioning and Learning*, stated unequivocally that autonomically mediated behavior could only be modified by classical, not operant conditioning.

However, in a discipline like psychology, assertions such as Kimble's often serve as challenges for others. For example, according to a review by Gatchel and Price (1979), case reports existed of individuals who reportedly could voluntarily alter autonomic functioning (see Lindsley & Sassaman, 1938; Luria, 1958; McClure, 1959; Ogden & Shock, 1939). Interestingly, Edmund Jacobson, the originator of progressive relaxation training (see Chapter 13), performed some of the earliest clinical biofeedback work in the 1930s using an oscilloscope to measure forearm tension in progressive relaxation trainees. However, since he used a raw electromyograph (EMG) signal, most people had difficulty understanding how to interpret the information, and Jacobson apparently discarded the method (Schneider, 1989). Following Kimble's published work, other researchers reported the use of operant conditioning of heart rate to avoid mild electrical shocks (Frazier, 1966; Shearn, 1962). Supporters of Kimble's may have argued, however, that these types of studies, in which changes in autonomically mediated responses (such as heart rate) were modified by responses under voluntary control (such as altered breathing), were actually consistent with a classical conditioning paradigm (Blanchard & Epstein, 1978).

Therefore, the animal studies of Miller (1969) and DiCara and Miller (1968a,b,c) in which laboratory rats were given injections of curare, a drug that produces complete muscle paralysis, provided additional and clearer support for the effect of operant conditioning of autonomic responses. These rats were kept alive via artificial respiration, and stimulation of an electrode implanted in the pleasure center of the hypothalamus served as a reinforcer. Using this research design, DiCara and Miller (1968a,b,c) successfully demonstrated operant conditioning of heart rate, blood pressure, and urine formation. Although later attempts to replicate these findings were not supported (Miller & Dworkin, 1974), this type of basic research, along with the pioneering work of other researchers such as Green, who built EMG, temperature, GSR, and EEG biofeedback equipment to assess self-control of the ANS (see Green & Green, 1977), helped to define and legitimize the field of biofeedback. In fact, in a review, Schwartz (1995) noted that "some professionals view biofeedback as essentially *instrumental* [italics added] conditioning of visceral responses" (p. 5).

Basmajian (1963), another originator in the field, reported on the ability of patients to control single motor-unit activity. In the late 1960s, Budzynski and Stoyva began utilizing behavioral therapy techniques to enhance efficacy of biofeedback protocols for general relaxation and for the treatment of tension headaches (see Stoyva & Budzynski, 1974, for an early review). The early work of Kamiya (1969) and Brown (1977) in EEG biofeedback gained widespread attention for applications in relaxation and alteration of consciousness, although it was Sterman's (1973; Sterman & Friar, 1972) work in clinical applications in the treatment of epilepsy that appeared to have the most clinical utility.

In recent years, biofeedback has shown potential applicability to a variety of clinical problems, including vasoconstrictive syndromes (Green & Green, 1989; Thompson et al., 1999), GI disorders (Leahy, Clayman, Mason, Lloyd, & Epstein, 1998; Whitehead, 1992), attention-deficit hyperactivity disorder (ADHD; Baumgaertel, 1999; Lubar, Swartwood, Swartwood, & O'Donnell, 1995) urinary incontinence (Burgio & Goode, 1997; Butler, Maby, Montella, & Young, 1999; Johnson & Ouslander, 1999; McGuire, 1996), migraine headaches (McGrath, 1999; Reid & McGrath, 1996) and rehabilitation (Miller & Chang, 1999; Richards & Pohl, 1999). Biofeedback in its present form is not a new endeavor; the technology for its use has been available for decades. This does not mean, however, that there is a current consensus regarding applications and terminology within the field (Blanchard, 1999). What is also new at the beginning of this millenium is the speed, precision, and range of applications available from today's computers in acquiring, storing, analyzing, and displaying data. Basmajian (1999) views biofeedback as part of the Third Therapeutic Revolution, serving as an adjunct to surgery and pharmacology in the treatment of human illness. The technology associated with virtual reality is likely to be a promising area to expand this revolution.

BIOFEEDBACK MODALITIES

In this section, we will briefly review several types of biofeedback, focusing on their nature and potential utility.

Electromyographic (EMG) Biofeedback

Description. Applied to biofeedback, the EMG instrument that is used is one in which electrical impulses are picked up through special sensors (electrodes), which are applied to the skin with electrode jelly used as a conducting medium. The impulse is amplified and processed by the machine in such a way as to produce numerical data, a display of lights, a deflection of a meter, a sound that correlates with the magnitude of the signal, or any combination of these. Since measurement is of electrical correlates of muscle contraction, the numerical display of data in EMG biofeedback is expressed in volts, or more specifically, in microvolts, one-millionth of a volt. The displayed data serve as information to be processed by the client in order to modify function—in this case, muscle tension.

The words *stress* and *tension* are often used interchangeably, and muscle tension itself is a very obvious component of the fight-or-flight response. When a threat is perceived, any muscle throughout the body may tense; however, some do so in a characteristic way. For example, the muscles in the back of the neck characteristically become tense, as if in an effort to keep the head erect to aid in vigilance. Back, shoulder, and jaw muscles tense when the individual perceives him- or herself as being threatened, or when he or she is under stress.

Because we are describing striated muscle, it would seem that control would be voluntary, and therefore easily subject to learning. The difficulty arises when the contraction increases so slowly and imperceptibly that the individual is not aware of increased muscle tension until the muscles are already in spasm. The EMG apparatus allows the individual to become aware of small increments of change in muscle tension, thus allowing him or her to learn to relax the muscles involved.

One can place the EMG electrodes over virtually any striated muscle available to either skin or needle electrodes. Frontalis muscle biofeedback has traditionally been used for low-arousal training (Stoyva & Budzynski, 1993). However, the effectiveness of frontalis placement for generalized relaxation has been questioned (Graham et al., 1986; Jones & Evans, 1981), and other evidence suggests that multiple- and reactive-site EMG biofeedback may be as effective as frontalis biofeedback in reducing sympathetic arousal (Mariela, Matt, & Burish, 1992).

Indications. For the purposes of this chapter, EMG biofeedback is used to treat the stress response in primarily two ways: first, it allows the patient to learn to relax a particular set of muscles (e.g., the masseter muscles in bruxism—teeth grinding), and second, it may be used to produce a more generalized state of relaxation and decreased arousal (e.g., frontalis muscle EMG biofeedback), thus affecting the stress response more centrally (see Stoyva & Budzynski, 1993; Mariela et al., 1992; see also Chapter 10, this volume).

Historically, the two most commonly encountered, specific muscle contraction problems have been muscle tension headaches and bruxism. Sharpley and Rogers (1984), Arena et al. (1995), Barrett (1996), and Rokicki et al. (1997) have noted the usefulness of EMG biofeedback in alleviating muscle contraction headaches. Of note, Arena and colleagues (1995) suggest that trapezius muscle placement may be even more efficacious in alleviating tension headaches than the more standard frontalis muscle placement. Moreover, Rokicki and associates (1997) conclude that it is the increase in self-efficacy engendered by EMG biofeedback that may account for the treatment's effectiveness. Biondi and Picardi (1998) have reported on the benefits of biofeedback in the treatment of bruxism. Also, in a recent meta-analysis, Crider and Glaros (1999) have reported on the practical application of biofeedback to tempromandibular disorders (TMDs), disorders of the jaw muscles often related to bruxism. Within the past decade, the use of EMG biofeedback for the treatment of urinary incontinence has expanded greatly. Using surface abdominal EMG, plevic floor EMG, and rectal pressure, patients with urinary incontinence have been shown to learn successfully how to strengthen pelvic floor muscles and inhibit abdominal muscle contractions (Butler et al., 1999; McDowell et al., 1999).

As noted in Chapter 6, and alluded to in this chapter, the frontalis muscles appear to have value in the treatment of the human stress response because of their potential ability to serve as an indicator of generalized arousal, for example, SNS arousal (Rubin, 1977), by virtue of what appears to be their dual neurological constituency, that is, alpha motor neuron innervation and sympathetic neural innervation (see Everly & Sobelman, 1987). When using the frontalis muscles as a means of engendering the relaxation response, it is important to keep in mind that it may first be necessary to have the patient learn to relax the frontalis specifically before expecting any generalizability to the ANS. That is to say, the frontalis muscles may serve as indicators of sympathetic activity only when they are in a relaxed state. Everly and Sobelman note other issues related to skin preparation and equipment specifications in the use of EMG biofeedback. The EMG biofeedback paradigm has demonstrated its scientific integrity and clinical utility in the hands of competent, well-trained professionals and should still be considered for it usefulness in the treatment of the human stress response (see Sharpley & Rogers, 1984, for a meta-analysis).

Temperature Biofeedback

Description. The use of temperature biofeedback is based on the fact that peripheral skin temperature is a function of vasodilatation and constriction. Thus, when the peripheral blood vessels are dilated and more blood flows through them, the skin is warmer. By measuring the temperature in the extremities, it is possible to get an indication of the amount of blood vessel constriction. Also, since constriction and dilation are controlled by the sympathetic portion of the ANS, one can get an indirect measurement of the amount of sympathetic activity.

The equipment used in thermal biofeedback has the same basic function as the EMG biofeedback equipment described earlier—that is, a sensor, a processor, and a display. The sensor is a thermistor, a small thermal sensing device that is usually attached to the subject's finger. Connected to a machine that transforms the electrical signal, the thermistor produces a signal that is amplified and processed in such a way that, once again, either lights, sounds, or a change in meter reading show small increments of rising or lowering temperature in varying time intervals. It seems obvious that skin temperature can be raised only to the theoretical high of core body temperature, 98.6 °F, although in early accounts, Fuller (1972) reported producing a higher than core body temperature. Change scores from baseline are often used to gauge success of thermal biofeedback; however, baseline skin temperature will affect the amount of change. For example, a patient with a baseline skin temperature of 75 °F will have a greater possible warming change than one with a baseline temperature of 94 °F.

Indications. Temperature feedback has been useful for treating individuals with functional vascular disease or circulatory problems, such as Raynaud's disease (Schwartz & Kelly, 1995; Sedlacek & Taub, 1996; Thompson et al., 1999), or advanced heart failure (Moser, Dracup, Woo, & Stevenson, 1997). It has also been used for patients with endocrine diseases, particularly diabetes (McGrady, Graham, & Bailey, 1996; Saunders, Cox, Teates, & Pohl, 1994), and in the treatment of migraine headaches in adults and children (Allen & Shriver, 1997; Herman, Blanchard, & Flor, 1997; Holroyd & Penzien, 1994), hypertension (Blanchard et al., 1996), and in those instances when control over sympathetic activity is sought (e.g., asthma; Meany et al., 1988). Thermal biofeedback has also been used in psychotherapy to help determine areas of prominent sympathetic arousal and to address the issue of treatment resistance. One minor difficulty involved in the interface between physiology and technology is the short but relevant delay of several seconds between the time of sympathetic discharge, vasoconstriction, and lowering of temperature in the extremity. This measurable reduction in temperature may be displayed several seconds after the event that caused the sympathetic discharge has passed.

Temperature biofeedback has a clear role in the treatment of the stress response in that it is a good indicator of general SNS arousal. Therefore, it is a useful teaching tool for general relaxation, because subjects are instructed to try to raise their skin temperature. This mode of therapy may be used alone, alternatively with EMG, or in combination with it. See Green and Green (1989), and Lehrer and colleagues (1994) for a practical review of thermal biofeedback.

Electroencephalographic (EEG) Biofeedback

Description. The brain's electrical activity is continuous, most likely the result of discharges at synapses. In 1924, Hans Berger developed a graphic method for recording that electrical brain-wave activity. What appears to be recorded by the EEG are those synapses closest to the surface of the brain. There are many ascending pathways to the cortex; however, it is believed that the most highly represented area on the outermost surface of the cortex is the reticular activating system (Guyton, 1987). These data are, however, difficult to analyze, because a single neuron may have as many as a thousand branchings in the cortex. Therefore, although data attained on the EEG are fairly nonspecific, it is generally agreed that various wave patterns do correlate with various states of consciousness and reflect activity, particularly in the reticular activating system.

Brain waves have been divided into four categories, depending on their predominant frequency and amplitude. The term *frequency* refers to the cycles per second, or per minute, and reflects the number of firings of neurons per unit of time. Brain-wave frequency on the surface of the scalp ranges from 1 every few seconds to 50 or more per second (Guyton & Hall, 1996). The *amplitude* refers to the amount of electricity generated and is a reflects the number of neurons firing synchronously.

Brain waves are classified as alpha, beta, theta, and delta waves. Alpha waves are characterized by a frequency of 8–13 cycles/sec and an amplitude of 20–100+µv. These rhythmic waves are related to an awake, relaxed state characterized by calmness and passive attention. Alpha waves do not occur when participants are asleep, or when they have their attention focused (Guyton & Hall, 1996). Beta waves occur at a frequency of 14 or more cycles per second to as high as 80 cycles per second and have low amplitude. They are characteristic of an awake, attentive state when the subject is focusing his or her thoughts, or is aroused or have tense. Theta waves occur at a frequency of 4–7 cycles/sec, with a usual amplitude of 20 µv or less. They are often considered part of the daydreaming state. Last, delta wave frequencies are from .5 to less than 4 cycles/sec and are associated with deep sleep. Thus, when one is resting, dominant EEG activity is in the alpha and theta ranges; however, excitement shifts brain-wave activity toward the beta range. It is also of note that as we grow older, the relative proportion of beta-wave activity increases, whereas theta-wave activity decreases (Lubar, 1991).

Indications. Predicated on the work of Sterman and colleagues (Sterman, 1973; Sterman & Friar, 1972) involving sensorimotor rhythm (SMR) training, which is thought to capture activity of the sensorimotor cortex, one of the first areas investigated for use of EEG biofeedback training occurred in an attempt to manage epileptic seizures (Seifert & Lubar, 1975). This research expanded to include treatment of hyperkinetic children, in which EEG biofeedback was used to increase SMR production and inhibit theta-wave production (Lubar & Shouse, 1976; Shouse & Lubar, 1978). Lubar and colleagues (see Lubar, 1991; Lubar & Deering, 1981) later added enhanced beta-wave production via EEG biofeedback in the treatment of ADHD. EEG biofeedback, which has received increased attention as a viable treatment option for ADHD (Alhambra, Fowler, & Alhambra, 1995), has recently been employed successfully to assist treatment of ADHD in a school setting (Boyd & Campbell, 1998). In fact, more than 300 organizations use EEG neurofeedback in the treatment of ADHD (Lubar, 1995). The premise behind the use of EEG neurofeedback is that ADHD is thought to be associated with neurological dysfunction at the cortical level, involving primarily the prefrontal lobes (Lubar, 1995). The use of EEG neurofeedback is thought to normalize cortical function, which leads to normalization of behavior and overall academic and social adjustment (Lubar, 1995). A practical issue worth noting is that for ADHD, it may take anywhere from 40 to 80 sessions for effective EEG treatment (Lubar, 1991) compared to 10–20 sessions for EMG biofeedback for tension headaches.

Also, Swingle (1998) has used psychotherapy and EEG biofeedback, which enhanced SMR and suppressed theta-wave activity, to treat 6 patients with pseudoseizure disorder. Case studies have shown EEG biofeedback to be effective in the treatment of Lyme disease (Packard & Ham, 1996), chronic fatigue syndrome (James & Folen, 1996), and depression (Baehr, Rosenfeld, & Baehr, 1997). Moreover, there has been increased experimental use of alpha–theta EEG neurofeedback therapy in the treatment of alcoholism (see Peniston & Kulkosky, 1999, for a review). Particularly relevant to this text has been the use of topographic EEG mapping of Benson's relaxation response on 20 novice subjects (Jacobs, Benson, & Friedman, 1996). Using a controlled, within-subjects design, the data revealed that elicitation of the relaxation response resulted in statistically significant reductions in frontal EEG beta activity, which reflects reduced cortical activation in anterior brain regions.

Sensor placement in neurofeedback is usually standardized based on the International 10–20 System of electrode placement. For the neurotherapy systems typically in use, an experienced therapist requires only about 2 minutes to connect the sensors to the scalp. Training sessions include a baseline assessment to determine the average microvolt level of the brain waves being investigated. Reward criteria are then established by an amplitude "window," which sets high and low microvolt levels that are reinforced or inhibited. For example, in the beta–theta training used in treating ADHD, beta thresholds may be raised $1 \mu v$ higher, or theta levels may be set $1–2 \mu v$ lower (Lubar et al., 1995). Rewards are often auditory and visual, and given today's advancements in computer software technology, the effects, as you can imagine, can be quite elaborate.

Electrodermal (EDR) Biofeedback

Description.   *Electrodermal* is a generic term that refers to the electrical characteristics of the skin. There are numerous measurement options available when considering this type of biofeedback. The oldest and most commonly used is the galvanic skin response (GSR); the name attributed to Galvani's discovery of electrical activity in nerves and muscles. Generally, variation of the skin's electrical characteristics appears to be a function of sympathetic neural activity; therefore, when using EDR biofeedback, the patient appears to be training to affect sympathetic neural arousal. More specifically, what is being measured is the conductance and resistance of sweat gland activity.

Indications.   The major use for EDR is to reduce levels of sympathetic tone and reactivity. It has been used in conjunction with other biofeedback modalities in the treatment of hypertension (Patel & Marmot, 1988) and asthma (Meany et al., 1988), and has also been used as an adjunct in

psychotherapy. For example, EDR has been used for systematic desensitization, the theory being that relaxation and arousal cannot happen concurrently, and that phobias and anxiety would respond to this type of
treatment. EDR has also been used as a tool for exploration in psychotherapy, and in "lie detector" equipment (Peek, 1995).

PRECAUTIONS

Several adverse reactions can occur as a result of using biofeedback.
The practitioner should be aware of the unfavorable conditions that may
be produced or potentially exacerbated by its use (see Chapter 10, this volume; see also Schwartz, 1995). Let us briefly review several of these issues.
First is the case of patients taking medication for any purpose. Some
patients may consider biofeedback a replacement for medication and
prematurely or mistakenly stop taking medication they have received for
some other purpose. Therefore, it is necessary to question patients closely
regarding their medication history and also be willing to work closely with
their physicians. The most dramatic example of this occurrence is diabetic
patients who are taking insulin. In these cases, inducing relaxation may
diminish the need for insulin, and the normal dosage that the patient had
been taking may now precipitate a hypoglycemic coma. Changes in blood
pressure as a result of efficacious biofeedback treatment are also an area
of valid concern for patients taking medication for hyper- or hypotension.
In addition, seizures have occurred in patients undergoing biofeedback
treatment for epilepsy.
Other problems may arise related to improper training of the patient
by the therapist. An example might be treatment of bruxism with unilateral
placement of EMG sensors, producing dislocation of the jaw through
imbalance of the muscles. Muscle imbalance is also a potential precaution
in the treatment of torticollis with biofeedback.
Practitioners may also want to exercise caution in the selection of
patients. For example, individuals experiencing psychosis, including hallucinations or delusions, and dissociative disorders are considered poor
candidates for biofeedback training.

ROLE OF THE THERAPIST AND OTHER FACTORS

From the information covered thus far in this chapter, a reasonable
conclusion may be that the major element in biofeedback is the machinery.
However, this is really not a valid statement. In fact, the clinician–patient
dyad is a far more important element in this form of therapy. More than

many types of therapies, biofeedback requires that the patient be motivated to get better and to practice between sessions what he or she has learned. Thus, his or her relationship with the therapist is quite important.

A decisive factor in biofeedback success appears to be the extent to which cognitive restructuring helps patients recognize the ways in which the mind and body interact. Again, this occurrence is dependent on the patient's relationship with his or her clinician to facilitate the process. Within this context, biofeedback may be considered an adjunct to a total therapeutic relationship. It is comparable to hypnosis, relaxation therapy, and so on, in that it is a tool used to treat a symptom complex, but only within the context of the total therapeutic relationship. Thus, clinicians may be thought of as theatrical directors: They set the stage for change to occur by giving useful hints, pointers, feedback, and encouragement, but they do not change patients themselves. Sometimes, for example, the therapist may not be present during certain portions of biofeedback training. However, clinicians facilitate change by using the therapeutic relationship to motivate patients and make it easier for them to experience success. Our original diagram of the biofeedback encounter (Figure 15.1) may now be modified as indicated in Figure 15.3.

Thus, the clinician receives information regarding the patient's functioning from both the instrument and the patient, then provides information to the patient, allowing the patient better to use data acquired from the instrument. Again, the clinician, although not directly responsible for therapeutic change, plays an important role in the biofeedback loop. His or her empathetic skills, clinical demeanor, and effectiveness as a health educator interact with other factors, such as office setting, room temperature, and type of equipment, to affect the outcome of clinical feedback. It would be naive to believe that personality factors do not affect biofeedback skills acquisition. As noted in Chapter 7, individuals bring

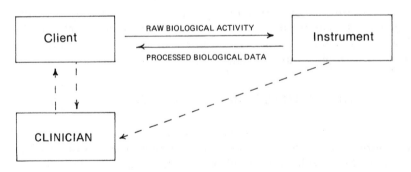

Figure 15.3.

various strengths, vulnerabilities, and reservations to the clinical encounter. Also, as noted in Chapter 8, issues of mastery, self-control, and self-efficacy are quite germane to the biofeedback paradigm. Bandura (1982a,b, 1997) has noted, however, that the perception of self-efficacy is even more salient than the degree of manifest self-efficacy. Once again, the clinician's function is paramount in assisting the patient to recognize meaningful acquisition in lieu of possible propensities for self-debasement, catastrophic ideation, or general pessimism.

In their reviews of the utilization and delivery of biofeedback within research and clinical applications, Shellenberger and Green (1986) and Schwartz and associates (1995) discuss some of the most common errors, in addition to ways of ensuring competence. The following errors have particular relevance to the use of biofeedback in the treatment of excessive stress:

1. Failure of the clinician to receive proper training and experience in the use of applied biofeedback equipment and modalities.

2. Failure of the inexperienced clinician to ask for and use prudent supervision.

3. Failure to provide the patient with the appropriate number of training sessions. In biofeedback, which represents a form of learning, individual differences account for a large preponderance of the variation. In other words, no consistent rule governs the rate of skills acquisition. Nevertheless, it is apparent that most people cannot acquire useful biofeedback skills in only two or three sessions. Moreover, recall that 40–80 sessions may be required when using EEG biofeedback to treat ADHD.

4. Failure to provide the patient with homework exercises that reinforce and extend the skills acquired within the office or laboratory setting. Again, one of the primary goals of biofeedback is to generalize the response to settings outside of the office.

5. Failure of the clinician to recognize and facilitate the social-psychological and clinical aspects of biofeedback. Some clinicians erroneously believe that biofeedback is immune to the usual clinical variables that affect other aspects of clinical psychology and psychiatry. Therefore, it is often useful to conceptualize some forms of biofeedback as biofeedback-assisted psychotherapy.

6. Failure of the clinician to recognize that the patient's formation of a sense of control or self-efficacy serves as one of the most relevant clinical aspects or powerful therapeutic forces within the biofeedback paradigm.

7. Failure of the clinician to allow the patient ample time to adapt or habituate to the physiological assessment process. Biofeedback, in addition to being a therapeutic intervention, is also an exercise in physiological assessment. In any such paradigm, the subject must be allowed to adapt

to the novel stimuli represented by the biofeedback training environment. Adaptation needs to occur within every training session.

8. Failure to take baseline measurements relevant to the biofeedback variables to be trained. In a sense, it is useful to consider the patient as the control within a single-subject research design and to structure the clinical paradigm with that in mind.

9. Failure of the clinician to train the clinical patient to mastery as opposed to initial skills acquisition. In other words, too many patients are prematurely terminated by biofeedback clinicians who lose sight of the need to have patients overlearn the acquired skills in self-regulation.

THE PAST AND FUTURE OF BIOFEEDBACK

As in the first edition of this text, the reader will undoubtedly detect our sense of optimism regarding the clinical utility of EMG, EEG, EDR, and temperature biofeedback. The successes of biofeedback applications in the past decade, along with the trend for increased use of alternative medical therapies (Eisenberg et al., 1998) and an enhanced focus on wellness and prevention, has helped to increase the acceptance and recognition of biofeedback. In fact, the recently introduced *Journal of Neurotherapy* addresses the growing interest in the area of EEG biofeedback. It is important to note, however, that the field of biofeedback as a clinical technology has not always been universally accepted by clinicians and researchers. Past criticisms and scrutiny have focused on the soundness and rigor of some of the research design and methodology (Schwartz, 1995), as well as the apparently exaggerated claims of applied applications and successes made by some practitioners. For a good review of the epistemological issues that affect the conduct of inquiry as it pertains to the investigation of the clinical efficacy of biofeedback, the reader is referred to Shellenberger and Green (1986, 1987) and Lehler et al. (1994). As the literature and computerized technology in this area continue to expand and attention is devoted to producing quality research and helping consumers evaluate outcome data, we hope that the biofeedback field has learned from its history and will continue its course toward a vibrant future.

SUMMARY

This chapter has explored biofeedback, the creation and clinical uti-lization of psychophysiological feedback loops for the purpose of treating excessive stress and/or its target-organ effects. Let us review the main points:

1. Biofeedback gives the patient access to learning paradigms that involve physiological functions not previously accessible to conscious alteration.
2. Biofeedback can be used directly to modify the stress response itself, through the elicitation of the relaxation response or the alteration of target-organ activity.
3. EMG, temperature, EEG, and EDR biofeedback are the most commonly used forms of clinical biofeedback. The use of EEG neurofeedback has blossomed in the past decade.
4. The clinican's impact on the biofeedback paradigm is so important that it can mean the difference between clinical success or failure. For this reason, the clinician should receive training in not only clinical psychophysiology but also the fundamentals of counseling or clinical psychology.
5. In understanding the process of therapeutic effect, one of the most important aspects of clinical biofeedback may be the creation of the perception of self-efficacy, as discussed by Bandura (1997) and supported by Rokicki and associates (1997) in the use of EMG biofeedback specifically.
6. For precautions that should be followed in using biofeedback, refer to Chapter 10.
7. Useful reviews of clinical biofeedback are found in Schwartz (1995), Shellenberger and Green (1986), and Basmajian (1989).

16

Physical Exercise and the Human Stress Response

It has been suggested (Chavat et al., 1964; Kraus & Rabb, 1961) that the "wisdom of the body" dictates that the human stress response should lead to physical exertion or exercise. Indeed, physical exercise appears to be the most effective way of ventilating, or expressing, the stress response in a health-promoting manner, once it has been engendered.

Having reviewed the psychophysiological nature of human stress in Part I, it seems reasonable to conclude that stress represents a psychophysiological process that prepares the body for physical action. The increased blood supply to the heart and skeletal muscles, coupled with increased neuromuscular tension, circulating free fatty acids and glucose, as well as the diminished blood flow to the GI system, all lead to the conclusion that the stress response prepares the organism for action (Benson, 1975; Cannon, 1914, 1929; Chavat et al., 1964; Kraus & Raab, 1961).

It also seems feasible to assume that, thousands of years ago, the highly active lifestyle of primitive humans afforded ample opportunity to express physically the arousal that resulted from the frustrations and dangers they encountered on a daily basis. Similarly, there was likely sufficient opportunity for our ancestors to develop many of the positive physical and psychological advantages known to accrue from regular physical exercise. Yet in developing from "physical beings" to "thinking beings," humans have fewer chances to ventilate frustrations, failures, and challenges in healthful physical expression. This need to ventilate and refresh our minds and bodies through exercise is apparently so important that some have suggested (Chavat et al., 1964; Greenberg, Dintiman, & Myers-Oakes, 1998; Kraus & Raab, 1961) that the lack of physically active somatomotor expression may lead to an increase risk of disease and dysfunction.

Predicated on information from the World Health Organization, Chavat et al. (1964) concluded that when the body is aroused for physical action but that physical expression is suppressed, a condition of strain or psychophysiological overload may be created. They note: "When in civilized man ... [stress] reactions are produced, the ... [physically motivating] component is usually more or less suppressed. ... What is obvious is that often repeated incidents of ... [suppressed somatomotor activity] must imply an increased load on heart and blood vessels" (pp. 130–131).

Similarly, Kraus and Raab (1961) proposed that suppressed physical expression has a preeminent role in the etiology of a variety of anxiety- and stress-related diseases, which they referred to as "hypokinetic diseases." This concept is said to have influenced President John F. Kennedy to promote physical fitness as a major national priority during the early 1960s. Former Surgeon General Dr. C. Evert Koop developed a Web site, where he actively promoted physical activity, particularly for our youth.

If, indeed, we have accurately interpreted the "wisdom of the body" as intending that the stress response be consumated in some form of physical somatomotor expression, then a rationale quickly emerges for the consideration of physical exercise as a powerful therapeutic tool in prevention, treatment, and rehabilitation programs for stress-related disease and dysfunction.

HISTORY OF THERAPEUTIC EXERCISE

It seems reasonable to assume that our ancient ancestors suffered from few stress-related "hypokinetic" diseases because of their physically demanding lifestyles. It also appears that ancient Greeks, at least for a period of time, had an appreciation of the need to create a balance between physical and intellectual ventures. Plato (as cited in Simon & Levisohn, 1987, p. 50), claimed that "physical exercise is not merely necessary to the health and development of the body, but to balance and correct intellectual pursuits as well. ... The right education must tune the strings of the body and mind to perfect spiritual harmony." Physical exercise likely gained the potential for therapeutic application when our physically active culture evolved into a more sedentary one.

Perhaps the earliest use of exercise in a therapeutic capacity, according to Ryan (1974), was in the fifth century B.C. It was during this time that the Greek physician Herodicus prescribed gymnastics for various diseases. In the second century B.C., Asclepiades prescribed walking and running in conjunction with diet and massage for disease, as well as for the ills of an "opulent" society.

In 16th-century Europe, Joseph Duchesne is thought to have been the first to use swimming as a therapeutic tool. He is said to have used such physical activity to strengthen the heart and lungs. As a result, exercise gained great popularity in Europe for its therapeutic and preventive applications.

In 1829, the *Journal of Health*, a monthly magazine published in Philadelphia and intended for the general population as well as the medical profession, covered topics such as the health effects of food, drink, atmospheric variables, minerals, hygiene, and exercise. Edward Hitchcock, a professor of chemistry and natural history at Amherst College, and the first professor of physical education in the United States, was a strong supporter of the journal. The publication advocated regular exercise, and Hitchcock considered walking the very best exercise for retaining health (Green, 1986). However, it was not until after the Civil War that exercise and fitness expanded to include all age groups in America.

Following World War I, therapeutic exercise and the study of exercise physiology gained momentum in the United States. According to Miller and Allen (1995), Hans Selye contended that regular exercise would better prepare someone to resist other stressors, and that stressful situations would not be as perilous to a physcially fit individual compared to someone who has led a sedentary lifetsyle. Physical fitness came into vogue for the lay public with the advent of the President's Council on Physical Fitness in 1956, and the urging of President Kennedy in the 1960s.

As more and more individuals began exercising, more data became available regarding its nature and effects. Physical fitness was promoted in occupational settings with the founding of organizations such as the American Association of Fitness Directors in Business and Industry, which actively and vigorously promoted the "Good health is good business" philosophy to millions at the job site.

Also in the 1960s, America experienced the advent of the urban "health spa." These urban/suburban facilities were centers for the promotion of a health-oriented culture; however, they were typically segregated by gender. The 1970s and the 1980s witnessed two revolutions in the pursuit of exercise that changed the gender separation. The first was the invention of exercise equipment, such as Nautilus, which made weightlifting easier, safer, and more efficient. Moreover, when practiced using the recommended protocol, it actually yielded the *potential* to facilitate skeletomuscular development while concurrently improving the efficiency of the cardiopulmonary system, thus achieving what exercise enthusiasts at the time considered the best of both worlds. Newer equipment, such as Cybex and Hammer Strength, has continued to refine this type of training.

The second revolution involved the image of physical exercise. As noted earlier, there existed two different psychologies of exercise, one for women and one for men. Under the influence of writers such as Kenneth Cooper (*The Aerobics Way: New Data on the World's Most Popular Exercise Program*, 1977) and Jimm Fixx (*The Complete Book of Running*, 1977), as well as the marketing and development of sophisticated exercise facilities that fostered social support, the social barriers to physical exercise fell. For the first time in American history, exercise became a social as well as physical activity that both men and women could pursue and enjoy together.

The 1980s also produced an escalation of scientific research interest in how exercise may be related to mental health (Rejeski & Thompson, 1993). Moreover, the 1980s, with stores such as the General Nutrition Center (GNC), proliferated the current multibillion dollar a year supplement industry that sold products claiming to provide sundry functions such as adding muscle, reducing fat, and accelerating metabolism. Two supplements, creatine and androstenedione, the latter made famous for its use by baseball player Mark McGuire, received considerable press at the start of the new millenium. The late 1980s also spawned the advent of step aerobics, which continues as a mainstay in fitness facilities. Current trends such as tae bo and hydroaerobics have demonstrated the interplay between aerobics and other sports. Today, exercise continues to enjoy tremendous popularity in the United States and, as noted earlier, remains a viable area of pursuit for health care professionals. This chapter examines exercise as a therapeutic tool for the treatment of excessive stress.

MECHANISMS OF ACTION

Exercise itself represents an intense form of stress response, yet it differs greatly from the stress response implicated in the onset of psychosomatic disease. Why then is the stress of exercise health promoting, in most instances, and the emotionally related stress of living in a competitive urban environment, for example, health eroding? We now examine the mechanisms that may answer this question.

Three therapeutic mechanisms of action serve to explain the clinical effectiveness of exercise in the treatment of excessive stress.

1. Mechanisms active during exercise
2. Mechanisms active shortly after exercise
3. Long-term mechanisms

The therapeutic mechanisms at work during the acute process of exercising are manifest in the propensity for such physical activity healthfully to utilize the potentially harmful constituents of the stress response. The stress-responsive gluconeogenic hormones (primarily cortisol) begin to break down adipose tissue for energy during the stress response. In this process, a form of fat, called *free fatty acid* (FFA), is released into the bloodstream (Ganong, 1997). During the stress of physical exercise, FFA levels actually decline, because the FFA is utilized for energy by the active muscles. In contrast, however, during emotionally related stress, FFA is not utilized as rapidly because of the sedentary nature of this type of stress. The FFA persists in the bloodstream and is converted to triglycerides and, ultimately, to low-density lipoproteins (LDLs). LDLs are considered a major source of atherosclerotic plaque associated with premature coronary artery disease (Berne, Levy, Koeppen, & Stanton, 1998).

A second factor to consider during the stress response is the significant demand placed on the cardiovascular and cardiorespiratory systems. Cardiac output (heart rate × stroke volume), blood pressure, and resistance to peripheral blood flow all increase. Also, breathing rate increases and bronchial tubes dilate during the stress response. By the use of moderate physical activity, however, these factors are utilized in a healthful form. Although cardiac output must increase, the rhythmic use of the striated muscles actually assists the return of blood to the heart (increase of venous return). Moreover, physical training allows the body to redistribute blood from less active tissues, such as digestive organs and kidneys, to active muscles, and even to the skin for heat dissipation (Sharkey, 1990). Blood pressure must increase during exercise as well but not so dramatically as is seen when one remains inactive when stressed (e.g., as when sitting in a traffic jam). Regarding respiratory and O_2 transport, physical activity and training improve the efficiency of breathing muscles, allowing greater lung capacity. Thus, a moderately active individual uses fewer breaths to move the same amount of air, which improves diffusion of O_2 into the lungs.

Third, during the stress response, the hormones epinephrine and norepinephrine are released. Research (Dimsdale & Moss, 1980; Fibiger & Singer, 1984; Hoch, Werle, & Weicker, 1988) has shown that during the stress of exercise, norepinephrine is preferentially released, whereas during emotion-related stress, epinephrine is preferentially released. McCabe and Schneiderman (1984) concluded that circulating epinephrine represents the greatest risk to the integrity of the heart muscle, because the ventricles are maximally responsive to epinephrine, not norepinephrine. In an individual suffering from heart ischemia, they conclude that high levels of epinephrine could induce a lethal arrhythmia. Also, during the stress response, the resistance of blood flow to the skin and other peripheral aspects increases. During the stress of exercise, resistance of blood flow in the skin actually decreases, which has implications for cooling the body and lowering blood pressure (see Ganong, 1997, for a discussion of cardiovascular dynamics). Overall, exercise seems to fine-tune the body's secretions and response to hormones, leading to a more efficient use of energy sources (Sharkey, 1990).

The preceding examples are indicative of the different ways the body responds to the stress of exercise in contrast to the stress response that we undergo if we remain static or inactive. Clearly, the acute strain on the body is quite different if one undergoes a stress response in an active rather than inactive state. Although physical activity is capable of using the constituents of the stress response in a constructive manner, the therapeutic reactions may persist beyond the acute period of exercise.

The short-term therapeutic mechanisms associated with exercise entail the initiation of a state of relaxation following the physical activity. In most circumstances, plasma catecholamines return to resting levels within minutes of acute exercise (Peronnet & Szabo, 1993). Clearly, exercise itself represents a powerful ergotropic response mediated by the SNS; however, according to Balog (1978), on completion of exercise, the organism may undergo psychophysiological recovery by initiating a trophotropic response mediated by the PNS. According to de Vries (1966), gamma motor neural discharge may also be inhibited during recovery from physical activity. The gamma motor system is a complementary connection from the cerebral cortex to the striated musculature. The result of such inhibition is said to be striated muscle relaxation.

The muscle-relaxant qualities of exercise have important implications for short-term declines in diffuse anxiety and ergotropic tone in autonomic as well as striated muscles. It has been demonstrated that striated muscle tension contributes to diffuse anxiety and arousal in striated and autonomic musculature through a complex feedback system (Gellhorn, 1964, 1967; Jacobson, 1978). This system involves afferent (incoming) proprioceptive stimulation from striated muscles to the limbic emotional centers, the hypothalamus and cerebral cortex. Therefore, reduction in striated muscle tension should lead to a generalized decrease in ergotropic tone throughout the body, as well as a decrease in diffuse anxiety levels. These results have been demonstrated empirically by Gellhorn (1958), and de Vries (1968, 1981), and the notion that exercise leads to decreased skeletal muscle tension now appears readily accepted (Foss & Keteyian, 1998).

Several theoretical rationales have been generated to explain the physiological benefits of physical exercise in reducing stress and anxiety. These include the endorphin hypothesis, which suggests that it is the release and binding of morphine-like endogenous opioids, such as beta endorphin, that affect feelings such as euphoria that have been associated with the anecdotal reports of a runner's high. Another hypothesis is the monoamine neurotransmitter theory, or norepinephrine hypothesis, which that suggests that the affective benefits of exercise may derive from increased levels of norepinephrine. The thermogenic hypothesis contends that the elevation in body temperature that occurs during exercise leads to decreased stress (Tuson & Sinyor, 1993). Although these theories are readily accepted in this field of study, it is worth noting that none has received conclusive empirical support.

The most significant long-term mechanisms of health promotion inherent in exercise appear to emerge when exercise is aerobic and practiced for a minimum of at least 1 month. One of the areas most positively affected is the ability to use O_2 more efficiently. Exercise training of an aerobic nature increases maximum ventilatory O_2 uptake by increasing both maximum cardiac output (the volume of blood ejected by the heart per minute, which determines the amount of blood delivered to the exercising muscles) and the ability of muscles to extract and use O_2 from blood (Fletcher et al., 1996). In addition to reduced cardiovascular responses to stress, which lead to long-term, reduced risk of clinical manifestations of coronary heart disease (CHD), recent data suggest that physical activity may help in the prevention and treatment of osteoporosis and certain cancers, most notably colon cancer (Fletcher et al., 1996; Lee, 1994).

Within the past 10 years, a surge of research has investigated the effects of exercise on improved psychological functioning, particularly in the areas of anxiety, depression, and self-esteem. The bulk of the data in the area of stress and anxiety, however, has not been generated from controlled experimental investigations with accurately diagnosed individuals (Tkachuk & Martin, 1999). In a review of studies on the affective benefits of acute aerobic exercise, Tuson and Sinyor (1993) reported that four of the five studies with sound methodological rigor revealed reductions in self-reported anxiety following exercise. In a comprehensive review of exercise as a coping strategy for stress that included preexperimental, quasi-experimental, and experimental designs, Rostad and Long (1996), again acknowledging that design and conceptual problems limit some of the conclusions drawn from the studies, did suggest that the accumulated evidence indicates a postive trend to support the use and efficacy of an exercise program as a coping strategy for stress.

In a recent controlled investigation (Broocks et al., 1998), a 10-week protocol of running or walking a 4-mile route at least three times per week was compared to the prescription drug clomipramine and to placebo in the treatment of patients diagnosed with moderate to severe panic disorder with or without agoraphobia (based on DSM-III-R criteria). At the end of the 10-week period, results revealed that exercise and clomipramine were found to be more effective than placebo in reducing scores on clinician- and self-rated measures of anxiety, panic, agoraphobia and global improvement. Comparing the two active treatments at the end of 10 weeks revealed equal effectiveness in the primary outcome measures except in the rater version of global improvement, where clomipramine was higher.

Comparable to the work in the fields of anxiety and stress, research efforts have also focused on the long-term benefits of exercise in the treatment of depression (Noth, McCullagh, & Tran, 1990), self-esteem (McDonald & Hodgdons, 1991), and self-efficacy (Marcus, Eaton, Rossi, & Harlow, 1994). Similar to the conclusions derived for exercise and anxiety, a review of the data on exercise and depression suggests that more controlled investigations are warranted. However, tentative conclusions suggest that aerobic exercise seems to be as effective as other forms of psychotherapy in the treatment of mild to moderate forms of unipolar depression (Martinsen & Morgan, 1997). Of added clinical interest is the consistent finding that patients without physiological gains in fitness reported psychological benefits in subjective mood comparable to those of patients with improved aerobic fitness. Sonstroem (1997) has suggested that the level of physical activity is probably better associated with the constructs of physical self-concepts (which are components of the global construct of self-esteem). As with exercise and depression, he also notes that self-concept changes as a result of physical activity seem to be independent of increases in physical fitness. In a recent controlled experimental study that assessed a number of psychological variables, DiLorenzo and associates (1999) reported that exercise-induced increases in aerobic fitness using a stationary bicycle resulted in improved short- and long-term effects on the psychological variables anxiety, depression, self-concept, and vigor.

Collectively, it may well be that the long-term physiological and psychological mechanisms of action that support the use of exercise in the treatment and prevention of stress-related disease represent a higher level of physical and psychological fitness and, therefore, a higher level of stress resistance. This higher level of fitness may then aid the individual, both psychologically and physically, in withstanding the potentially injurious effects of excessive stress. One might consider such a level of fitness as a buffer to excessive stress reactivity (Rejeski & Thompson, 1993). Based upon the work of Sime (1984), Weller and Everly (1985), Sharkey (1990), Seraganian (1993), Weyerer and Kupfer (1994), Haskell (1995), and Blair et al. (1996), we suggest that the stress-resistant aspects of sustained, chronic exercise include the following:

1. Improved cardiorespiratory efficiency
2. Improved glucose utilization
3. Reduced body fat
4. Reduced resting blood pressure

5. Reduced resting muscle tension
6. Decreased ANS reactivity
7. Increased steroid reserves to counter stress
8. Reduced trait anxiety
9. Improved self-concept
10. Improved sense of self-efficacy, physical self-concept, and self-control

All of these potential alterations are relevant in that they contribute to the individual's ability to tolerate high levels of stress, and, therefore, decrease the likelihood of developing stress-related pathology.

RESEARCH SUPPORTING THERAPEUTIC EXERCISE FOR STRESS

A review of the following current and past literature on the clinical use of exercise in the treatment of excessive stress and stress-related disease provides ample support and rationale for the application of exercise:

1. A review by Donoghue (1977) supports the relationship between habitual exercise and improved work performance.
2. Twenty minutes of walking (about 100 cal) reduce the risk of coronary artery disease by approximately 30% (Sharkey, 1990).
3. Regular, strenuous activity (greater than 7.5 cal/min) for at least 3 hours per week resulted in lower incidence of heart attacks in active compared to inactive individuals or those who did not exercise vigorously (Paffenbarger, Hyde, & Wing, 1986).
4. In a review by Blair and colleagues (1996), moderately fit male nonsmokers had a 41% lower all-cause death rate than those in the corresponding low fit category. Also, moderately fit female nonsmokers had a 55% lower all-cause death rate than those who were low fit. Moreover, high fit men with two or three other risk-factor predictors had a 15% lower death rate than did low fit men with none of the predictors. High fit women with two or three other risk factors had a 50% lower death rate than did low fit women with none of the predictors.
5. Exercise, in the form of cycling, has been shown to reduce subjective anxiety elevated by ingesting 1,200 mg of caffeine (Youngstedt, O'Conner, Crabbe, & Dishman, 1998).
6. Tai chi chuan, used as an alternative form of exercise, was demonstrated to promote muscle relaxation in older adults (Chen & Sun, 1997).

7. In a recent meta-analysis of 37 studies investigating the effects of exercise on depression, Craft and Landers (1998) reported that individuals who exercised were −0.72 standard deviation less depressed than individuals who did not exercise.

8. Graded exercise was shown to produce improvements in functional work capacity and fatigue in 96 patients diagnosed with chronic fatigue syndrome (Wearden et al., 1998).

9. After adjusting for demographics and lifestyle factors (e.g., cigarette smoking, alcohol use), adults judged to be in excellent aerobic fitness (as assessed by a step test and 3-minute recovery test) had less than one-half the risk of elevated serum cholesterol compared to adults with poor fitness levels (Tucker & Bagwell, 1991).

10. Exercise has also been shown to improve mood, decrease distress, and increase body cell mass and lean body mass in HIV-positive men (Wagner, Rabkin, & Rabkin, 1998).

11. Approximately 12% of all deaths in the United States are attributable to lack of regular physical activity (McGinnis & Foege, 1993).

12. Sedentary men and women have nearly twice the risk of developing colon cancer compared to those who are physically active (Lee, 1995).

This section on research may be summarized cogently by the conclusion drawn by Sime (1984) more than 17 years ago: "If stress is defined in the traditional fight-or-flight terminology, then exercise is a classic method of stress management through its active, dynamic release of physiological preparedness" (p. 502).

EXERCISE GUIDELINES

Once the decision to exercise has been made, the issue of how much exercise is enough to promote health and better cope with stress needs to be addressed. An acronym often used to account for the ingredients of exercise prescription is FITT, which stands for Frequency, Intensity, Time (duration), and Type (Foss & Keteyian, 1998). Before beginning an exercise program, it is wise to consider some type of screening or medical evaluation that includes a comprehensive history; a physical exam, including a measure of resting heart rate and blood pressure; blood analysis for fasting blood sugar and cholesterol levels; a measurement of expired gases; a 12-lead resting electrocardiogram (ECG); and an exercise tolerance or stress test with ECG monitoring (American College of Sports Medicine, 1995). Exercise tolerance tests include the Harvard Step Test, the Cooper 12-Minute Test, the Rockport One-Mile Fitness Walking Test, the YMCA

Table 16.1. Estimated Maximum Heart Rates and
Exercise Training Heart Rates by Age for Normal Persons[a]

Age	Maximum	Percent		
		70	60	50
21–30	195	159	147	135
31–40	185	152	141	130
41–50	175	145	135	125
51–60	165	138	129	120
61–70	155	131	123	115

[a]Values are listed in beats per minute (bpm), computed using a heart rate of
75 bpm (adapted from Foss & Keteyian, 1998).

protocol, and the Astrand–Ryhming test. These evaluations are useful in determining fitness levels, target heart rates, and maximal aerobic power, and screening for latent abnormalities that may only be evident during physical exertion.

Returning to the question of how much exercise is enough, the American College of Sports Medicine (ACSM) has been providing minimum guidelines for enhancing cardiopulmonary efficiency since 1975. These recommendations have been based on data on dose–response improvements in performance capacity, especially in maximal aerobic power (maximum O_2 consumption) for otherwise healthy adults with unremarkable physical exams. Following these guidelines, Pate and his colleagues (1995) from the Centers for Disease Control and Prevention (CDC) and the ACSM, in a special communication in the *Journal of the American Medical Association* (JAMA), suggested the following physical exercise criteria for enhanced cardiopulmonary fitness:

1. Duration: 20–60 minutes of moderate- to high-intensity endurance exercise.
2. Intensity: 60–90% of maximum heart rate (estimated to be 220 − age in years) (see Table 16.1) or 50–85% of maximal aerobic power.
3. Frequency: three or more times per week.

According to Ribisl (1984), exercise sessions for enhancing cardiopulmonary efficiency should be structured using a format that contains a warm-up phase, an exercise phase, and a cool-down phase. In an exercise session lasting 60 minutes, 10–20 minutes should be devoted to warm-up, 20–40 minutes to the actual aerobic exercise, and 10–20 minutes to cool-down. The benefits of the warm-up phase, according to Ribisl (1984) and Foss and Keteyian (1998) include the following:

1. Facilitation of enzymatic activity due to an increase in body and muscle temperature.

2. Increased metabolic activity.
3. Improved blood flow and oxygen delivery.
4. Decreased peripheral resistance.
5. Increased speed of nerve conduction.

Another important component of the warm-up phase is not to begin by immediately stretching a cold muscle. Time should first be taken to do the sport activity at a slow, mild pace for 4–5 minutes. Foss and Keteyian (1998) suggest that this provides the most physiological benefits and minimizes muscle injuries, such as tears.

The actual aerobic activity itself may include walking, jogging, dance or step aerobics, rollerblading, cycling, and swimming, among others. If these exercise activities are performed according to appropriately pre-scribed FITT standards, then improved cardiopulmonary efficiency and increased resistance to stress should result. It is important to emphasize that to gauge intensity, standards should be based on heart rate instead of the myth that one must experience pain in order to receive the benefits of training.

The cool-down phase is also extremely important, especially for adults, since it facilitates venous return. This prevents pooling of blood in the extremities, which reduces the possibility of muscle soreness and cardio-vascular strain, and the likelihood of becoming dizzy. The cool-down phase also enhances the removal of lactic acid and other metabolic waste prod-ucts. This phase, which is the one most likely to be forgotten, is just as important as the two preceding phases for healthful, safe exercising.

Again, these recommendations are for aerobic fitness training, the type of exercise training most often associated with improved cardiovascu-lar health. However, the components of muscular strength and flexibility, most often associated with anaerobic fitness or resistance training, should also be considered for their potential health benefits. Exercises such as weightlifting, speed skating, and rapid sprinting that require short bursts of "all-out" effort are examples of anaerobic activities. During these types of activities, the body demands more O_2 then can be supplied by the cardio-vascular system. Therefore, anaerobic (without O_2) exercises, which rely on energy being generated within the muscle by adenosine triphosphate (ATP), creatine phosphate, and the lactic acid (anaerobic glycolysis) sys-tem (Greenberg et al., 1998), cannot be performed indefinitely.

Although anaerobic activities rely on intensity, frequency, and dura-tion of effort to achieve benefits, intensity (how hard one exercises) is con-sidered the most important factor. Anaerobic performance enhancement typically relies on a process known as interval training, which incorporates the concept of the overload principle. As the name implies, the overload principle requires near maximal intensity in the performance of a series of repeated exercises known as work intervals or sets (e.g., rate, distance, number of repetitions) alternated with periods of relief (e.g., amount of time at rest between intervals, or the performance of some sort of light activity between sets). The number of intervals and periods of relief vary depending on the type of anaerobic activity and the goal of training; however, Fletcher and colleagues (1996), in a statement from the American Heart Association, recommend using "eight to 10 different exercise sets with 10 to 15 repetitions each (arms, shoulders, chest, trunk, back, hips, and legs) performed at a moderate to high intensity (form example, 10 to 15 pounds of free weight) for a minimum of 2 days per week" (p. 859). Also worth noting is that most aerobic activities can be performed anaerobically by increasing the intensity of effort to approximately 85% or more of the heart rate reserve (Miller & Allen, 1995).

Pate and his colleagues (1995) note that some potential benefits of anaerobic activities, it may include reduced risk of developing back pain, and improved balance, coordination, and agility. Muscular strength and endurance training have also been associated with improved body image and enhanced self-concept (Greenberg et al., 1998), which, along with the other benefits, serve to enhance an individual's resistance to stress.

An additional consideration in developing exercise guidelines concerns adherence issues. Obviously, just providing a fitness program is not enough. The availability of the most modern exercise facilities does not significantly improve exercise adherence. As Dishman (1994) notes, the worldwide dropout rate for supervised exercise programs has remained at around 50% for the past 20 years. Dishman and Buckworth (1997) have more recently summarized the major factors affecting exercise adherence:

1. Access to facilities
2. Perceived availability of time
3. Social support or reinforcement
4. Moderate exercise intensity
5. Self-motivation

This variety of different factors clearly suggests the multidimensional nature of physical activity determinants in establishing and sustaining exercise adherence.

In their 1995 article, Pate and his colleagues also provided a formal and distinctly separate statement regarding *physical activity* and *health*. It is important to note that most exercise regimens have traditionally focused primarily on exercise recommendations and prescriptions for fitness (i.e., cardiovascular fitness). However, the current prescription for improved *general health* states that every U.S. adult should accumulate 30 minutes or more of moderate-intensity physical activity on most—and preferably all—days of the week. Moderate-intensity activities (40% to 60% of maximal O_2 intake, or enough to expend approximately 200 calories per day) include walking briskly (3–4 mph), cycling at a leisurely pace (<10 mph), golfing, fishing (standing/casting), gardening, raking leaves, or pushing a stroller (Foss & Keteyian, 1998; Pate et al., 1995). This statement on physical activity for improved health is not meant to detract from the previous exercise recommendations for fitness. Rather, these current suggestions, based on a comprehensive review of the literature, expand the opportunity for Americans simply to be more active solely for health purposes.

What should be even more appealing to the 25–60% of U.S. citizens who do not engage in the recommended amount of physical activity (Caspersen, Merritt, & Stephens, 1994) is the report of the benefits of accumulating the suggested 30 minutes of moderate activity throughout the course of the day. With respect to health improvements, the body is apparently not particular about how the calories are expended, or how the exercise is accumulated. In other words, a combination of short-term actions, such as climbing stairs, walking a longer distance from a parking lot, mowing the lawn, or chasing the children, that expend moderate-intensity energy may suffice. However, we must acknowledge that what constitutes an acceptable duration of short-term activity is not well defined, although Pate and his colleagues (1995) have suggested that it should last at least 8–10 minutes or more.

EXERCISE FOR STRESS MANAGEMENT

It remains generally accepted that exercise designed for stress management should meet the following three criteria:

1. Exercise should generally be aerobic compared to anaerobic (Koltyn, Raglin, O'Conner, & Morgan, 1995) in nature; however, as noted earlier, anaerobic training may also be related to increased stress resistance.

2. Exercise should contain rhythmic, coordinated movements rather than random, uncoordinated movements that might place excessive strain on joints or connective tissue.

3. Exercise, from a psychological perspective, should entail a sense of being egoless; that is, it should either avoid competitive paradigms or allow one to win on every occasion. Part of a stress management strategy may include helping the individual define what winning means. Ideally, exercise for stress management should be exercise for the sake of exercise. Its goals should be intrinsic—self-improvement, ventilation, long-range

improvement in somatomotor coordination and motoric skill, and the like. Whenever exercise and self-evaluation or self-esteem become intertwined, the healthful characteristics of exercise become questionable.

ADDITIONAL CAVEATS ABOUT PHYSICAL EXERCISE

In this chapter, physical exercise has been discussed as a tool in assisting in stress management. The guidelines are offered *not* as an exercise prescription, but as a model to demonstrate to the clinician the therapeutic considerations associated with exercise. Readers interested primarily in exercise prescription should refer to the American College of Sports Medicine (1995), Fletcher et al. (1996), and Pate et al. (1995). However, we still offer the following considerations.

- Physical exercise is a potent stressor. Intense exercise stresses both the cardiopulmonary and the musculoskeletal systems.
- Physical exercise has the potential to evoke a greater stress response than any imaginable psychosocial stressor. Although physical exertion does appear to divert most of the potential pathogenic qualities associated with psychophysiological arousal, the abrupt quantity of arousal during physical exercise can be overwhelming to the cardiopulmonary system. There are many documented cases of individuals who die from cardiac failure while exercising for their health.
- The musculoskeletal system is also vulnerable to the strain of physical exercise. Numerous joint and connective-tissue problems are related to excessive physical exercise. Therefore, it is recommended that persons use only proper equipment and technique when exercising.
- Exercise is an individualistic, unique activity; what works for some may not be right for others. It is always a reasonable idea to have a family physician assess an individual's physiological readiness to participate in an exercise program and then suggest appropriate guidelines.
- The success of an exercise program depends on its consistent utilization. Therefore, the question of motivation arises. It is important for the participant to find an exercise program that is not aversive. A common mistake is that eager individuals overdo an exercise program. The results are, typically, soreness, injuries, or the realization that the program too lofty a time commitment. Therefore, people should engage in programs that they will continue. Emphasis should be placed on patience and the need to integrate the exercise program into one's lifestyle. It may help to locate an exercise partner, one with whom the person can exercise, not compete.

• The cardiovascular, pulmonary, and weight-reducing aspects of an exercise program will become manifest within several weeks. The therapeutic psychological effects will likely take longer to realize. Therefore, patience is again required.

SUMMARY

In this chapter, the use of physical exercise has been considered for its utility as an instrument in the treatment of excessive stress and its pathological correlates. Let us review the main points:

1. There is ample evidence to suggest that the stress response is nature's way of preparing the human species for muscular exertion. Physical exercise may then represent nature's prescription for how to ventilate healthfully and utilize the initiated stress response.
2. There is also evidence that suppression of the intrinsic need for somatomotor expression that accompanies the stress response may well be pathogenic itself, hence the concept of hypokinetic diseases and related concepts.
3. The idea that exercise can be therapeutic dates back to the fifth century B.C. and the Greek physician Herodicus.
4. In American society, regular exercise is now accepted as a regular part of the lifestyle for both men and women.
5. Regular exercise appears to be therapeutic by virtue of: for the following reasons:

    • During exercise, constituents of the stress response such as lactic acid, free fatty acid, and epinephrine are utilized in a healthful manner.
    • Upon short-term cessation of exercise, a rebound relaxation effect occurs, which results in feelings of reduced muscle tension and increased feelings of tranquility.
    • Exercise promotes the development of physical and psychological characteristics that appear to facilitate a certain degree of stress resistance, for example, reduced adipose tissue, electrical stabilization of the myocardium, an improved lipoprotein profile, and improved myocardial strength and physical self-concept.

6. Several theoretical rationales have been proposed to explain the physiological benefits of exercise in reducing stress and anxiety, including the endorphin hypothesis, the epinephrine hypothesis, and the thermogenic hypothesis.

7. The major criteria in designing exercise protocols to enhance fitness involve the acronym FITT—Frequency, Intensity, Time, and Type. Generally accepted, minimum exercise guidelines to achieve fitness for normal healthy adults include performing an exercise at a minimum of 60% of maximum heart rate for at least 20 minutes, at least three times per week.

8. Actual exercise sessions should contain warm-up, exercise, and cool-down periods. If exercise is not convenient, supported, and perceived as reinforcing, it will most likely not be sustained.

9. Anaerobic activities may also have stress-resistant benefits.

10. The American College of Sports Medicine, the Centers for Disease Control and Prevention, and the American Heart Association have issued statements suggesting that health benefits can be attained from the accumulation of 30 or more minutes of daily, moderate-intensity exercise.

In summary, there is ample research evidence to conclude that physical exercise can promote psychological and physical alterations that are antithetical to the pathogenic processes of excessive stress. It may well be that physical exercise activates a form of coping mechanism unlike that of any other stress management intervention—ventilation/utilization of the stress response before it leads to disease, as depicted in the introduction to Part II.

17

The Pharmacological Management of Stress Reactions

Jason M. Noel, Pharm, D. and Judy L. Curtis, Pharm, D.

The use of drug therapies in the management of acute stress reactions and chronic stress-related disorders has emerged as understanding of the pathophysiology of these conditions has become better understood. The general approach to treatment has evolved from the use of predominantly rapid-acting sedative agents for the treatment of acute anxiety attacks, to the more frequent use of agents to control the underlying anxiety disorder.

With most psychiatric conditions, conservative strategies for treatment should be employed before more restrictive interventions, such as drug therapies, are used. In the case of stress arousal, relaxation therapies that promote the development of the client's own response mechanisms should be attempted if his or her condition is responsive to such techniques. Cognitive-behavioral therapies, neuromuscular relaxation, structured breathing, and clinical hypnosis (see Chapters 9, 12, 13, and 14) are generally preferred over drug therapy in situations where clients respond to these treatments, because these methods avoid the potential dependency problems and adverse effects of pharmacological agents.

However, there are instances in which drug therapy is appropriate for treatment of excessive stress. Drug therapy is a useful adjunct for the treatment of panic attacks associated with panic disorder and social phobia, increased arousal and traumatic recall associated with PTSD, and anxiety and compulsive behaviors associated with obsessive–compulsive disorder (OCD).

The present chapter reviews the major classes of pharmacological agents used in the treatment of pathological stress arousal states.

Indications and target symptoms (i.e., desired therapeutic effects) are discussed, along with potential problems associated with these agents—adverse effects, dependency liabilities, and drug interactions. We begin with a basic discussion of psychotropic drug pharmacology.

PHARMACOLOGY

Psychotropic drugs exert various effects in the CNS. Most currently available psychotropic medications modulate the activity of neurotransmitters in the brain. Neurotransmitters are small molecules or peptides that carry signals between neurons. Receptors located on pre- and postsynaptic neuronal membranes are the targets for the activity of neurotransmitters and certain drugs.

Norepinephrine, for example, is a monoamine neurotransmitter that has important functions in both the central and peripheral nervous systems. In the brain, several noradrenergic neuronal tracts have been identified, most of which originate in the locus ceruleus. These noradrenergic pathways modulate mood, attention, energy, motor movements, and autonomic functions such as blood pressure control and perspiration. Peripherally, norepinephrine plays a major role in the somatic manifestations of the acute stress response. Elevations in heart rate and urinary retention are mediated by noradrenergic projections from the spinal cord.

Serotonin is an abundant neurotransmitter derived from the dietary amino acid tryptophan. Cell bodies for the serotonergic neurons in the brain are concentrated in the raphe nuclei. Projections from the raphe nuclei are involved in the regulation of mood, motor activity, appetite, sleep, and sexual functioning. Anxiety and panic are also regulated by CNS serotonergic projections. Serotonin release is controlled, in part, by its interactions with norepinephrine, which can either enhance or inhibit serotonin release through interconnecting pathways in the brain stem and the cortex.

Gamma-aminobutyric acid (GABA) is an amino acid derivative that serves as the major inhibitory neurotransmitter in the CNS. It has several functions associated with CNS inhibition, including anxiolytic activity, anticonvulsant activity, sleep promotion, and muscle relaxation. Upon ligand signaling to the GABA-ergic neuron, a very rapid neuronal inhibition is produced. The operation of this mechanism may play an important role in mediating the sensation of anxiety and the initiation of the relaxation response.

Many specific biochemical abnormalities have been identified in psychiatric illnesses. For example, an excess of dopamine neurotransmission in the mesolimbic tract has been correlated with the presence of positive symptoms (e.g., hallucinations and delusions) in patients with schizophrenia. Major depression is felt to be due, in part, to a relative deficiency of serotonin, norepinephrine, and dopamine. Similarly, anxiety states have been associated with an excess of norepinephrine discharge in the locus ceruleus and a relative deficiency of GABA neurotransmission. It is important to note, however, that the identification of these neurotransmitter abnormalities does not necessarily suggest any underlying pathology. In fact, most mental illnesses develop as a result of a combination of genetic, neurodevelopmental, environmental, and social factors.

Current drug therapy, while not always addressing the underlying causes for these mental illnesses, can symptomatically treat these disorders through its effects on the various neurotransmitter systems. There are several mechanisms by which drugs can modulate neurotransmission in the CNS:

1. Direct agonist activity at pre- and postsynaptic receptors.
2. Facilitation of the release of stored neurotransmitters.
3. Inhibition of presynaptic neurotransmitter reuptake.
4. Inhibition of enzymatic neurotransmitter degradation.
5. Inhibition of neurotransmitter synthesis and storage.
6. Alteration of feedback mechanisms modulating neurotransmitter release.
7. Alteration of receptor or ion channel binding sites, leading to facilitation or inhibition of neurotransmission.

With the exception of the sedatives–hypnotics, therapeutic effects of psychotropic drug therapy generally occur after several weeks of continuous dosing. Changes in synaptic neurotransmitter concentration tend to lead to altered sensitivity and concentrations of the postsynaptic receptors. These changes occur over the course of several weeks, resulting in the delay in clinical response. Since adverse effects of psychotropic agents are usually most severe at the onset of therapy, a delayed therapeutic response significantly compromises patient adherence to treatment. This is an especially significant consideration when dealing with manifestations of excessive stress, when the patient needs immediate relief from the discomfort associated with the disorder and has little tolerance for side effects. Fortunately, there are many agents available, and while not being optimal for long-term treatment, they can provide a faster onset of symptom resolution.

Many CNS depressants, including sedatives–hypnotics, have a more direct mechanism of action, leading to a more immediate therapeutic effect. While this type of pharmacological profile may be more desirable to patients, problems with dependence and adverse effects associated with CNS depression make the agents most useful for short-term intervention.

The following sections of this chapter review the classes of drugs used in the treatment of disorders characterized by excessive stress. The mechanisms of action, indications, adverse effects, expected therapeutic outcomes, and relevant drug interactions are described. Our objective is to provide a basic familiarity with the concepts and the role of drug treatment for stress.

Benzodiazepines

Benzodiazepines are the most widely used medications for the treatment of anxiety disorders and stress reactions. This class of drugs includes diazepam (Valium®), lorazepam (Ativan®), oxazepam (Serax®), alprazolam (Xanax®), clorazepate (Tranxene®) and chlordiazepoxide (Librium®). Other drugs in this class that are used primarily for sleep disturbances include triazolam (Halcion®), flurazepam (Dalmane®), estazolam (ProSom®) and temazepam (Restoril®). They are considered less toxic and addictive than older agents such as the barbituates, meprobamate, chloral hydrate, gluthethimide and ethchlorvynol.

The benzodiazepines are all identical in their mechanism of action, and the only differences among them lie in their pharmacokinetic properties (half-life, absorption, metabolism, and excretion) (Grimsley, 1995). Table 17.1 lists pharmacokinetic differences and usual therapeutic doses. The benzodiazepines work by enhancing GABA in the brain. These agents have four therapeutic effects—antianxiety, sedative–hypnotic, muscle relaxant, and anticonvulsant. Typically, sedative effects are seen at lower doses. Anxiolytic, muscle relaxant, and anticonvulsant effects are seen at moderate doses. At high doses, benzodiazepines can be used to induce sleep.

In the treatment of anxiety, benzodiazepines are most appropriately used for the treatment of acute panic attacks. Certain longer acting benzodiazepines (e.g., clonazepam, diazepam) are approved for long-term use in the prevention of anxiety symptoms such as those seen in panic disorder and generalized anxiety disorder. However, chronic use may lead to tolerance, the phenomenon whereby a certain fixed dose loses its effectiveness over time. Patients may try to counteract this by increasing their own dose, potentially leading to physical dependence, addiction, and abuse. Continued use of the drugs may also result in more difficult withdrawal.

Choice of agents depends on the clinical state of the individual for whom they are prescribed. Benzodiazepines with shorter half-lives, such as lorazepam, alprazolam, and oxazepam, may be most useful for persons requiring limited treatment for acute anxiety due to a stressful situation. Those with longer half-lives, such as diazepam, clonazepam, clorazepate,

Table 17.1. Comparative Characteristics of Benzodiazepines

Drug	Dosage range (mg/day)	Duration of action ($t_{1/2}$) in hours	Onset of action (oral absorption)
Alprazolam (Xanax®)	0.25–4.0	12–15	Intermediate
Clonazepam (Klonopin®)	0.5–12.0	18–50	Intermediate
Clorazepate (Tranxene®)	7.5–60.0	Metabolite dependent Desmethyldiazepam (30–200) Oxazepam (3–21)	Fast
Chlordiazepoxide (Librium®)	10–100	5–30 Demoxepam (14–95) Desmethylchlordiazepoxide (18)	Intermediate
Diazepam (Valium®)	5–60	20–50 Desmethyldiazepam (30–200) 3-Hydroxydiazepam (5–20) Oxazepam (3–21)	Fastest
Lorazepam (Ativan®)	2–16	10–20	Intermediate
Oxazepam (Serax®)	15–60	3–21	Intermediate

and chlordiazepoxide, may be better for persons requiring longer therapy for chronic anxiety. Shorter acting agents may also be preferred for the elderly or those with impaired liver function, because they are less likely to accumulate and produce oversedation (Brown et al., 1993).

Side effects of the benzodiazepines include sedation, confusion, amnesia, unsteady gait, and lethargy. They are relatively safe on overdose except when combined with other CNS-depressant drugs such as alcohol or other sedatives–hypnotics. The most serious problem with benzodiazepine therapy can be withdrawal, the result of physical dependence. Physical dependence may occur after 4–6 months with usual doses or more rapidly, 2–3 weeks, with high doses (Brown et al., 1993). Withdrawal symptoms are frequently the opposite of the usual therapeutic effects of the benzodiazepines. Psychological symptoms include irritability, insomnia, feelings of apprehension, and dysphoria. Physical symptoms may include tremor, palpitations, dizziness, muscle spasm, and sweating. Perceptual symptoms include hypersensitivity to sound, light, and touch, and depersonalization. In severe situations, seizures may occur. Withdrawal symptoms can be minimized by using a slow taper (4–16 weeks, depending on the starting dose), and adjunctive therapy may be needed, such as beta-blocking agents or sedating antidepressants. These drugs should never be discontinued abruptly unless serious side effects warrant the risk of withdrawal.

Antidepressants

Antidepressant agents are so named because drugs possessing the common pharmacology of these agents are traditionally used in the treatment of depressive disorders. All currently available antidepressants facilitate neurotransmission of serotonin, norepinephrine, and/or dopamine. However, the exact neuronal targets (e.g., enzymes, reuptake pumps, and autoreceptors) differ from class to class. It is interesting to note, however, that despite the wide array of mechanisms of action of the antidepressants, no agent or class of drugs has been shown to be more consistently efficacious in the treatment of depression. Drug choice is based on presenting symptoms and adverse effect profile, among other clinical factors. However, in the treatment of anxiety states, the pharmacological profiles of the agents determine which spectrum of disorders for which the drugs are likely to be effective.

Antidepressant-associated increases in serotonin (5-HT) and norepinephrine (NE) neurotransmission may have effects other than their direct benefits in affective and somatic manifestations of depression and anxiety. Increasing evidence suggests that by increasing NE and 5-HT neurotransmission in the neurons of the hippocampus, the nerve damage induced by chronic stress can be reversed. The expression of neurotrophic factors that serve to promote neuronal survival and growth in the CNS is decreased during stress. Antidepressant treatment may reverse these changes by upregulating neurotrophic-factor expression (Duman, Malberg, & Thome, 1999).

The antidepressant drugs are classified by pharmacological mechanism or chemical structure (see Table 17.2). The monoamine oxidase inhibitors (MAOIs) and the tricyclics were the first classes of antidepressants developed. The selective serotonin reuptake inhibitors (SSRIs) and various other agents with novel mechanisms of action were later introduced to address the tolerability issues of the earlier drugs.

Monoamine Oxidase Inhibitors (MAOIs). The agents in the classes phenelzine (Nardil®) and tranylcypromine (Parnate®) work by irreversibly inhibiting the enzyme that degrades monoamine neurotransmitters. As a result, the concentration of NE and other catecholamines is increased in the synaptic cleft, thereby facilitating neurotransmission.

The benefits of MAOI therapy in the treatment of depression and stress-related disorders are significant. These agents are considered to be very effective in the prevention of panic attacks associated with panic and social

Table 17.2. Trade Name, Usual Dosage, and Indicated Uses of Antidepressants

Generic name	Trade name	Usual daily dosage (in milligrams)	Indications	
MAO Inhibitors				
Phenelzine	Nardil	45–90	MDD, PD	Used only as last-line agents due to drug interactions
Tranylcypromine	Parnate	20–50	MDD, PD	
TCAs and Related Agents				
Amitriptyline	Elavil	100–300	MDD, PD, pain, insomnia, enuresis	May have severe anticholinergic and cardiovascular side effects
Amoxapine	Asendin	200–600		
Desipramine	Norpramin	100–300		
Doxepin	Sinequan	100–300		
Imipramine	Tofranil	100–300		
Maprotiline	Ludiomil	150–225		
Nortriptyline	Pamelor	50–200		
Protriptyline	Vivactil	20–60		
Trimipramine	Surmontil	100–300		
Clomipramine	Anafranil	100–250	OCD	Higher risk of seizures
SSRIs				
Citalopram	Celexa	20–60	MDD, PD, SP, PTSD, OCD, bulimia	Lower doses effective for depressive disorders; higher doses generally needed for anxiety disorders
Fluoxetine	Prozac	10–80		
Fluvoxamine	Luvox	100–300		
Paroxetine	Paxil	20–60		
Sertraline	Zoloft	50–200		
Others				
Mirtazapine	Remeron	15–45	MDD	Sedating effects only at lower doses
Nefazodone	Serzone	300–600	MDD	
Trazodone	Desyrel	200–600	MDD	Used primarily as a hypnotic
Venlafaxine	Effexor	75–375	MDD, GAD	

Note: MDD—major depressive disorder, PD—panic disorder, OCD—obsessive–compulsive disorder, SP—social phobia, PTSD—Posttraumatic stress disorder, GAD—generalized anxiety disorder.

anxiety disorder. In clinical trials, 60–70% of patients with panic and social anxiety disorder show significant decreases in the frequency of panic attacks after 8–12 weeks of MAOI therapy (Spiegel, Wiegel, Baker, & Greene, 2000).

However, due to significant food and drug interactions associated with treatment, MAOIs are not currently employed as first- or second-line agents. By irreversibly inhibiting monoamine oxidase, MAOIs subject the patient to a prolonged inability to metabolize tyramine, an amino acid found in aged cheeses, red wines, and cured meats. Elevated levels of tyramine can cause a life-threatening syndrome of elevated blood pressure, palpitations, and hyperthermia. These effects may be avoided by adopting a diet with very low levels of tyramine and avoiding the use of drugs with sympathomimetic effects (e.g., over-the-counter decongestants); however, most clinicians prefer to first use drugs with a better safety profile, avoiding these concerns, unless absolutely necessary.

Tricyclic Antidepressants (TCAs).   The TCAs are a fairly large group of structurally and pharmacologically similar drugs. The therapeutic effects of these agents are thought to be due to their activity as inhibitors of presynaptic NE and 5-HT reuptake. A variety of other receptor effects that differ from drug to drug impact clinical utility and adverse effect profiles.

The TCAs have been found to be consistently effective for panic disorder and generalized anxiety disorder. Imipramine (Tofranil®) has been shown to have efficacy comparable to that of alprazolam in suppressing panic attacks associated with panic disorder. In generalized anxiety disorder, imipramine has been shown to significantly improve symptoms in 60–70% of patients, again, comparable to the response seen with benzodiazepines (Spiegel et al., 2000). However, for all disorders, the effects may only be seen after 3–4 weeks of continuous treatment and tend to disappear after drug discontinuation. Clomipramine (Anafranil®), nortriptyline (Pamelor®), desipramine (Norpramin®), and other agents in this class may produce similar effects at therapeutic doses.

In the treatment of OCD, clomipramine has a level of efficacy not seen with other TCAs. This is thought to be due to this agent's more potent effects in inhibiting serotonin reuptake. About half of clomipramine-treated patients demonstrate moderate improvement (35% reduction in symptoms) in obsessive thoughts and compulsive behaviors (Spiegel et al., 2000).

Several significant liabilities with TCA therapy severely limit their utility. They are associated with anticholinergic side effects such as constipation, urinary retention, and blurred vision. Many of these agents are very sedating due to antihistamine effects. Small doses of amitriptyline (Elavil®) and doxepin (Sinequan®) have been used as adjuncts for sleep disorders. TCAs may cause cardiovascular effects such as arrythmias and postural hypotension. There are also the risks of seizures, weight gain, light sensitivity, and cognitive impairment associated with TCA therapy. Because of these effects, this agent is usually an alternative to the newer, safer drugs for nonresponders.

Selective Serotonin Reuptake Inhibitors (SSRIs). The selective serotonin reuptake inhibitors—fluoxetine (Prozac®), fluvoxamine (Luvox®), paroxetine (Paxil®), sertraline (Zoloft®), and citalopram (Celexa®)—are a structurally heterogeneous group of compounds that primarily exert their effects as inhibitors of presynaptic serotonin reuptake. Their relative lack of noradrenergic activity does not seem to reduce their antidepressant efficacy significantly. However, these agents have significant advantages in that their relative absence of anticholinergic and antihistaminic effects provides improved tolerability profiles.

The SSRIs have been shown to have a broad spectrum of activity in the treatment of anxiety disorders and other psychiatric conditions (Kent, Coplan, & Gorman, 1998). Drugs in this class have been approved for use in panic disorder, social phobia, OCD, and PTSD. In most cases, the SSRIs are considered the drugs of choice for these disorders. In panic disorder and social phobia, the SSRIs have shown consistent reductions in frequency of panic attacks after 10–12 weeks of treatment. As with clomipramine, SSRI therapy can reduce the symptoms of obsessions and compulsions associated with OCD. In PTSD, SSRIs have displayed benefits in reducing avoidance, arousal, and depressive symptoms. These agents have also been used to treat eating disorders, impulse control disorders, and premenstrual dysphoric disorder.

It appears that the efficacy for the treatment of anxiety disorders is similar for all SSRIs. However, there are subtle differences between them. When choosing from among the SSRIs the clinician should consider the drugs' CNS-activating properties and the potential for drug interactions. Side effects include jitteriness (a significant problem for people with anxiety disorders), GI discomfort, sexual dysfunction, tremors, and headaches. Fluvoxamine and fluoxetine tend to have a high rate of CNS-activating effects. Paroxetine, less activating than the other agents in the class, does exhibit mild anticholinergic effects not seen with the other SSRIs. Fluvoxamine and fluoxetine exert potent inhibitory effects on the liver metabolism of many drugs, including many benzodiazepines. Citalopram appears to be relatively free of liver enzyme inhibitory effects.

Other Antidepressants. Venlafaxine (Effexor®), an inhibitor of NE, 5-HT, and dopamine reuptake, is an accepted treatment for generalized anxiety disorder. It can reduce the constant symptoms of anxiety associated with this disorder within the first few weeks of treatment. It is associated with dose-related increases in blood pressure, GI discomfort, and sexual dysfunction.

Nefazodone (Serzone®), a 5-HT–NE reuptake inhibitor, may prove to be useful in the treatment of some anxiety disorders due to its antagonist activity at serotonin 5-HT$_2$ receptors. Antagonism of this receptor subtype confers advantages not seen with other serotonin reuptake inhibitors. Nefazodone is associated with fewer acute anxiety symptoms and less sexual dysfunction that the SSRIs and venlafaxine. However, it may be quite sedating and may cause postural hypotension. Mirtazapine (Remeron®) is a facilitator of NE and serotonin neurotransmission that shares the 5-HT$_2$ blockade profile with nefazodone. This may also become a viable treatment for anxiety in the future. Mirtazapine may cause excessive sedation, weight gain, and postural hypotension.

Buspirone

Buspirone (BuSpar®), an anxiolytic, is structurally unrelated to benzodiazepines and antidepressants. It functions as a treatment for generalized anxiety in certain patients but is largely ineffective for most anxiety disorder subtypes, including panic disorders. It is a partial agonist at serotonin type 5-HT$_{1A}$ receptors. Anxiolytic effects of this agent are thought to be due to long-term adaptations that take place with neurotransmitter receptors (Stahl, 2000). Buspirone therefore requires continuous therapy for several weeks to achieve complete resolution of generalized anxiety.

As a chronic therapy, buspirone has advantages over traditional sedatives–hypnotics that clinicians may find useful. Unlike the benzodiazepines, buspirone is not associated with CNS depression, dependence, and withdrawal symptoms upon discontinuation. This profile may make buspirone useful for the elderly and for individuals with a substance abuse history. However, anxiety sufferers may not be able to tolerate the 2- to 4-week latency to clinical effect. Indeed, patients with generalized anxiety disorder who have a history with benzodiazepine treatment tend not to be affected by buspirone therapy. Adverse effects of buspirone are mild and include headache, nausea, dizziness, and insomnia.

MISCELLANEOUS AGENTS

Beta-Adrenergic Blocking Agents

This group of medications include popranolol (Inderal®), metoprolol (Lopressor®), nadolol (Corgard®) and atenolol (Tenormin®). These drugs are used to treat the physical manifestations of anxiety or stress, such as tremor and increased heart rate. They are not as effective as the benzodiazepines at treating anxiety. Beta-adrenergic blocking agents are effective in treating the acute physical reactions to a stressful event such as stage fright and public speaking. These drugs do not alter consciousness.

Beta-adrenergic agents should be used with caution in people who have asthma, since they can exacerbate the disorder. They should also be avoided in people with diabetes, since they can mask a hypoglycemic event. Side effects of the beta-adrenergic blocking agents include lethargy, sedation, low blood pressure, decreased heart rate, dizziness, tiredness, insomnia, and depression in susceptible individuals with chronic use (American Hospital Formulary Services, 2000; Grimsley, 1995).

Antihistamines

The most commonly used antihistamine is hydroxyzine (Vistaril®, Atarax®); diphenhydramine (Benadryl®) has also been used. These medications do not have anxiolytic properties. They both possess significant sedative properties. There is no evidence that they are useful in primary anxiety disorders, but they may be useful in periodic and short-term use for insomnia. These agents also have potent anticholinergic effects and can cause side effects such as confusion, constipation, cognitive impairment, and nausea. Elderly patients, especially those who have dementia or are medically ill, are particularly susceptible to these side effects (Grimsley, 1995).

Barbiturates and Nonbarbiturate Sedative–Hypnotics

Barbiturates such as phenobarbital should be used very sparingly, if at all, due to their side effects and abuse potential. These drugs are profoundly sedating and cause cognitive difficulty. They are also potentially lethal in overdose. Nonbarbiturates include meprobamate (Miltown®, Equanil®), glutethimide (Doriden®), and ethchlorvynol (Placidyl®). The primary effect of these drugs is also sedation, and these agents are potentially lethal in overdose and may be no more effective than placebo in treating anxiety due to stressful events.

Antipsychotic Medications

This group of drugs includes agents such as haloperidol (Haldol®), thioridazine (Mellaril®), chlorpromazine (Thorazine®), thiothixene (Navane®), mesoridazine (Serentil®), and others. Newer antipsychotic medications include risperidone (Risperdal®), olanzapine (Zyprexa®), quetiapine

(Seroquel®) and clozapine (Clozaril®). These drugs are largely ineffective in treating anxiety- or stress-related disorders (Grimsley, 1995). Due to potentially serious side effects, such as tardive dyskinesia, sedation, cognitive difficulties, blood problems (clozapine), decreased blood pressure, and extrapyramidal symptoms (parkinsonian symptoms), their use is also discouraged for treatment of anxiety.

SUMMARY

The armamentarium of available pharmacological agents for the treatment of stress-related syndromes and anxiety disorders is evolving as safer alternatives to the CNS-depressant drugs become available. Let us review some of the main points covered in this chapter:

1. Symptomatic improvement of the symptoms of acute stress can be addressed with a short-term course of CNS depressants, such as benzodiazepines. Use of benzodiazepines for longer term therapy has the liabilities of development of tolerance, dependence, and withdrawal symptoms. However, the benzodiazepines do represent a significant improvement in drug safety over barbiturates and non-barbiturate sedatives–hypnotics.
2. Situational anxiety may respond to as-needed treatment with beta-adrenergic blocking agents. These drugs directly antagonize the NE-mediated peripheral manifestations of the stress response.
3. Antihistamines may also be used episodically for sedation.
4. Over the long-term, most anxiety disorders are most appropriately treated with antidepressant drugs. Because these agents work by inducing long-term alterations in neurotransmitter receptor function and sensitivity, response may take several weeks of continuous treatment. However, improvements in the safety profiles of the newer antidepressants make these agents viable choices in the treatment of anxiety disorders.

III

Special Topics in the Treatment of the Human Stress Response

The purpose of the third and final section of this volume is to address specific issues that are uniquely relevant to treatment of the human stress response.

Chapter 18, entitled "Religion, Spirituality, and Stress," provides an overview of the stress-related issues and putative mechanisms of action and research associated with spiritual and religious beliefs. The goal of the chapter is to sensitize the reader to the impact that religious beliefs may have on emotional and physical health, as well as how to incorporate these beliefs into a clinical practice.

Considering that people have generally become increasingly attuned to the association between diet, nutrition, and health, we present an examination of the relationship between energy sources—carbohydrates, fats, and proteins—and stress in Chapter 19, "Nutrition and Stress." We also address the association between serotonin and antioxidants and the stress response, as well as introduce the concept of psychoneuronutritional medicine.

Chapters 20 and 21 address the topic of posttraumatic stress disorder (PTSD). This psychiatric disorder remains the most florid stress-related disorder directed toward the mind as the target organ. Chapter 20 entitled, "Posttraumatic Stress Disorder" presents the two-factor theory of PTSD, which addresses both the neurological and psychological hypersensitivity associated with the disorder. Treatment issues, including reviews of psychopharmacotherapy and Eye Movement Desensitization and Reprocessing (EMDR), are also covered in Chapter 20.

Chapter 21, entitled "Management of Acute Distress through a Comprehensive Model of Crisis Intervention for Mass Disasters and Terrorism" addresses how the multifaceted intervention system of CISM, which encompasses the full temporal spectrum of a crisis (i.e., precrisis through acute crisis, and into postcrisis phases), can be used to prevent or mitigate the impact of traumatic stress. Research findings supporting the use of CISM are presented.

Chapter 22, "Hans Selye and the Birth of the Stress Concept," by Dr. Rosch provides a unique historical account and rare glimpse of the man considered to be the "father of stress research."

Chapter 23 employs, for a final time, the phenomenological model as a graphic tool to summarize the treatment of the human stress response. A general treatment model is reviewed within this summary chapter as a means of integrating and summarizing the essence of this volume: treatment of the human stress response.

After providing the summation in Chapter 23, an appendix section presents microdiscussions of selected topics of interest in the treatment of excessive stress arousal. Although far more lengthy and comprehensive discussions of the topics are available elsewhere, our goal in this section is to provide a brief, practical introduction to these "special clinical considerations."

18

Religion, Spirituality, and Stress

> Science without religion is lame; religion without science is blind.
>
> ALBERT EINSTEIN (1879–1955)

In Chapter 11, we reviewed the process of meditation as a treatment for human stress. The reader will recall that the history of meditation is grounded firmly in religion. Let us take a closer look at religion and spirituality, over and above their meditative components, as tools for the reduction or amelioration of stress and disease.

A relevant and actively debated question involves whether or not religion is beneficial to one's health. Within the past 20 years, objective empirical data have explored the relationship between spiritual and religious involvement and physical and emotional health. Even with the accumulation of methodologically sound data, the debate over religion's role in health is far from resolved. The purpose of this chapter is to provide a brief review of some of the pertinent literature in this area, particularly relative to stress.

Before addressing some of the possible mechanisms of action and the research literature, it may be helpful to define and clarify the terms *spiritual* and *religious*. Not surprisingly, the terms are interrelated; however, Richards and Bergin (1997) have differentiated them in the following way: "Religious expressions tend to be denominational, external, cognitive, behavioral, ritualistic, and public. Spiritual experiences tend to be universal, ecumenical, internal, affective, spontaneous, and private. It is possible to be religious without being spiritual and spiritual without being religious" (p. 13).

MECHANISMS OF ACTION

Herbert Benson, the originator of "the relaxation response," has investigated and written extensively on how beliefs and expectancies, including religious beliefs, have a positive impact on one's physical and emotional health. He introduced the term *remembered wellness* in an attempt to replace the term *placebo effect*, which he felt had a rather negative connotation. *Remembered wellness* is a term designed to capture the powerful healing and empowering force of individual beliefs in promoting and enhancing treatment and curative effects. Benson (1996) further described the combination of the physiological powers of the relaxation response and the construct of remembered wellness as the "faith factor." He provides an example of this combination by suggesting that the influence of religious rituals practiced in childhood may actually have the potential to regenerate neural pathways that are related to faith and well-being in later adulthood.

Benson (1996) further suggests that belief in God, in whatever transcendent form an individual chooses to manifest it, may serve as an influential source of strength and healing. Moreover, he acknowledges that worship services may possess certain therapeutic effects, including the chance to listen to soothing music in a pleasant environment, to be distracted from daily pyschosocial stressors and socialize with others, to perform comfortable and familiar rituals, and to reflect, pray, and learn. Other proposed therapeutic effects associated with religion include finding a sense of meaning (Spilka, Shaver, & Kirkpatrick, 1985), prescribing to a healthier lifestyle (Bergin & Payne, 1993), and achieving a sense of control (Pargament et al., 1987). To elaborate, Koenig (1997) notes that religious beliefs can provide a sense of control over one's destiny when a person puts his or her complete trust in a personal God and asks for forgiveness. Moreover, he suggests that relief may occur:

> There is no sin or mistake in life that cannot be confessed and forgiven. Thus, no matter what a person has done in the past, he or she can start fresh again by recommitting one's life to God. Guilt, which religion itself can provoke, is erased by the simple act of asking for forgiveness. Not surprisingly, such beliefs may have powerful psychological consequences, and may indeed bring comfort to those who are lonely anxious, discouraged, or feeling out of control. (p. 68)

Harris, Thoresen, McCullough, and Larson (1999) have recently provided suggestions for therapeutic application and applied research in the use of forgiveness-based interventions.

Regarding physical health, religious individuals may be more likely to perceive their bodies as "temples of the Holy Spirit" (Koenig, 1997) and to adhere to medical regimens. Furthermore, Koenig notes that religious individuals may be less likely to be involved in activities that adversely affect physical health, such as smoking cigarettes, drinking alcohol, and engaging in risky sex practices.

RESEARCH

Despite the fact that the bulk of empirical evidence on the benefits of religious beliefs has been gathered from cross-sectional and correlational studies, there has been no shortage of recent articles and books describing the techniques and virtues of religious and/or spiritual therapy. For example, it is interesting to note that about 40% of medical schools in the United States now offer at least one course related to the role of spiritual and religious factors in health and medical practice (Puchalski & Larson, 1998).

Emotional Health

Available data are generally supportive of the benefits of religious beliefs relative to many outcome measures of emotional and social adjustment. Donahue (1985) noted that people who use religion as an end in itself (i.e., the intrinsically religious) seem to do better emotionally than those who use religion as a means to achieving some other end (i.e., the extrinsically religious). Religious factors have been associated with reduced alcohol, cigarette, and drug use, as well as improved quality-of-life measures for patients suffering from cancer (Matthews, Larson, & Barry, 1993).

Koenig and his colleagues have done considerable work examining the general health benefits of religion. For example, in a sample of 298 patients admitted consecutively to the general medical services at Duke University Medical Center, 40% ranked religion as the most important factor that enabled them to cope with the stress of their illness (Koenig, 1997). In a separate, earlier study, Koenig, Kvale, and Ferrel (1988) reported that elderly individuals, regardless of gender, age, race, or physical health, who acknowledged being more deeply religious (attending church, praying, reading the Bible) experienced higher scores on a standardized measure of well-being. Moreover, Koenig and associates (1995) reported that higher religious beliefs as assessed by the Religious Coping Index (RCI) were associated with lower cognitive symptoms (anhedonia, boredom, social withdrawal, and feeling sad, blue, or hopeless), but not necessarily fewer somatic symptoms (weight loss, sleep disturbance, fatigue, loss of energy, psychomotor retardation) of depression in a sample of 832 men, with an average age of 70 years, admitted to a VA hospital.

Additional treatment outcome data in the area of religion have been gathered when readily accepted psychotherapeutic interventions have been modified to include a spiritual component. For example, Pargament (1990) adapted Lazarus's cognitive model of stress and coping (see Chapter 9) to include religious thoughts and behaviors, and reported success when applying this model therapeutically. Efficacy studies have also compared spiritually focused cognitive-behavioral therapy (CBT) with standard CBT. In the most well-controlled of these investigations, Propst, Ostrom, Watkins, Dean, and Mashburn (1992) reported that Christian participants who received CBT with religious content had significantly less depression at the end of treatment compared to participants in the regular CBT group or a wait-list control group. Other studies have not, however, demonstrated similar differences between groups (Johnson, DeVries, Ridley, Pettorini, & Peterson, 1994). Researchers recognize the need to explore how diversity of religious beliefs and lack of religious beliefs in both participant and therapist could affect the outcome of studies employing religious themes in CBT interventions.

Physical Health

The data on religion and physical health are more abundant and in many ways more impressive than those relating to mental health (Richards & Bergin, 1997). In general, recovery rates from illness, including surgery, are better for religious people (Larson & Larson, 1994). Furthermore, approximately 90% of studies investigating the relationship between religious beliefs and blood pressure showed lower diastolic and systolic pressures for religiously active participants (who attended church more frequently and reported stronger convictions) compared to those not as religiously active (Koenig, 1997). Friedlander and associates (1986) stated that the risk of heart attack was four to seven times lower in religious men compared to those who were not religious. Again, these differences remained after consideration of normal risk factors for heart disease.

Oxman, Freeman, and Manheimer (1995), who investigated mortality rates after elective, open-heart surgery for coronary artery disease or aortic valvular stenosis in 232 patients over the age of 55 years, reported that "patients receiving no strength and comfort from religion were over three times more likely to die after heart surgery" (p. 10). These results occurred even after controlling for history of previous surgery, functional impairment prior to surgery, and age.

Dean Ornish (1990) received considerable acclaim for well-designed research demonstrating that the progression of coronary atherosclerosis could be stopped or reversed in patients without the use of lipid-lowering drugs. Instead of medications, patients in the experimental group were prescribed an intensive lifestyle component that included diet, exercise, smoking cessation, and stress management. Also included in this program, and a factor that Ornish considered essential for success, was a spiritual component designed to help patients seek communion with God or a Higher Power. Ornish and his colleagues (1998) have recently reported on the continued improvement and success of the patients with heart disease who incorporated and adhered to these lifestyle changes for 5 years. For example, the average-percent diameter of stenosis in the experimental group decreased during the 5 years, whereas it increased for the control group that used lipid-lowering drugs. Moreover, the number of cardiac events (myocardial infarction, coronary angioplasty, coronary artery bypass surgery, cardiac-related hospitalizations) were significantly less in the experimental group compared to the lipid-lowering-drugs group.

In an intriguing yet controversial study, Byrd (1988) investigated the effects of intercessory prayer (praying for the benefits of others, also known as "distant prayer") on 393 patients admitted to the coronary care unit at San Francisco General Hospital over a 10-month period. In a psychometrically sound, well-controlled, prospective, double-blind study, patients were randomly assigned to either the intercessory prayer group or a nonprayer group. Byrd then randomly assigned anywhere from three to seven active, "devotional" Christians to pray for the 192 patients in the intercessory prayer group. The intercessors were given the patients' first names, diagnosis, general medical conditions, and updates. Prayer was done outside the hospital on a daily basis, until the patients were discharged. Although not instructed specifically on what to include in their prayers, intercessors were asked to pray daily for rapid recovery and prevention of complications and death, in addition to other areas that they thought would be helpful to the recovering patients.

The results of the study revealed that members of the prayer group did significantly better than the nonprayer group on a number of health-related measures during the course of their hospitalizations. A series of unpaired t tests and chi-square tests revealed that congestive heart failure, diuretic use, cardiopulmonary arrest, pneumonia, antibiotic use, and need for intubation/ventilation occurred less frequently in the intercessory prayer group. After mulivariate analyses were performed to correct for the large number of variables examined, fewer patients in the prayer group required diuretics, antibiotics, or intubation/ventilation. Additional analyses of hospital course (rated as good, intermediate, or bad) revealed that the prayer group had a better overall outcome.

Byrd acknowledged a potential weakness of his study: He did not attempt to limit the amount of prayer that the control group received from outside persons not associated with the study, or the amount of individual prayer or religiosity held by the participants. Regardless of these factors, these data remain impressive, although the mechanism of effect remains uncertain.

Sicher, Targ, Moore, and Smith (1998) recently provided a replication study on the use of intercessory prayer. In a double-blind, randomized trial of 40 patients diagnosed with advanced AIDS and matched by age, CD4+ count, and number of AIDS-defining diseases (ADDs), participants were informed that they had a 50-50 chance of receiving "distant healing" treatment. The 20 subjects in the prayer condition, unaware of the group in which they were placed, received intercessory prayer from 40 healers from various religious traditions, who each had an average 17 years' experience treating more than 100 patients from a distance. Ten different healers prayed for patients over the course of 10 weeks. Healers worked on their assigned patient for about 1 hr/day for 6 consecutive days and were told to develop an intervention of "health and well-being" for each patient.

The results, similar to the Byrd (1988) study, are noteworthy. At the 6-month study endpoint, the prayer group experienced significantly fewer outpatient visits (185 vs. 260), hospitalizations (3 vs. 12), and days in the hospital (10 vs. 68), and ADDs (2 vs. 12), and higher ratings of improved mood. Of note, there were no differences, however, between the two groups on CD4+ cell counts. Sicher and associates (1998) offer several possible secular explanations for their results but also recognize that these provocative data cannot be completely dismissed without considering other possible benefits of intercessory prayer. In a review of the Byrd study, Harris and associates (1999) acknowledged that the large number of individual, paired t tests may have influenced the error rate.

Shealy, Smith, Liss, and Borgmeyer (2000) have recently reported on some intriguing findings on the alteration of EEG brain maps (see Chapter 15) on 110 volunteers who received distant or absent "healing." In all instances, notable changes in EEG activity occurred within the first 5 minutes of receiving healing energy at distances ranging from 100 feet to 160 miles. Sometimes, however, the EEG alterations appeared most dramatically 20 minutes postintervention. The typical pattern evidenced was a marked increase in delta-wave activity, with concurrent, albeit less significant, changes in theta and alpha activity. The 50 participants who received directed energy (i.e., healing specifically aimed to frontal or occipital lobes of the brain) all demonstrated increased EEG activity in the part of the brain receiving directed energy, along with alterations in other lobes.

INCORPORATING SPIRITUAL AND RELIGIOUS BELIEFS INTO PRACTICE AND THERAPY

Interest in the relationship between counseling and religion has grown and prospered substantially over the past decade. For example, as of 2002, the American Association of Christian Counselors (AACC) had more than 40,000 active members (personal communication with Jim Clinton, January 28, 2002); it had 2,000 members in 1993 (Worthington, Kurusu, McCullough, & Sandage, 1996).

The use of spiritual themes and religion in intervention and counseling is not a new phenomenon. For example, 12-step programs or fellowships, most notably, Alcoholics Anonymous (AA), which has an estimated membership of about 1.7 million worldwide (Alcoholic Anonymous World Services, 1990), have as their base the relevance of spiritual processes in clinical outcomes. The emphasis of the AA model is that success requires surrendering to a Higher Power, along with an acknowledgment of the need for God's assistance. Given the success of the AA model, other spiritually based, 12-step programs have been developed (e.g., Gamblers Anonymous and Narcotics Anonymous).

Richards and Bergin (1997) have suggested a number of religious and spiritual factors that they consider relevant for success within an integrative, multidimensional, psychotherapeutic approach. For patients willing to pursue this strategy, they define the following goals:

1. Helping clients experience and affirm their spiritual identity and divine worth.
2. Working with clients to explore the impact that their spiritual and religious convictions may have on their presenting problems and general life.
3. Discovering ways to incorporate religious or spiritual tools to help with coping and healing.
4. Helping to explore and resolve spiritual concerns related to patients' problems and to decide how they want to incorporate spirituality and religion into their lives.
5. Continuing to work on spiritual growth and well-being.

SUMMARY

This chapter has provided a general overview of the relationship between stress and spirituality. Let us review the main points of this chapter:

1. We began with a differentiation of the terms *religious*, which is considered to be external, denomination, and public, and *spiritual* which is thought to be ecumenical, internal, and private.
2. Various mechanisms of action regarding the potential psychological benefits of religion were then proposed. Herbert Benson's more recent work.on the "faith factor" and therapeutic benefits of worship services was covered, as well as other psychological benefits, such as increased sense of meaning and control, and asking for forgiveness.
3. Potential physical benefits of religion include perceiving the body as a "temple of the Holy Spirit" (Koenig, 1997), increased medical adherence, and less smoking and drinking.
4. Research has shown a positive relationship between religious practice, including the use of intercessory prayer (distant prayer), and emotional and physical health.
5. Spiritual themes have been used in interventions such as Alcoholics Anonymous, Gamblers Anonymous, and Narcotics Anonymous.
6. Finally, Richards and Bergin (1997) suggest a number of religious and spiritual factors that may be incorporated during psychotherapy.

19

Nutrition and Stress

Kristy Kelly, Jeffrey Lating, and George S. Everly, Jr.

This text has emphasized the body's adaptive mechanisms that attempt to maintain homeostasis in response to physical and psychosocial stressors (see Chapter 2 for a detailed explanation). However, as we have noted, intense stress can deplete and weaken the body, including, for example, the SNS response to inhibit digestion. As Whitney, Hamilton, and Rolfes (1990) note, "Much of the disability imposed by prolonged stress is nutritional" (p. 13). The purpose of this chapter is to briefly review how some of the basics of nutrition are involved in the stress response. We then discuss how serotonin and antioxidants, two chemicals found in our bodies and in the foods we eat, are associated with stress. We conclude this chapter by introducing the concept of psychoneuronutritional medicine.

ENERGY-YIELDING NUTRIENTS

When responding to stress, our bodies rely primarily on three classes of energy-yielding nutrients to cope: carbohydrates, fats, and proteins. Although in reality most foods contain a mixture of nutrients, we frequently classify them according to one of these three primary constituents.

Kristy Kelly • Department of Psychology, Loyola College in Maryland, Baltimore, Maryland 21210-2699.

Carbohydrates

Carbohydrates in foods provide about half of our body's energy source. There are two general types of carbohydrates, simple and complex. Simple carbohydrates (monosaccharides and disaccharides) or sugars, come from fruits and vegetables (e.g., glucose, fructose, maltose, and sucrose) and from milk or milk products (lactose and galactose). Simple carbohydrates are especially concentrated in sweeteners such as table sugar, confectioner's sugar, brown sugar, honey, and molasses. Complex carbohydrates (polysaccharides), mainly starches, are found in grains such as rice, wheat, rye, barley, and oats. Another important source of starch is legumes such as peanuts, beans, peas, and soybeans. Potatoes, yams, and cassava (a tropical American plant with a starchy root from which tapioca is derived) are yet other sources of starches. Complex carbohydrates are metabolized or broken down more slowly than simple carbohydrates and serve as our major source of vitamins (except B_{12}) and minerals. Fiber is considered the indigestible portion of complex carbohydrates (Greenberg et al., 1998). Although it is not considered a nutrient because it is not used in metabolism, fiber facilitates the process of digestion.

Fats

Despite receiving considerable, albeit understandable, "bad press" in contemporary dieting literature, fats serve as very important energy sources for the body. The body's fat (adipose) cells contain large stores of triglycerides that meet ongoing energy needs. When we are resting, our muscles expend little energy; therefore, it is not necessary to produce adenosine triphosphate (ATP) rapidly. Instead, the body's oxygen system, which uses carbohydrates, fats, and proteins as energy sources, provides the required ATP for the resting physiological processes (Williams, 1999). More specifically, carbohydrates and fats combine with oxygen in the cells to provide the major sources of energy during rest (Williams, 1999). In fact, in a normal diet, fat supplies about 60% of the body's resting energy requirement (Eschelman, 1996; Groff, Gropper, & Hunt, 1995). However, during potential periods of food deprivation, such as those occurring during prolonged stressful circumstances, fat stores are likely to contribute an even higher percentage of our energy needs (Whitney, Cataldo, & Rolfes, 1998). Red meats, whole milk, cheeses, peanut butter, ice cream, butter, bacon, avocados, chocolate, and nuts are examples of foods containing an appreciable quantity of fat. Although fat provides the body with a concentrated source of energy, unused fat from the food we eat is also easily converted to body fat, or adipose tissue, which has an essentially unrestricted storage capacity

(Whitney et al., 1990). Consider for example, that "the energy liberated from each gram of carbohydrate as it is oxidized to carbon dioxide and water is 4.1 Calories and that liberated from fat is 9.3 Calories" (Guyton & Hall, 1996, p. 889). Therefore, it is worth noting that even though fat may be very helpful during a period of prolonged stress, a small amount of fat in the body typically goes a long way, particularly during periods of low stress.

Proteins

Proteins are found in most foods and are used to rebuild, repair, and replace cells. Animal products such as eggs, milk, beef, and fish are very high in protein, as are plant-derived foods such as rice, corn, soybeans, nuts, and seeds. The principal constituents or building blocks of proteins are amino acids. Some amino acids are produced in the body if not gathered from food sources (nonessential amino acids), whereas others (essential amino acids) must be acquired through food for normal protein metabolism to proceed (Greenberg et al., 1998). Twenty of these amino acids are particularly relevant to human nutrition (Guyton et al., 1996). Essentially, "the role of protein in food is not to provide body proteins directly, but to supply the amino acids from which the body can make its own proteins" (Whitney et al., 1990, p. 140). The energy liberated from metabolism of protein is about 4.3 calories per gram.

ENERGY SOURCES AND STRESS

Previously, we addressed the percentage of fat used as an energy source within the body; however, an additional consideration is the energy potential or energy value of food itself. According to Eschelman (1996), in a typical American diet, "the energy value of food is 48% from carbohydrate, 35% from fat, and 14% to 18% from protein" (p. 123). Particularly relevant for the purposes of this chapter is that under low or mildly stressful conditions, the body gives preference to carbohydrates and fats as its energy source. In fact, carbohydrates and fats are often referred to as "protein sparers." However, during periods of severe, excessive stress, when hunger may be suppressed and digestion may be working inefficiently, the body may begin to consume protein stores rapidly for energy, often at six to seven times the typical rate, once carbohydrates and fats have been depleted. When this process occurs, dietary protein, along with lean muscle tissue throughout the body (including major organs such as the heart), is converted to glucose to supply energy for the nervous system. Obviously, if this process occurs for prolonged periods, then it may jeopardize one's health.

Therefore, if you are able to eat during a period of stress, do so, of course. You may discover, however, that it is prudent to limit your caloric intake per meal, although you may try to eat more frequently. Also, the body, which does conserve fluids during stress, will also excrete what it does not need. Therefore, drink fluids, especially water (our most essential nutrient), which will enable your kidneys to help reestablish homeostasis. Although we do not obtain energy directly from water, vitamins (e.g., A, B, C, D, E, and K), which are organic chemicals, or minerals (e.g., calcium, iron, phosphorous, potassium, zinc, copper, iodine, magnesium, and fluoride), which are inorganic substances, "these nutrients provide important components for the metabolic processes that produce the energy required for growth, development, and all life functions" (Brehm, 1998, p. 186). In converting nutrients to energy, vitamins may also produce hormones and break down waste products and toxins. It is also worth noting that the best way to obtain necessary vitamins and minerals is from the diet, not from supplements.

It is also important to note that when excessive stress begins to subside and homeostasis is being reestablished, we should take the opportunity to replenish ourselves with a healthy balance of foods and exercise (see Chapter 16) to restore both lean and fat tissue. Also, it may be helpful during this time of recuperation to recognize the difference between the constructs of hunger and appetite. When we are physically hungry, our bodies crave the nutrients found in the calories, vitamins, and minerals of food. Appetite, which is often described as "psychological hunger," is associated with a desire for specific foods. Fortunately, for most of us, the episodes of sustained, intense, debilitating, stress described earlier occur infrequently. Instead, we are generally accustomed to coping with recurrent episodes of mild to moderate psychosocial stressors on a regular, often daily, basis.

As most of us are all too aware, mild to moderate and sometimes even high psychosocial stressors can trigger our appetites. According to Macht (1996), when this occurs, we may crave sweet and starchy foods, and both our stress level and coping abilities dictate when and how much food we eat. Polivy and Herman (1999) suggest that people disguise their life-related distress by overeating in order to associate their stress with binge eating rather than with the more uncontrollable areas of their lives. When we overeat, we blame ourselves for being weak and lacking self-control, but recent research suggests that overeating is not necessarily an issue of willpower. According to Wurtman and Suffes (1997), the hunger we experience when under variable to high levels of psychosocial stressors is biologically rooted, and this is why our cravings do not subside until sated and intensify when denied.

Macht (1996) discusses the possible relationship between stress and the consumption of low-energy foods heavy in fat, salt, and sugar. He concludes that a person's emotional stress level heightens when he or she eats food that provide little energy, and this increase in anxiety can then lead to an increase in his or her desire to eat. Low-energy foods such as cheese, potato chips, and cookies are generally deficient in the natural chemicals that moderate stress, whereas a diet that includes high-energy foods such as cereals, beans, raw vegetables, and fruit is helpful in mitigating the stress and cravings we experience. These low-energy foods are those that are mainly composed of sweet and starchy carbohydrates.

SEROTONIN, STRESS, AND EATING

The neurochemical, serotonin, found in carbohydrates is a neurotransmitter that plays a role in both eating and emotions. Wurtman and Suffes (1997) suggest that people with a deficiency of serotonin in their brains, which is associated with depression, are also those who binge most frequently. When serotonin levels are low, the brain sends signals to notify the body that serotonin is needed, and this is when we have an impulse to eat. When the food we eat (carbohydrates in particular) is digested, insulin is secreted from the pancreas into the bloodstream, which delivers glucose to the cells, to be used as an energy source. Because the serotonin we receive from carbohydrates is not activated until 30 minutes after digestion, we may tend to overeat because we consume our food quickly and do not stop until we feel full. If our bodies lack adequate amounts of serotonin, the food cravings we experience are intense; we binge on fatty, salty, and sweet food until we feel uncomfortable. A diet that includes carbohydrates with every meal will supposedly maintain our serotonin levels, and therefore we will not be overwhelmed with impulses to eat junk food (see Wurtman & Suffes, 1997, for additional details). Markus and colleagues (1998) report a relationship between college students and stress, and conclude that the high amounts of stress student's experience are due to a serotonin deficiency in the brain. They believe that eating carbohydrates can prevent this neurochemical degeneration. The relevant physical influence of serotonin supports the existence of a carbohydrate–stress connection in the human body.

ANTIOXIDANTS

Antioxidants, which play a key role in maintaining our physiological well-being, are another group of neurochemicals associated with diet and stress, and have become very popular as supplements in the past several years. In general, antioxidants (vitamin E, vitamin C, selenium, beta-carotene, and other carotenoids) defend our bodies from an imbalance in the production of free radicals, which are by-products of active aerobic metabolism. Since all cells in the human body use O_2 to break down the energy sources of carbohydrates, fats, and proteins, free radicals are formed when O_2 molecules lose an electron during this metabolic process. The free radicals (technically O_2 molecules now with a missing electron) will then attempt to stabilize themselves by indiscreetly stealing an electron from any nearby molecule, whether the molecule is a protein, fat, or another chemical, such as nucleic acids. Unfortunately, free radicals may attach to and subsequently damage these chemicals in their stabilization quest. An excess of free radicals, along with its damaging effects, has been referred to as oxidative stress and is implicated in the formation of heart disease (Faggiotto, Poli, & Catapano, 1998; Hodis et al., 1995; Pratico, Tangirala, Rader, Rokach, & Fitzgerald, 1998; Pryor, 2000), cancer (Ames, Gold, & Willett, 1995; Halliwell, 1998), cataracts (Knekt, Heliovaara, Rissanen, Aromaa, & Aaran, 1992; Taylor, Jacques, & Epstein, 1995), age-related macular degeneration (Goldberg, Flowerdew, Smith, Brody, & Tso, 1988), and even Alzheimer's disease (Morris et al., 1998; Sano et al., 1997). For example, cancer has been thought to occur and proliferate when free radicals, in their search for available electrons, attack and in turn alter our DNA (our cells' genetic material).

The body's cells produce antioxidants that serve to limit the activity and repair the damage caused by free radicals. Research, for example, has demonstrated that vitamin E, found in foods such as vegetable oils, nuts, sunflower seeds, and wheat germ, may function as a "chain-breaking" antioxidant that prevents the propagation of low-density lipoprotein (LDL) cholesterol, which is related to heart disease. Given the growing interest in antioxidant use, the Food and Nutrition Board of the Institute of Medicine (2000) recently provided recommended antioxidant intake for healthy people. For vitamin E, the Recommended Daily Allowance (RDA) for both men and women is 15 mg/day. For vitamin C, which is found in citrus fruits as well as broccoli, asparagus, peppers, and spinach, the RDA is 90 mg/day for adult men and 75 mg/day for adult women. Because smoking increases oxidative stress and metabolic turnover of vitamin C, the Board recommends an additional 35 mg/day of vitamin C for smokers. The RDA of selenium, which is found in egg yolks, tuna, chicken, liver, and whole grains, for both men and women is 55 µg/day.

Compelling observational and epidemiological data have related higher consumption of carotenoid-containing fruits (e.g., yellow fruits such as apricots and peaches), vegetables (e.g., dark green, yellow, and orange), and higher plasma concentrations of several carotenoids (including beta-carotene) with lower rates of lung cancer (Ziegler, Mayne, & Swanson, 1996), cervical cancer (Batieha et al., 1993), and oral cavity, pharyngeal, and laryngeal cancers (Mayne, 1996; Mayne & Goodwin, 1993). Based in part on these data, the Food and Nutrition Board of the Institute of Medicine (2000) recommends eating five or more servings of fruits and vegetables per day, which would provide 3–6 mg/day of beta-carotene. However, no upper limit has been set for carotenoid consumption, partly because it is unclear whether the observed health benefits are due specifically to the carotenoids or to other substances found in carortenoid-rich foods. Also, despite the growing correlational evidence, three large, well-controlled, randomized clinical trials using various high-doses of beta-carotene supplements (20 or 30 mg/day or 50 mg every other day) for a period of 4–12 years produced no significant results for any of the previously described cancers (Hennekens et al., 1996). Given these data, the Food and Nutrition Board of the Institute of Medicine (2000) concluded that beta-carotene supplements, while valuable, for example, in populations with inadequate vitamin A nutrition, are currently not advisable for the general population. Additional data are clearly needed from intervention trials in order to determine further the putative mechanisms involved and the recommended dietary and supplemental intakes.

PSYCHONEURONUTRITIONAL MEDICINE

Modern science has heightened our attention to the importance that diet has in mental and physical wellness. From the ample data gathered on stress, neurochemistry, and diet, a paradigm known as psychoneuronutritional medicine has been developed and advanced (Bland, 1995). Psychoneuronutritionists focus on the interface and relationships between sensory organs, nervous systems, psychology, nutrition, and neurobiology when treating patients. According to Bland, our diets affect the synthesis and regulation of neurotransmitters, which in turn affect our mood and ability to cope with stress. A proper diet mediates neurochemical activity, guards against neurotoxins, and improves emotional reactions to stress.

SUMMARY

This chapter has presented a brief overview of how diet and nutrition are associated with the human stress response. Let us review the following main points:

1. Our bodies rely on carbohydrates, fats, and proteins as primary energy sources when responding to stress.

2. Of two general types of carbohydrates, simple and complex, simple carbohydrates (monosaccharides and disaccharides), or sugars come primarily from fruits, vegetables, and milk (or milk products), and are found in many different sweeteners (e.g., table sugar, honey, molasses). Complex carbohydrates (polysaccharides) are found in grains (e.g., rice, wheat, rye, barley, and oats), legumes (e.g., peanuts, peas, beans), and potatoes.

3. Fat provides the body with a concentrated energy source that may be especially relevant during periods of intense stress. Red meats, whole milk, cheeses, butter, bacon, chocolate, and nuts provide a large quantity of fat.

4. Proteins, composed of amino acids (nonessential and essential), are used to repair, rebuild, and replace cells. Eggs, milk, beef, fish, rice, corn, and soybeans are foods high in protein.

5. During periods of excessive stress, the body, which usually conserves protein as its energy source, may begin to consume protein stores rapidly for energy when carbohydrates and fats are depleted.

6. Appetite is an important trigger during psychosocial stressors of varying intensities. There is a relationship between stress and consumption of certain types of low-energy foods that are heavy in fat, salt, and sugar.

7. The neurotransmitter serotonin is an important component in both eating and emotions.

8. Antioxidants (vitamin E, vitamin C, selenium, beta-carotene, and other carotenoids), also associated with diet and stress, have been implicated in illnesses such as heart disease, cancer, cataracts, age-related macular degeneration, and Alzheimer's disease. A report from the Food and Nutrition Board of the Institute of Medicine (2000) recently provided recommended daily allowances (RDA) for different antioxidants.

9. Psychoneuronutritional medicine is a multidisciplinary field that focuses on the interface between psychology, neurobiology, and nutrition.

20

Posttraumatic Stress Disorder

The posttraumatic stress syndrome has been recognized for decades (Freud, 1921). Even systematic empirical inquiry dates back to the 1940s (Kardiner, 1941). Yet it was not until 1980 that the now highly recognizable posttraumatic stress syndrome was officially catalogued within the official nosological compendium of the American Psychiatric Association, the *Diagnostic and Statistical Manual of Mental Disorders*, third edition (DSM-III; American Psychiatric Association, 1980). With this recognition of the syndrome as an official mental disorder came a surge of research efforts designed to lead to better diagnostic refinement as well as improved treatment.

Whereas once the syndrome was viewed almost exclusively as a result of armed combat, now posttraumatic stress disorder (PTSD) has been found to result from not only war-related situations but also a host of non-combat-related experiences as well. In 1987, and again in 1994 and 2000, the American Psychiatric Association revised its official nosology (1987, 1994). Are we coming closer to a comprehensive understanding of PTSD, or are we just beginning to scratch the surface of what may be a uniquely complex interaction of pathophysiological and psychopathological constituents? The purpose of this chapter is to review current evidence on the nature of PTSD as well to as offer an integrating phenomenological hypothesis regarding this disorder, which appears to be playing more and more a role in Western society.

THE PREVALENCE OF TRAUMA AS A PUBLIC HEALTH PROBLEM

What is the magnitude of risk for experiencing a significant psychological trauma that might yield a significantly adverse impact upon one's mental health? Is the risk minimal, or does it represent a significant public health issue? To review Chapter 1, the reader will recall:

- Recent evidence suggests that 90% of adults in the United States will be exposed to a traumatic event during their lifetime (Breslau et al., 1998).
- The rate of trauma exposure for children and adolescents has been estimated to be about 40% (see Bureau of Justice Statistics, 1996).
- United States citizens age 12 years or older experienced 37 million crimes in 1996 (Bureau of Justice Statistics, 1997).
- The lifetime prevalence of criminal victimization was assessed among female HMO patients and found to be about 57% (Koss et al., 1991).
- The prevalence of PTSD was found to be 13% in a sample of suburban law enforcement officers (Robinson et al., 1997).
- Of the clinical health care staff sampled, 62% reported being exposed to a traumatic stressor at work (Caldwell, 1992).
- The prevalence of PTSD ranged from 15% to 31% for samples of urban firefighters based on a traumatic exposure prevalence ranging from 85% to 91% (Beaton et al., 1996).

Clearly, trauma has reached epidemic proportions in the United States! It seems clear that such crisis events represent a "clear and present danger" to the psychological health of Americans.

DIAGNOSTIC SYMPTOMATOLOGY

In 1941, Kardiner (1941) described five consistent clinical features of the syndrome now referred to as PTSD:

1. Constriction of personality functioning
2. Exaggerated startle reflex and irritability
3. Psychic fixation upon the trauma
4. Atypical dream experiences
5. A propensity for explosive and aggressive reactions

In 1942, Gillespie described an acute "war neurosis" as having as an important clinical feature an increased startle reaction characterized by increased and generalized muscular tension, palpitations, and a "sinking feeling," thus emphasizing a distinct autonomic nervous system (ANS) component to this posttrauma syndrome.

In 1980, the American Psychiatric Association described PTSD as a form of anxiety disorder:

> The essential feature is the development of characteristic symptoms following a psychologically traumatic event that is generally outside the range of usual human experience.... The characteristic symptoms involve re-experiencing the traumatic event; numbing of responsiveness to, or reduced involvement with, the external world; and a variety of autonomic, dysphoric, or cognitive symptoms. (p. 236)

The specific criteria are listed in Table 20.1.

PTSD was described in subvariations as well:

1. "Acute," in which the onset of symptoms occurred within 6 months of the trauma and lasted less than 6 months.
2. "Chronic or delayed," in which either or both of the following applied: duration of the symptoms for 6 months or more (chronic) and/or the onset of symptoms at least 6 months after the trauma (delayed).

In 1987, the American Psychiatric Association revised its criteria for PTSD (American Psychiatric Association, 1987). In doing so, the traumata giving rise to PTSD were somewhat better defined. Once again, the notion

---

Table 20.1. Diagnostic Criteria for Posttraumatic Stress Disorder, DSM-III

A. Existence of a recognizable stressor that would evoke significant symptoms of distress in almost everyone
B. Reexperiencing the trauma as evidenced by at least one of the following:
  1. Recurrent and instrusive recollections of the event
  2. Recurrent dreams of the event
  3. Suddenly acting or feeling as if the traumatic event were reoccurring, because of an association with an environmental or ideational stimulus
C. Numbing of responsiveness to or reduced involvement with the external world, beginning some time after the trauma, as shown by at least one of the following:
  1. Markedly diminished interest in one or more significant activities
  2. Feeling of detachment or estrangement from others
  3. Constricted affect
D. At least two of the following symptoms that were not present before the trauma:
  1. Hyperalertness or exaggerated startle response
  2. Sleep disturbance
  3. Guilt about surviving when others have not, or about behavior required for survival
  4. Memory impairment or trouble concentrating
  5. Avoidance of activities that arouse recollection of the traumatic event
  6. Intensification of symptoms by exposure to events that symbolize or resemble the traumatic event

---

of a psychologically distressing event outside the normal range of human experience was emphasized. Yet specific instances were cited:

> a serious threat to one's life or physical integrity; a serious threat or harm to one's children, spouse, or other close relatives and friends; sudden destruction of one's home or community; or seeing another person who has recently been, or is being, seriously injured or killed as a result of an accident or physical violence. In some cases the trauma may be learning about a serious threat or harm to a close friend or relative. (pp. 247–248)

Table 20.2 describes the specific criteria requisite for the PTSD diagnosis.

In 1994, the American Psychiatric Association once again changed the diagnostic criteria for PTSD as contained within the revised nosological compendium (DSM-IV; American Psychiatric Association, 1994). The DSM-IV criteria (see Table 20.3) represented major alterations in the official criteria for PTSD, and even recognized a more acute variant of the posttraumatic syndrome, acute stress disorder (ASD; see Table 20.4).

The major changes in the DSM-IV formulation of PTSD reside in the definition of the traumatic event. While DSM-III and DSM-III-R defined the traumatic stressor as an unusually distressing event, the DSM-IV actually restricted the nature of the stressor by limiting it to events that involve actual or threatened death or serious injury to oneself or others. The DSM-IV-R stressor of the sudden destruction to one's home or community, in the absence of injury or death, was now omitted. This restriction in the nature of the traumatic stressor was not well received by many individuals who work in mass disaster venues.

While restricting one aspect of the traumatic criterion (Criterion A), the DSM-IV actually broadened another aspect of the traumatic stressor by including a subjective distress criterion.

Are these diagnostic criteria of equal phenomenological import? Or are certain elements more important than others? Let us take a closer look at the posttraumatic stress concept with an appreciation for reformulation. Figure 20.1 presents a phenomenological algorithm that provides a hierarchical structure to the constituent elements.

As the algorithm indicates, posttraumatic stress represents a dynamic "process" rather than a monothetic formulation. Figure 20.1 emphasizes the etiological role that subjective interpretation of the traumatic stressor can play in the determination of the amplitude and chronicity of the posttraumatic stress response. This view is in concert with the model utilized throughout this text as the overarching framework for understanding the human stress response. At the same time, Figure 20.1 argues that much

Table 20.2. Diagnostic Criteria for Posttraumatic Stress Disorder, DSM-III-R

A. The person has experienced an event that is outside the range of usual human experience and that would be markedly distressing to almost anyone (e.g., serious threat to one's life or physical integrity; serious threat or harm to one's children, spouse, or other close relatives and friends; sudden destruction of one's home or community; or seeing another person who has recently been, or is being, seriously injured or killed as the result of an accident or physical violence)

B. The traumatic event is persistently reexperienced in at least one of the following ways:
1. Recurrent and intrusive distressing recollections of the event (in young children, repetitive play in which themes or aspects of the trauma are expressed)
2. Recurrent distressing dreams of the event
3. Suddenly acting or feeling as if the traumatic event were recurring (includes a sense of reliving the experience, illusions, hallucinations, and dissociative [flashback] episodes, even those that occur upon awakening or when intoxicated)
4. Intense psychological distress at exposure to events that symbolize or resemble an aspect of the traumatic event, including anniversaries of the trauma

C. Persistent avoidance of stimuli associated with the trauma or numbing of general responsiveness (not present before the trauma), as indicated by at least three of the following:
1. Efforts to avoid thoughts or feelings associated with the trauma
2. Efforts to avoid activities or situations that arouse recollections of the traumas
3. Inability to recall an important aspect of the trauma (psychogenic amnesia)
4. Markedly diminished interest in significant activities (in young children, loss of recently acquired development skills such as toilet training or language skills)
5. Feeling of detachment or estrangement from others
6. Restricted range of affect (e.g., unable to have loving feelings)
7. Sense of a foreshortened future (e.g., does not expect to have a career, marriage, or children, or a long life)

D. Persistent symptoms of increased arousal (not present before the trauma), as indicated by at least two of the following:
1. Difficulty falling or staying asleep
2. Irritability or outbursts of anger
3. Difficulty concentrating
4. Hypervigilance
5. Exaggerated startle response
6. Physiological reactivity upon exposure to events that symbolize or resemble an aspect of the traumatic event (e.g., a woman who was raped in an elevator breaks out in a sweat when entering any elevator)

E. Duration of the disturbance (symptoms in B, C, and D) of at least one month

of the depressive avoidance, numbing, and withdrawal that is replete in the posttraumatic stress constellation may, indeed, be but a second-order symptom manifestation.

While acknowledging the important role that subjective interpretation plays in the traumatic response, Figure 20.2 is presented as a means of understanding the variable impact of subjective interpretation upon the spectrum of traumata.

Table 20.3. Diagnostic Criteria for Posttraumatic Stress Disorder, DSM-IV

A. The person has been exposed to a traumatic event in which both of the following were present:
1. Event or events that involved actual or threatened death or serious injury, or a threat to the physical integrity of self or others.
2. The person's response involved intense fear, helplessness, or horror. *Note*: In children, this may be expressed instead by disorganized or agitated behavior.

B. The traumatic event is persistently reexperienced in one (or more) of the following ways:
1. Recurrent and intrusive distressing recollections of the event, including images, thoughts, or perceptions. *Note*: In young children, repetitive play may occur in which themes or aspects of the trauma are expressed.
2. Recurrent distressing dreams of the event. *Note*: In children, there may be frightening dreams without recognizable content.
3. Acting or feeling as if the traumatic event were recurring (includes a sense of reliving the experience, illusions, hallucinations, and dissociative flashback episodes, including those that occur on awakening or when intoxicated). *Note*: In young children, trauma-specific reenactment may occur.
4. Intense psychological distress at exposure to internal or external cues that symbolize or resemble an aspect of the traumatic event.
5. Physiological reactivity on exposure to internal or external cues that symbolize or resemble an aspect of the traumatic event.

C. Persistent avoidance of stimuli associated with the trauma and numbing of general responsiveness (not present before the trauma), as indicated by three (or more) of the following:
1. Efforts to avoid thoughts, feelings, or conversations associated with the trauma
2. Efforts to avoid activities, places, or people that arouse recollections of the trauma
3. Inability to recall an important aspect of the trauma
4. Markedly diminished interest or participation in significant activities
5. Feeling of detachment or estrangement from others
6. Restricted range of affect (e.g., unable to have loving feelings)
7. Sense of a foreshortened future (e.g., does not expect to have a career, marriage, children, or a normal life span)

D. Persistent symptoms of increased arousal (not present before the trauma), as indicated by two (or more) of the following:
1. Difficulty falling or staying asleep
2. Irritability or outbursts of anger
3. Difficulty concentrating
4. Hypervigilance
5. Exaggerated startle response

E. Duration of the disturbance (symptoms in Criteria B, C, and D) is more than 1 month

F. The disturbance causes clinically significant distress or impairment in social, occupational, or other important areas of functioning.

Specify if:
   Acute: if duration of symptoms is less than 3 months
   Chronic: if duration of symptoms is 3 months or more

Specify if:
   With Delayed Onset: if onset of symptoms is at least 6 months after the stressor

---

Source: *Diagnostic and Statistical Manual of Mental Disorders*, Fourth Edition. Copyright © 1994 American Psychiatric Association. Reprinted with permission.

Table 20.4. Diagnostic Criteria for Acute Stress Disorder, DSM-IV

A. The person has been exposed to a traumatic event in which both of the following were present:
  1. The person experienced, witnessed, or was confronted with an event or events that involved actual or threatened death or serious injury, or a threat to the physical integrity of self or others.
  2. The person's response involved intense fear, helplessness, or horror.
B. Either while experiencing or after experiencing the distressing event, the individual has three (or more) of the following dissociative symptoms:
  1. A subjective sense of numbing, detachment, or absence of emotional responsiveness
  2. A reduction in awareness of his or her surroundings (e.g., "being in a daze")
  3. Derealization
  4. Depersonalization
  5. Dissociative amnesia (i.e., inability to recall an important aspect of the trauma)
C. The traumatic event is persistently reexperienced in at least one of the following ways: recurrent images, thoughts, dreams, illusions, flashback episodes, or a sense of reliving the experience; or distress on exposure to reminders of the traumatic event.
D. Marked avoidance of stimuli that arouse recollections of the trauma (e.g., thoughts, feelings, conversations, activities, places, people).
E. Marked symptoms of anxiety or increased arousal (e.g., difficulty sleeping, irritability, poor concentration, hypervigilance, exaggerated startle response, motor restlessness).
F. The disturbance causes clinically significant distress or impairment in social, occupational, or other important areas of functioning or impairs the individual's ability to pursue some necessary task, such as obtaining necessary assistance or mobilizing personal resources by telling family members about the traumatic experience.
G. The disturbance lasts for a minimum of 2 days and a maximum of 4 weeks and occurs within 4 weeks of the traumatic event.
H. The disturbance is not due to the direct physiological effects of a substance (e.g., a drug of abuse, a medication) or a general medical condition, is not better accounted for by Brief Psychotic Disorder, and is not merely an exacerbation of a preexisting Axis I or Axis II disorder.

Source: Diagnostic and Statistical Manual of Mental Disorders, Fourth Edition. Copyright © 1994, American Psychiatric Association. Reprinted with permission.

Let us take a closer look at posttraumatic stress through the utilization of a factorial taxonomy (i.e., a two-factor model of posttraumatic stress), including the notion of subjective appraisal. The A (2) criterion of the DSM-IV notes that the individual's response to the traumatic event must involve "intense fear, helplessness, or horror." This alteration has engendered some concern from victims' advocacy groups in that acknowledgment of the subjective aspects of the traumatic stressor may lead to a "blame the victim" attitude. Yehuda (1998) raised this issue and stated, "The stipulation in DSM-IV that individuals must experience a subjective response to an event now makes the study of risk factors necessary rather than inappropriate" (p. 3).

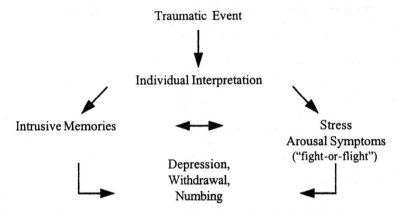

Figure 20.1. As described by Everly and Lating (1995), the manifestation of the three symptom clusters consisting of intrusive memories, stress arousal symptoms, and withdrawal, depression, and numbing are predicated upon a complex interaction between the traumatic event and the individual experiencing the event.

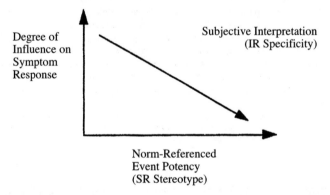

Figure 20.2. As noted in Figure 20.1, the nature and degree of manifest posttraumatic symptomatology is a function of the nature of the traumatic event and the individual experiencing the event. So as not to misinterpret this concept as reason to "blame the victim," the role of the victim's subjective interpretation is portrayed in overall event potency (severity). Traumatic events will vary in their normative severity, or potency. This is called stimulus–response (SR) stereotype and simply means that "mild" stressors usually engender "mild" responses, while "severe" stressors usually engender "severe" responses. Automobile accidents are less severe than torture. Thus, as the norm-referenced severity of the stressor event increases, the less a role subjective interpretation, called individual response (IR) specificity, plays in determining the severity of the manifest symptom response. Thus, subjective interpretation plays less of a role in shaping the traumatic response to torture than it might to an automobile accident.

The DSM-IV also acknowledges the potential for PTSD to be associated with"…a change from the individual's previous personality characteristics" (American Psychiatric Association, 1994, p. 425). In recognizing that PTSD could alter something as concretized as personality, a new realm of psychological and biological phenomenological possibilities emerges.

A TWO-FACTOR THEORY OF POSTTRAUMATIC STRESS

Everly (1993; Everly & Lating, 1995) has analyzed the posttraumatic stress disorder construct and found it to reveal two key factors, or constituents:

1. Neurological hypersensitivity
2. Psychological hypersensitivity (Everly, 1993; Everly & Lating, 1995)

Neurological Hypersensitivity

It is clear that the posttraumatic stress syndrome possesses a significant neurological constituency.

Kolb (1987) has suggested that the PTSD symptoms fall within four categories: (1) impaired perceptual, cognitive, and affective functions; (2) symptoms of released activation; (3) reactive affect and avoidance; and (4) restitutive symptoms and behaviors.

Yet Kolb argues that the symptoms of released activation are the "constant" symptoms of the condition: the exaggerated startle reaction, irritability, hyperalertness, nightmares, and related psychophysiological expressions of ANS hyperfunction.

Similarly, Foy et al. (1984), in a comparison of methods for the concurrent discrimination of PTSD, found that self-report indices of anxiety and ANS arousal alone were capable of correctly identifying more than 90% of the study's subjects. The investigation employed 21 Vietnam veteran PTSD patients and 22 Vietnam veterans with other psychiatric complaints.

In a review of three psychophysiological investigations into PTSD, Kolb (1984, 1987) concluded that indices of sympathetic nervous system (SNS) arousal were capable of differentiating PTSD from non-PTSD subjects.

PTSD subjects showed more autonomic arousal in response to trauma-related stimuli than did non-PTSD subjects. Thus, Kolb (1987) concluded that "psychophysiological assessment offers strong potential not only for diagnostic identification…but also for assessment of severity of the disorder" (p. 991).

Finally, Horowitz, Wilner, Kaltreider, and Alvarez (1980) investigated the signs and symptoms of PTSD. Using a multi-inventory battery of self-report indices, they investigated the three major PTSD clusters: (1) intrusive reexperiencing of the trauma, (2) numbing/avoidance reactions, and (3) anxiety/stress reactions. The authors concluded that intrusive thinking and general symptoms of distress were of primary clinical prevalence and importance in the PTSD phenomenon. They added that the numbing and avoidance signs and symptoms are best understood as efforts of the PTSD patient to control the primary PTSD symptomatology.

From an anatomical perspective, in concert with the formulation of MacLean (1949), Gray (1982) has identified the septal–hippocampal complex as the neuroanatomical epicenter for the integration of exteroceptive as well as interoceptive, proprioceptive, and cognitive stimuli (Seifert, 1983; Van Hoesen, 1982). More specifically, Gray argues, as do Reiman et al. (1986), that the noradrenergic system within the septal–hippocampal nuclei bears primary responsibility for integrating and responding, via hypothalamic efferent mechanisms, to novel and unpleasant stimuli, and furthermore, that stimulation of these projections results in a heightened sensitivity and reactivity within all innervated regions, including neuroendocrine effector mechanisms, to environmental cues seen in any way as novel, threatening, or otherwise aversive. Similarly, Madison and Nicoll (1982) found that noradrenergic neurons from the locus ceruleus to the hippocampus serve to impair the ability of the septal–hippocampal region to accommodate to excitatory stimuli.

Reiman et al. (1986) have demonstrated through positron emission tomography that the septal–hippocampal complex plays a major role in panic attacks. They further conclude that via the septal–amygdalar complex, the septal–hippocampal nuclei can initiate a hypothalamically mediated stress response (see Aggleton, 1992; Cullinan et al., 1995; Le Doux, 1995).

Gloor (1986) has reported that the hippocampus plays a major role in memory and fear reactions. Electrophysiological investigations of awake patients having surgery for epilepsy found that activation of the hippocampus was capable of engendering "flashbacks," affective lability, perceptual distortions, fear, worry, and even guilt reactions (see also Post, 1986; Seifert, 1983).

In summary, to this point, a wide range of evidence indicates that residing with the confines of the septal–hippocampal–amygdalar complex are nuclei responsible for engendering all of the major symptoms of PTSD, including intrusive recollections and flashbacks (Gloor, 1986), neurological hypersensitivity, hyperstartle reactions, and inhibited stimulus accommodation (Gray, 1982; Madison & Nicoll, 1982), panic-like responses (Reiman et al., 1986), fear, rumination, worry, guilt-like reactions (Gloor, 1986), and affective lability (Post, 1986). Cooper, Bloom, and Roth (1982) have suggested that the role of the locus ceruleus is to act as a general orienting system rather than as a specific organizing epicenter for panic and related dysfunction (see also Charney et al., 1995).

More recently, the amygdala has been ascribed a preeminent role in the anatomical foundations of PTSD (Charney et al., 1993). Consistent with the survival orientation of the "fight-or-flight" response, the amygdala appears to possess a specialized mechanism for processing emotional, especially fear-related, memories (LeDoux, 1992). LeDoux has argued that the amygdala may process emotional memories in such a way that "memories established through the amygdala are indelible" (p. 342). This may help us understand the persistence of traumatic memories; that is, the maintenance of fear-related memories may serve as a means of assuring continued survival, especially if coupled with autonomic mobilization, hypervigilance, and explosive reactivity or withdrawal and avoidance behaviors (the fight-or-flight response).

If, indeed, the anatomical basis for PTSD is in the septal–hippocampal–amygdalar system, what extraordinary physiology serves to sustain the phenomenon? The hypersensitivity formulations of van der Kolk et al. (1985) and Kolb (1987) as generically extended within this text and elsewhere (Everly, 1985b, 1993; Everly & Benson, 1989) seem reasonable. Using the disorders of arousal model described earlier, it may be argued that PTSD represents a limbic-system-based condition of neurological hypersensitivity, where a pathognomic propensity for limbic hyperreactivity is related to intraneuronal alterations that result from and lead to further neural hypersensitivity/hyperexcitability.

The neurological hypersensitivity proposed as a factorial constituent of PTSD may possess several pathognomonic and sustaining mechanisms (see Everly, 1995, for a review):

1. Increased excitatory neurotransmitter activity within the limbic circuitry (Black et al., 1987; Post, 1985; Post & Ballenger, 1981; Post, Weiss, & Smith, 1995; Post et al., 1986; Sorg & Kalivas, 1995).
2. Declination of inhibitory neurotransmitters and/or receptors (Cain, 1992; see Everly, 1993).
3. Augmentation of micromorphological structures (especially amygdaloidal and hippocampal dendritic branching) (Cain, 1992; Post et al., 1995; see Everly, 1993).

4. Changes in the biochemical bases of neuronal activation, for example, augmentation of phosphoproteins and/or changes on the transduction mechanism *c-fos* so as to change the genetic message within the neuron's nucleus (Cain, 1992; Horger & Roth, 1995; Sorg & Kalivas, 1995).

5. Increased arousal of neuromuscular efferents, with resultant increased proprioceptive bombardment of the limbic system (especially amygdaloidal, and hippocampal nuclei) (Gellhorn, 1964, 1968; Malmo, 1975; Weil, 1974).

6. Repetitive cognitive excitation (Gellhorn, 1964, 1968; Gellhorn & Loofbourrow, 1963; Post et al., 1986).

While examining the physiological bases of PTSD, a more specific look at the neurochemistry seems in order. It is clear that excitatory neurotransmitter activity is an essential component of the presentation of PTSD. Specifically, central amino acids such as glutamate and aspartate are implicated in hyperarousal as well as excitotoxic effects (Everly, 1995). Corticotropin-releasing factor (CRF), endogenous opioids, vasopressin, and oxytocin, are also implicated in extreme stress arousal (Selye, 1976; Rossier et al., 1980; Rochefort et al., 1959). Finally, there is evidence that serotonin, dopamine, and certainly norepinephrine play significant roles in extreme stress (Kolb, 1987; Sorg & Kalivas, 1995; van der Kolk et al., 1985).

The excitatory processes inherent in PTSD are not limited to the CNS. The mobilization of neuroendocrine and endocrine pathways carries the posstraumatic stress response throughout the human body. Especially implicated are the sympathoadrenomedullary (SAM) (Everly, 1990) and the hypothalamic–pituitary–adrenal (HPA) systems (Yehuda et al., 1995). Figure 20.3 summarizes some of the key elements involved in the biology of PTSD.

Psychological Hypersensitivity

Psychological hypersensitivity is thought to arise from a violation of some deeply held belief, referred to as a worldview, or *Weltanschauung* (Everly, 1993, 1994, 1995). Thus, according to this perspective, a traumatic event is predicated upon some situation that violates a deeply held and important worldview. Most commonly, we think of the traumatic event as a life-threatening event—a violation of the assumption of safety discussed by writers such as Maslow (1970). But there appear to be at least five universally traumatogenetic themes:

1. Violation of the belief that the world is "just" or "fair". For example, why does an infant die in a motor vehicle accident?

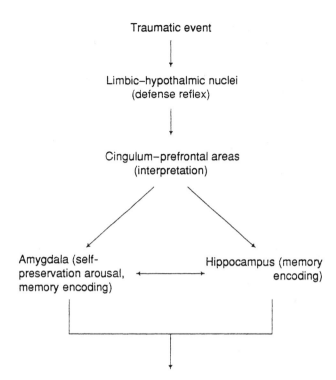

Traumatic event

Limbic–hypothalmic nuclei
(defense reflex)

Cingulum–prefrontal areas
(interpretation)

Amygdala (self-
preservation arousal,
memory encoding)

Hippocampus (memory
encoding)

1. Sympatho–adrenal–medullary augmentation (increased catecholamines)

2. Gonadatropin alteration (increased testosterone in males, and possible progesterone and/or estrogen dysfunction in females)

3. Potential hypothalmic–anterior–pituitary adrenal–cortical augmentation (fluctuations in cortisol; increased endogenous opioids)

Figure 20.3. Neurobiology of posttraumatic stress disorder.

2. Violation of a sense of who you are by having not done something you should, or by having done something you should not have done.
3. Abandonment, betrayal, violation of trust.
4. Violation of a universal sense of safety.
5. Disruption of a religious or spiritually based belief.

Within his construct of "psychotraumatology," Everly (1993, 1994, 1995) discusses these issues in greater detail.

THE PSYCHOLOGICAL PROFILE OF
POSTTRAUMATIC STRESS DISORDER

The work of Keane and his colleagues is preeminent in the search for the psychological PTSD prototype. Using patients evaluated with the Minnesota Multiphasic Personality Inventory (MMPI) and 100 patients with other psychiatric diagnoses, Keane, Malloy, and Fairbank (1984) were able to identify an MMPI profile capable of correctly classifying 74% of all patients. The MMPI decision rule was $F \geq 66$, Depression (2) ≥ 78, Schizophrenia (8) ≥ 79 (using T scores). Item analysis led to the creation of a 49-item MMPI PTSD subscale that correctly identified 82% of the patients studied. On this MMPI subscale, patients who scored 35 out of 49 had an 87% chance of possessing a valid PTSD diagnosis, whereas patients who scored above 40 had a 90% chance of a true positive PTSD diagnosis.

In a cross-validation of the aforementioned MMPI PTSD subscale, Fairbank, McCaffrey, and Keane (1985) found that patients with a T score above 88 on the F scale were most likely to possess a factitious disorder. Thus, the F decision rule became $66 \leq F \leq 88$ and correctly identified 93% of the sample studied when combined with the previous (2) ≥ 78 and (8) ≥ 79.

The work of McDermott (1987) sought to extend the psychometric diagnosis of PTSD beyond the MMPI. Using the Millon Clinical Multiaxial Inventory (MCMI), McDermott evaluated 22 Vietnam combat veterans, 11 of whom had been diagnosed with PTSD. The results of his study indicate that PTSD patients may present elevations on the MCMI schizoid and avoidant scales ($x > 80$), with a concomitant depression on the histrionic scale.

The MCMI-III contains a scale (R) that purports to assess PTSD with a 53% sensitivity and a positive predictive power of 73%. But the MCMI-III aggregate configural profile may take several forms:

1. Aggregate elevations on Schizoid, Avoidant, and Negativistic (passive–aggressive) scales are often viewed as the withdrawing "flight" variant of the MCMI posttraumatic stress profile.
2. Aggregate elevations on the Narcissistic, Aggressive, and Antisocial scales may be viewed as the aggressive "fight" variant of the MCMI posttraumatic stress profile.
3. Aggregate elevations on the Negativistic, Self-Defeating, Schizoid/Avoidant, Aggressive, and Borderline scales may be viewed as the affectively labile profile that is often characteristic of "complex PTSD" (i.e., indicative of early developmental trauma, abuse, and/or neglect).

Based on Kolb's (1987) hypothesis that PTSD represents a partial cognitive deficit, in combination with the belief that PTSD resides within the hippocampal complex, Everly and Horton hypothesized that there would be a short-term memory deficit among PTSD patients. Using 15- and 30-second trials of the Peterson Memory Paradigm, these authors found that 9 out of 14 (65%) non-combat-related PTSD patients failed to meet the 55% correct cutting-line criterion for the 15-second trials, and 11 out of 14 (79%) patients failed to meet the 45% correct cutting-line criterion for the 30-second trials. These data served to support the hypothesis that PTSD patients are likely to possess a cognitive deficit that manifests as an impairment to immediate and short-term memory function. Long-term memory was unimpaired in these subjects.

Finally, it should be noted that despite the growing interest in PTSD, as Brett and Ostroff (1985) have suggested, PTSD remains underrated and underdiagnosed. They conclude that PTSD patients are likely to be misdiagnosed as substance abusers, alcohol abusers, antisocial personalities, and malingerers (Silverman, 1986). It is clear that although our database is growing, there remains much to learn about PTSD. Special care should be taken to expand our PTSD subject pools. Currently, most of what we know about PTSD is based on Vietnam veteran studies. We may significantly increase our risk of false-negative diagnoses unless we gather additional data on non-combat-related PTSD.

TREATMENT OF POSTTRAUMATIC STRESS DISORDER

This chapter has presented posttraumatic stress as a quintessential example of psychological and biological factors combining in an inextricable integration. Our two-factor model of PTSD implies that the recovery from posttraumatic stress is predicated upon improvement in both domains. This is not to say that every patient who suffers from PTSD requires medication, but it does suggest that the more severe the manifest symptomatology, the more psychotropic medications should be considered as an addition to the therapeutic mix. It is doubtful, however, that any PTSD patient has ever recovered on the basis of psychotropic medication alone. Because the "injury" is a psychological one, recovery will be based upon some alteration in the "psychological domain." That psychotherapeutic improvement may be greatly facilitated, indeed, by the addition of psychopharmacological agents. In instances when the amplitude of the neurological pathology has become self-sustaining, psychopharmacological agents will be mandatory. Let us take a look at current issues in the treatment of posttraumatic stress.

Psychopharmacotherapy

A wide variety of psychopharmacological agents have been used in the treatment of PTSD. As van der Kolk (1987) has stated, "Psychotherapy is rarely helpful as long as the patient continues to respond to contemporary events and situations with a continuation of physiological emergency reactions" (p. 75).

A recent review of the pharmacological treatment of PTSD has been offered by Platman (1999) and lists psychotropic agents for consideration by virtue of the symptoms they tend to target:

Learned helplessness—clonidine, benzodiazepines, tricyclics (TCAs), and monoamine oxidase inhibitors (MAOI)
Hyperstartle response—clonidine
Intrusive ideation—selective serotonin reuptake inhibitors (SSRIs), TCAs, and MAOIs
Panic—alprazolam, clonazepam
Depressed mood and avoidance—SSRIs
Impulsive rage—lithium and carbamazepine
Sleep disturbance—trazodone

In 1999, the *Journal of Clinical Psychiatry* published findings from its Expert Consensus Panel for the Treatment of PTSD (Foa, Davidson, & Frances, 1999). The Panel recommended that psychopharmacological intervention either follow or be used in combination with psychotherapy for both acute and chronic PTSD. The medications of choice were the SSRIs. If no response was achieved, the Panel recommended that nefazodone or venlafaxine be initiated. If a partial positive response was achieved, it recommended a mood stabilizer in addition to the SSRI.

Given that some researchers consider severe posttraumatic stress a form of kindling, or subcortical ictus, the question of the utilization of mood stabilizers (carbamazepine, divalproex) as a primary medication becomes a relevant issue.

Psychotherapy

The Expert Consensus Panel for the Treatment of PTSD (Foa, Davidson, & Frances, 1999) has recognized the superordinate role that psychotherapy initially plays in the therapeutic arsenal. The report notes that anxiety management, psychoeducation, and cognitive therapy appear to be the safest and most acceptable psychotherapeutic interventions. The work of Meichenbaum (1977, 1994) stands as a most significant contribution. His treatise on the treatment of PTSD from a cognitive-behavioral perspective represents a powerful multidimensional approach to this complex and challenging disorder (Meichenbaum, 1994; also see Foy, 1992).

Other valuable resources in the area of treatment formulation for PTSD include the work of Foa, Keane, & Friedman (2000) and Flannery (1992). Wilson, Friedman, and Lindy (2001) offer an updated integrative perspective on the treatment.

Group therapy interventions have shown significant promise and have been summarized by van der Kolk (1987). The rationale for the use of group psychotherapy for PTSD includes the provision of peer support, a safe venue for therapeutic abreaction, consensual validation, and the minimization of regression and avoidance.

Neurocognitive Strategic Therapy for Posttraumatic Stress

Everly (1993, 1994, 1995) has posited that posttraumatic stress represents a two-factor phenomenon (i.e., two inextricably intertwined factors that make up its core essence): (1) neurological hypersensivity and (2) psychological hypersensitivity. We reviewed their respective constituencies earlier in this chapter, so we shall not reiterate them here. It may be argued that treatment should be the natural corollary of phenomenology. If so, then treatment formulations for posttraumatic stress reactions, including ASD and PTSD, should parallel, or match, their phenomenology. To put it another way, the treatment of posttraumatic stress reactions, including ASD and PTSD, should possess a two-factor constituency so as to match the two-factor phenomenology of the disorder.

Everly (1994, 1995) has proposed that a neurocognitive strategic treatment formulation for posttraumatic stress is likely to prove the most effective and is clearly the most theoretically sound. By way of explanation, it is clear that numerous therapies are effective for posttraumatic stress. In that it is unclear that any given "brand name" tactic is always superior to any other given tactic, Everly offers a strategic formulation for the treatment of posttraumatic stress rather than recommending a specific tactical approach. This strategic formulation recommends a phenomenologically driven *approach* to therapy rather than a specific *technique* for therapy. Thus, Everly suggests that *neurological desensitization* techniques should be used to address the neurological sensitivity of posttraumatic stress and be combined with techniques that address the *cognitive schemas* that have been threatened or destroyed by the traumatic event. Techniques for neurological desensitization might include meditation, Yoga, physical exercise, massage, neuromuscular relaxation techniques, hypnosis, psychotropic medications, imagery, and so on. Techniques to address the endangered cognitive schemas might included cognitive therapy, cognitive-behavioral therapy, dynamic therapies, group therapy, behavior therapy, and so on.

One relatively recent therapy called Eye Movement Desensitization and Reprocessing (EMDR) may represent a unique example of an integrated neurocognitive therapy in that it may address both the neurological hypersensitivity and the cognitive schemas within the same therapeutic paradigm, virtually simultaneously.

Eye Movement Desensitization and Reprocessing (EMDR)

No discussion of the treatment of posttraumatic stress would be complete without mentioning the most noteworthy of recent therapeutic innovations: Eye Movement Desensitization and Reprocessing (EMDR). EMDR is a therapeutic method originated by Francine Shapiro in 1987, when she indiscriminately discovered that recurring, disturbing thoughts rapidly and permanently disappeared when she engaged in rapid, saccadic eye movements (Shapiro & Solomon, 1995). Shapiro first published her work in 1989 as EMD and reported on the successful controlled treatment of 22 rape/molestation victims and Vietnam veterans, using a one-session application that included as part of the protocol having the participant follow the repeated side-to-side movement of her fingers (Shapiro, 1989). The impressive treatment gains were maintained at a 3-month follow-up. The results of Shapiro's initial work generated tremendous excitement in area of PTSD treatment; however, it also raised considerable skepticism because of the lack of validated PTSD measures employed and the possibility of placebo effects, including demand characteristics (Feske, 1998).

The intense research scrutiny that resulted from the introduction of EMDR led in a relatively short period of time to numerous applied studies. However, the overall results of early studies of EMDR were largely equivocal due primarily to flawed methodology, poor experimental design, and inadequate treatment delivery (i.e., inexperienced or minimally trained therapists providing the treatment) (Shapiro, 1999). Others have proposed that the negative findings may have been due to the EMDR technique itself (see Rosen, 1999, for a critical review). Within the past several years, controlled studies on the effectiveness of EMDR have been conducted by independent research teams using subjects who experienced a single traumatic episode that led to PTSD. For example, the results of four rigorously controlled studies of 107 patients found that 84–100% of participants no longer had PTSD symptoms after 4–5 hours of treatment (Marcus, Marquis, & Sakai, 1997; Rothbaum, 1997; Scheck, Schaeffer, & Gillette, 1998; Wilson, Becker, & Tinker, 1995, 1997). Moreover, a recent meta-analysis of various PTSD intervention treatments (Van Etten & Taylor, 1998) found EMDR to be not only effective but also more efficient than other treatments, including behavior therapy.

The reported success of EMDR in about three to five sessions raises the question of putative mechanism of effect, particularly that of underlying neurophysiological processes. A neuroimaging study (Levin, Lazrove, & van der Kolk, 1999) using EMDR with PTSD participants demonstrated increased activity in the anterior cingulate gyrus and the left frontal lobe. Increased activity in these brain areas is thought to provide patients with a way to differentiate more comfortably between real and imagined threat.

As noted by Rosen (1999), "The short but eventful history of EMDR has captured the attention of psychologists who work in the area of posttraumatic stress" (p. 181). In fact, Rosen's quote is from an article in the Special Issue of the *Journal of Anxiety Disorders* (Vol. 13, No. 1–2) devoted solely to the topic of EMDR. Despite a relative neoteric status as a PTSD intervention, the process and procedures of EMDR have undergone several variations. In order to better understand EMDR, the reader is referred to Shapiro (1995) for a complete description of the current procedural elements and eight phases of treatment.

According to Shapiro (1999), it is important to acknowledge that EMDR is "an integrated form of therapy incorporating aspects of many traditional psychological orientations and one that makes use of a variety of bilateral stimuli besides eye movement" (p. 37). In fact, treatment effectiveness has been reported for bilateral auditory stimulation therapist (e.g., snaps fingers nearer one ear of the patient than the other) and bilateral tactile stimulation (e.g., participant rests palms on his or her knees and therapist alternatively taps the palms) (Lipke, 2000). Therefore, the emphasis on eye movements is actually a misconception, but one that is certainly understandable given the name of the process. Shapiro is also quick to emphasize that other quite salient, nonspecific elements account for therapeutic success (Shapiro, 1995, 1999). She proposes that the general model of EMDR is predicated on the notion of accelerated information processing, which states that "there is an innate physiological system that is designed to transform disturbing input into an adaptive resolution and a psychologically healthy integration" (Shapiro, 1995, p. 53).

In the final analysis, as suggested by Horowitz (1974), psychotherapy should be directed toward cognitive control, improving self-image and interpersonal relationships, decreasing stress, and working through the "meaning" of the trauma. As noted by writers such as Janoff-Bulman (1992), addressing the "meaning" of the trauma becomes a pivotal aspect of the recovery process. This is clearly consistent with the two-factor model of PTSD introduced in this chapter, and also with the overarching formulation of the human stress response as used throughout this text, in that the "interpretation," or meaning, of the stressor event serves to contribute to the intensity and chronicity of the stress response itself.

Obviously, the treatment of PTSD needs to be tailored to the specific needs of the individual patient. Not only must the clinician consider the manifest symptomatology, but he or she must also strive to understand the "meaning" of the traumatic event. Once the symptoms have been stabilized and no longer represent a barrier to psychotherapy, the focus of the therapeutic process should most likely turn to the endangered or compromised belief about the world, or oneself, that lies at the foundation of the post-traumatic repsonse (Everly, 1993, 1994, 1995).

SUMMARY

This chapter has addressed the subject of PTSD, one of the most underrated and underdiagnosed of the psychiatric disorders. Historically, in its more severe forms, PTSD has led to permanent partial disabilities. In some cases, permanent total disabilities have resulted. Because of the prevalence and propensity to remain undiagnosed for protracted periods of time, this stress-related disorder has been included in the present volume. Let us review the main points:

1. PTSD is generally thought to possess four key phenomenological constituents: (a) the presence of stressful experience generally acknowledged as being outside the usual realm of human experience; (b) intrusive, recollective experiences; (c) ANS hyperactivity; and (d) avoidance and numbing symptoms.

2. Within this chapter, we have argued that the "essence" of PTSD is the intrusive, recollective experience in combination with the ANS hyperfunction. The avoidant and numbing symptoms have been reformulated as attempts by the patient to control the pathological syndrome. Exposure to a stressor remains a necessary but insufficient diagnostic criterion.

3. Once viewed in the context of a combat-related syndrome, PTSD is now recognized as having the potential to arise out of virtually any life-threatening experience. Recent evidence has even suggested that PTSD can arise out of an accumulation of stressor experiences; exposure to certain solvents, toxins, and stimulants; and the experience or observation of traumatic, but not necessarily life-threatening, events such as the loss of personal property and/or physical injury.

4. Once suggested as residing within the hindbrain, PTSD has been reformulated from a physiological perspective as residing primarily as a condition of neurological hypersensitivity within the noradrenergic projections

of the septal-amygdalar-hippocampal complexes. Potential causes of the neuronal hypersensitivity include an augmentation of tyrosine hydroxylase, an increase in beta-1 postsynaptic excitatory receptors, a decrease in alpha-2 presynaptic inhibitory receptors, and an increase in postsynaptic dendritic spines.

5. Attempts to identify the psychological profile of the PTSD patient have focused upon the use of the MMPI. The $66 \leq F \leq 88$, $(2) \geq 78$, and $(8) \geq 79$ decision rule for the MMPI seems a useful starting point. Other research utilizing the MCMI has found elevations on the Schizoid and Avoidant subscales, coupled with a diminution of the Histrionic subscale to be useful in identifying PTSD patients. Research has also found an impairment of short-term memory among PTSD patients. Finally, it should be noted that PTSD patients may frequently be misdiagnosed as sociopathic, hypochondriacal, and/or as substance abusers.

6. From a treatment perspective, PTSD, especially in its chronic forms, may require a combination of psychotherapeutic and pharmacological efforts to be truly effective. Antidepressants and anticonvulsants appear to be promising agents for the cases wherein psychotherapy alone seems insufficient.

7. Strategically, Everly (1993, 1994, 1995) has offered a two-factor neuro-cognitive strategic formulation for conceptualizing the treatment of posttraumatic stress.

21

Management of Acute Distress through a Comprehensive Model of Crisis Intervention for Mass Disasters and Terrorism

In the previous chapter, we reviewed the most severe form of human stress, posttraumatic stress disorder (PTSD). Over 50% of adults in the United States will be exposed to a traumatic event during the course of a lifetime! One of the factors that may determine whether such exposure develops into a disabling mental disorder (e.g., PTSD) is the availability and provision of emergency psychological "first-aid," historically referred to as crisis intervention. Whether working in response to mass disasters or terrorism responding to a crisis at a business or industrial venue, or treating clients in hospital, clinic, or private practice settings, every provider of mental (behavioral) health services will periodically encounter a person in acute, yet severe, psychological decompensation (i.e., a crisis).

This chapter is dedicated to the provision of emergency psychological services to those in the midst of a psychological crisis. In contradistinction to psychotherapy, these interventions are characteristically (1) brief in total duration, (2) concrete and uncomplicated, (3) provided relatively early, (4) provided wherever and whenever the intervention services are needed and best suited, and (5) provided with the expectation that the services will be focused, goal directed, and relatively brief in duration. The goals of these crisis intervention services may be clearly articulated as (1) the acute stabilization of signs and symptoms of distress, and (2) the facilitation of a

---

Portions of this chapter have been published in the *International Journal of Emergency Mental Health*. Used with permission.

return to adaptive, independent functioning, or (3) the facilitation of access to a higher, or more continuous, level of care, if necessary.

MASS DISASTERS AND TERRORISM

Mass disasters, such as floods, earthquakes, and fires, may create significant psychological distress because of their massive course of devastation and the enormous amount of time, energy, and money required to recovery from that devastation. The devastation is further compounded if there is a loss of human life. Generally speaking, however, natural disasters take less of a psychological toll than do human-induced disasters (Baum & Posluszny, 1999). It may be argued that the most pathogenic variant of mass disasters is terrorism. Our extant principles of emergency mental health are built mostly upon incidents that were not terrorism related. The terrorist bombing of the Oklahoma Federal building on April, 19, 1995 and the terrorist attacks against the World Trade Center in New York City and the Pentagon in Washington, DC on September 11, 2001 were both large-scale mass disasters that have caused us to rethink previous mental health dogma. For example, we typically expected about 9% of those exposed to a DSM-IV traumatic stressor to develop PTSD; now in response to a mass act of terrorism, our expectation has climbed to be in excess of 35% (U.S. Department of Health and Human Services, 1999). The specific impact of September 11 may push those expectations even higher. Similarly, much of the mental health community typically held a "wait-and-see" attitude when considering a mental health response to mass disasters. Fueled largely by concerns about interfering with natural psychological recovery mechanisms, this hesitancy to respond has been challenged by the widespread and intense acute distress in evidence in the wake of the terrorism of September 11. But what is terrorism?

Terrorism may be thought of as the actual or threatened use of unlawful violence or force against persons or property so as to cause a state of psychological distress with the intent of coercing those persons, or their government, to alter social, political, military, and/or economic actions. There can be little doubt that terrorism can engender psychological morbidity, perhaps more so than other mass disasters; in fact, that is the intention. The destruction of buildings, the contamination of water supplies, and the murder of innocent civilians are not the terrorist's goals. These things are but means to the intermediate goal of inducing a state of terror, consistent with the ultimate goal of coercive change. The intensity of the psychological impact of terrorism appears to be amplified by several factors: the targeting of innocent civilians, the targeting of women and children, the targeting of national or religious symbols, the unpredictable nature of the attacks, the omnipresent nature of the threat, the departure from traditional methods of warfare (e.g., suicide bombing), the use of moral or religious justification subsequent to the terrorist act, the difficulty in body recovery after the use of highly lethal or toxic weapons, the intense media coverage, and the extraordinary amount of time associated with rescue, recovery, rebuilding, and dealing with the criminal justice system, if applicable.

THE BATTLEFIELD OF THE MIND

Any effective response to mass disasters especially terrorism, must, include psychological as well as physical intervention. The Defense Against Weapons of Mass Destruction Act of 1996 (Senators Nunn, Lugar, and Domenici) mandates the enhancement of domestic preparedness and response capabilities in the wake of an attack against the United States using weapons of mass destruction (WMD). Unfortunately, Myers (2001) estimates that only 5% of federally sponsored courses on responding to WMD include disaster mental health related topics.

It seems clear that the emergency mental health response to critical incidents, mass disasters, and terrorism must be an integrated seamless continuum of care consisting of a functional integration of multiple and diverse emergency mental health interventions. Such has been recommended by a select workgroup of international experts on mass disasters (U.S. Department of Defense, 2001).

The Critical Incident Stress Management (CISM, Everly & Mitchell, 1999) intervention system represents an integrated multicomponent crisis intervention that may be applied to well-circumscribed critical incidents, or mass disasters including terrorism. The CISM system was employed on a wide scale subsequent to the events of September 11. In this chapter, we

Table 21.1. A Brief Historical Timeline for Crisis Intervention

As any field evolves, "milestones" mark events that are significant to the evolution of that field. The field of crisis intervention represents an endeavor characterized by the provision of urgent and acute psychological "first-aid." Some of the most important milestones in the development of this important area of applied mental health are as follows:

1906—National Save-a-Life League for suicide prevention.
World War I—The first empirical evidence that early intervention reduces chronic psychiatric morbidity.
World War II—The processes of immediacy, proximity, and expectancy are identified as important "active ingredients" in effective emergency psychological response.
1944—Lindemann's observations of grief reactions to the Coconut Grove Fire begin "modern era of crisis intervention.
Late 1950s—Community suicide prevention programs proliferated.

(Continued)

Table 21.1. (*Continued*)

1963/64—Caplan's three tiers of preventive psychiatry are implemented within the newly created Community Mental Health System (i.e., primary prevention, secondary prevention, tertiary prevention).

Late 1960s/early 1970s—Crisis intervention principles are applied to reduce the need for hospitalization of potentially "chronic" populations.

1980—Formal nosological recognition of PTSD in DSM-III "legitimizes" an examination of crisis and traumatic events as threats to long-term mental health.

1982—Air Florida 90 air disaster in Washington, D.C. prompts reexamination of psychological support for emergency response personnel; first use of group crisis intervention Critical Incident Stress Debriefing (CISD).

1986—"Violence in the workplace" era begins with death of 13 postal workers on the job.

1989—International Critical Incident Stress Foundation (ICISF) formalizes an international network of over 350 crisis response teams trained in a standardized and comprehensive crisis intervention model (CISM); ICISF gains United Nations affiliation in 1997.

1992—American Red Cross initiates formal training for the establishment of a nationwide mental health disaster capability; Hurricane Andrew tests the new mental health function.

1993—Social Development Office (Amiri Diwan), ICISF, Kuwait University, and others implement a nationwide crisis intervention system for postwar Kuwait.

1994—DSM-IV recognizes acute stress disorder.

1995—Bombing of the Federal Building in Oklahoma City underscores need for crisis services for rescue personnel, as well as civilians.

1996—TWA 800 mass air disaster emphasizes the need for emergency mental health services for families of the victims of traumas and disasters.

1996—OSHA 3148-1996 recommends comprehensive violence/crisis intervention programs in health care and social service agencies.

1997—Gore Commission recommends crisis services for airline industry.

1997—AFI 44153 mandates establishment of crisis programs for U.S. Air Force bases worldwide.

1998—OSHA 3153-1998 recommends crisis intervention programs for late-night retail stores.

1998—Based on Defense Against Weapons of Mass Destruction Act of 1996, the Metropolitan Medical Response System's Field Operations Guide is published.

1999—COMDINST 1754.3 requires the establishment of a CISM team for each U.S. Coast Guard region.

1999—Department of Defense Directive 6490.5 establishes policy and responsibilities for developing Combat Stress Control (CSC) programs throughout the U.S. military.

1999—Mass casualties in Colorado high school shooting leads to a reexamination of youth and school violence issues, and an increase in the establishment of school crisis response programs.

2000—Yemen. Terrorist attack on USS *Cole* kills 17 sailors. US Navy SPRINT teams employ integrated multicomponent crisis intervention response.

2001—New York City. Two hijacked airliners crash into World Trade Center killing over 3000.

2001—Washington, DC. Hijacked airlines crashes into Pentagon.

2001—Washington, DC, New York City, New Jersey. Anthrax is sent through the mail; causes several deaths.

2002—U.S. and Allied military forces invade Afghanistan causing collapse of Taliban, but not before Taliban calls for destruction of America and a worldwide "holywar."

will review the CISM approach to acute distress intervention. Before detailing the CISM mechanisms, we shall review key terms and concepts.

BASIC TERMS: ON THE NATURE OF A
PSYCHOLOGICAL CRISIS AND CRISIS INTERVENTION

One of the founding fathers of psychosomatic medicine, George Engle, noted that rational discourse is predicated upon the consistent use of terms. T. S. Eliot even noted that words decay with imprecision. It seems that effective clinical practice is guided by a firm conceptual foundation. As da Vinci once said, "First study the science, then practice the art." In order to guide the reader, we begin with a brief introduction to the terms that recur throughout this chapter.

Crisis—An acute response to an event wherein the following occur:

1. Psychological homeostasis has been disrupted.
2. One's usual coping mechanisms have failed.
3. There are signs and/or symptoms of distress, dysfunction, impairment (Caplan, 1961, 1964).

Cognitive Errors in Crisis—It has commonly been observed that individuals in crisis routinely exhibit an acute cognitive dysfunction. This phenomenon has been referred to by terms such as *cognitive distortion, cortical inhibition syndrome,* and even the "dumbing down" effect. It may be useful for the crisis interventionist to know that the person in crisis is commonly cognitively compromised, which explains many of the "irrational," or "illogical" things people do in a crisis. In attempting to better understand the crisis response, it may be helpful if the crisis interventionist notes that *a common cognitive error made by primary victims is a failure to understand the consequences of their actions while in a crisis state;* thus, people in crisis may be seen to act quite impulsively and often self-defeatingly. Similarly, those interventionists who commonly work with *secondary victims* (i.e., rescue workers, police and fire personnel, emergency medical personnel, and disaster workers) may benefit from the recognition that these professionals are often likely to make *a cognitive error of faulty self-attribution; that is, they are likely to blame themselves for adverse outcome when no such causal attribution is appropriate.* For example, it has been estimated that cardiopulmonary resuscitation (CPR) is successful less than 20% of the time when the patient is in full cardiac arrest. Yet many individuals who perform CPR expect that almost every patient will recover if the CPR is done correctly. The corollary of this assumption is that individuals who perform unsuccessful CPR believe that the patient died because they performed the CPR incorrectly. In short, the patient died because they made a mistake. The ramifications of such an attribution can obviously be devastating.

Critical Incident—A stressor event that appears to cause, or be most associated with, a crisis response; an event that overwhelms a person's usual coping mechanisms (Everly & Mitchell, 1999).

Trauma—An event outside the usual realm of human experience that would be markedly distressing to anyone who experienced it. In the fourth edition of the *Diagnostic and Statistical Manual of Mental Disorders* (DSM-IV; American Psychiatric Association, 1994) a trauma is defined exclusively in terms of the exposure to human suffering (i.e., personal or vicarious exposure to severe injury, illness, or death). A trauma, therefore, may be seen as a more narrow form of critical incident.

Crisis Intervention—Urgent and acute psychological support sometimes thought of as "emotional first-aid." The hallmarks of crisis intervention have historically been *immediacy* (early intervention), *proximity* (intervention within close physical proximity to the critical incident), *expectancy* (both the person in distress and the interventionist have the expectation that the intervention will be acute and directed toward the goal of symptom stabilization and reduction, not cure), *simplicity* (relatively concrete, uncomplicated intervention strategies that avoid complex psychotherapy-oriented tactics), and *brevity* (the total duration of the intervention is short, typically consisting of one to three contacts). The goals of crisis intervention are as follows:

1. Acute stabilization of symptoms and signs of distress and dysfunction (to keep things from getting worse).
2. Facilitation of symptom reduction (intervening so as to reduce acute distress and dysfunction).
3. Facilitation of a restoration of acute, adaptive independent functioning (successful reduction of impairment).
4. Facilitation of access to a higher, or more continuous, level of care, if needed (Caplan, 1961, 1964; Everly & Mitchell, 1999).

Table 21.1 provides a brief list of milestones in the evolution of the field of crisis intervention.

CRITICAL INCIDENT STRESS MANAGEMENT (CISM)

CISM is a comprehensive, integrated, multicomponent crisis intervention system (Everly & Mitchell, 1999; Flannery, 1998). Flannery's model of CISM has been recommended by the Occupational Safety and Health Administration (OSHA), while other variations of CISM have been utilized by organizations such as the U.S. Air Force, the U.S. Coast Guard, the Airline Pilots' Association, the U.S. Navy, the Bureau of Alcohol, Tobacco, and Firearms (ATF), the Federal Bureau of Investigation (FBI), the Australian Army and Navy, the Hospital Authority of Hong Kong, and numerous law enforcement agencies, fire departments, school systems, employee assistance programs, and hospitals throughout North America, Scandinavia, Europe, Australia, and Asia (see Everly & Mitchell, 1999).

Just as a good golfer would never play a round of golf with only one golf club, a good crisis interventionist would never attempt the complex task of intervention in a crisis or disaster with only one crisis intervention technology. As noted earlier, CISM is an integrated, multicomponent crisis intervention system, whose core crisis intervention components are outlined in Table 21.2 and described as follows:

1. *Preincident preparation.* Preincident preparation may be thought of as a form of psychological "immunization." The goal is to strengthen potential vulnerabilities and enhance psychological resilience in individuals who may be at risk for psychological crises and/or psychological traumatization. One important aspect of preincident preparation is the provision of information. Sir Francis Bacon once noted, "Information itself is power." Many crises and traumas result from a violation of expectancy; thus, setting realistic expectations serves to protect against violated assumptions. But preincident preparation also consists of behavioral response preparation and rehearsal, including familiarization with common stressors, stress management education, stress resistance training, and crisis mitigation training for line personnel as well as management.

2. *Disaster or large-scale crisis intervention programs, including demobilizations, staff advisement, and crisis management briefings* (CMBs). The *demobilization* is an opportunity for temporary psychological "decompression" immediately after exposure to a critical incident. This technique was originally developed for use by emergency services personnel. *Staff advisement* refers to the provision of psychological consultations to command staff (emergency services personnel, military, disaster response teams), as well as management personnel in business and industrial settings. The *CMB*, which refers to a four-step crisis intervention for large groups of individuals (up to 300 at one time), is ideal for school crises, business and industrial crises, community violence, and mass disasters (see Everly, 2000a; Newman, 2000).

3. *Defusing.* This is a three-phase, 45-minute, structured, small-group discussion provided within hours of a crisis for purposes of assessment, triaging, and acute symptom mitigation. In some cases, the defusing may do much to foster psychological closure after a critical incident.

4. *Critical Incident Stress Debriefing.* CISD refers to the seven-phase, structured group discussion usually provided 1 to 14 days postcrisis

Table 21.2. Critical Incident Stress Management (CISM): The Core Components

	Intervention	Timing	Activation	Goal	Format
1	Precrisis preparation	Precrisis phase	Crisis anticipation	Set expectations Improve coping Stress management	Groups/ organizations
2a	Demobilizations and staff consultation (rescuers)	Shift disengagement	Event-driven	To inform, consult, and allow psychological decompression	Large groups/ organizations
2b	Crisis Management Briefing (CMB) (civilians, schools, business)	Anytime postcrisis		Stress management	
3	Defusing	Postcrisis (within 12 hours)	Usually symptom-driven	Symptom mitigation Possible closure Triage	Small groups
4	Critical Incident Stress Debriefing (CISD)	Postcrisis (1–10 days; 3–4 weeks mass disasters)	Usually symptom-driven; can be event-driven	Facilitate psychological closure Symptom mitigation Triage	Small groups
5	Individual crisis intervention (1:1)	Anytime, anywhere	Symptom-driven	Symptom mitigation Return to function, if possible Referral, if needed	Individuals
6	Pastoral crisis intervention	Anytime, anywhere	Whenever needed	Provide spiritual, faith-based support	Individuals/ groups
7a	Family CISM	Anytime	Either symptom- or event-driven	Foster support and communications	Families/ organizations
7b	Organizational consultation			Symptom mitigation Closure, if possible Referral, if needed	
8	Follow-up/ referral	Anytime	Usually symptom-driven	Assess mental status Access higher level of care, if needed	Individual/ family

Source: G. Everly & J. Mitchell (1999). *Critical Incident Stress Management (CISM): A New Era and Standard of Care in Crisis Intervention.* Ellicott City, MD: Chevron Publishing.

(although in mass disasters it may be used 3 weeks or more postincident), and designed to mitigate acute symptoms (Campfield & Hills, 2001; Deahl et al., 2000), assess the need for follow-up, and, if possible, provide a sense of postcrisis psychological closure (Mitchell & Everly, 2001). In fact, one of the great utilities of the CISD appears to be its facilitation of psychological reconstruction. Due to its structure, the CISD may take up to 2–3 hours to complete. It is sometimes used subsequent to the crisis management briefing and the defusing, and is almost always followed by intervention on an individual basis with those individuals who require help. Referral for more formal mental health intervention may then follow.

5. *One-on-one crisis intervention/counseling* or psychological support throughout the full range of the crisis spectrum (the most frequently used CISM intervention). Typically, this consists of one to three contacts with an individual in crisis. Each contact may last from 15 minutes to more than 2 hours, depending upon the nature and severity of the crisis. Although flexible and efficient, this form of crisis intervention lacks the added advantage of group process. Because of its extremely time-limited nature, it is especially important with this intervention, as with all crisis interventions, to avoid using paradoxical interventions, interpretation of unconscious processes, or confrontational techniques (see Everly & Mitchell, 1999).

6. *Pastoral crisis intervention* (Everly, 2000b), more than ministerial or chaplaincy services, represents the integration of traditional crisis intervention with pastoral-based support services. In addition to traditional crisis intervention tools, pastoral crisis intervention may employ scriptural education, prayer (personal, conjoint, intercessory), rituals and sacraments, and the unique ethos of the pastoral crisis interventionist. A specialized form of crisis intervention, pastoral crisis intervention may not be suited for all persons or all circumstances; nevertheless, it represents a valuable addition the comprehensive CISM matrix.

7. *Family crisis intervention,* as well as organizational consultation, represent crisis intervention at the systems level. Both family and organizational crisis intervention, when done most effectively, possess proactive (precrisis) and reactive elements.

8. *Follow-up and referral mechanisms for assessment and treatment,* if necessary. No crisis intervention system is complete without the recognition that some critical incidents are, by their very nature, so toxic that they require a more intense and formalized intervention, perhaps even psychotropic medications. Therefore, it is important to build in to any crisis intervention system a mechanism for follow-up assessment and treatment for those individuals for whom acute crisis intervention techniques prove insufficient. An important aspect of this element is the existence of a set of principles or guidelines for psychological triage (see Everly, 1999).

Table 21.2 further describes this crisis intervention system. Specific guidelines for these interventions may be found in Flannery (1998), Mitchell and Everly (2001), and Everly and Mitchell (1999).

The historical evolution of the CISM system has, unfortunately, created considerable semantic confusion. Initially, Mitchell (1983) authored a paper on crisis intervention as it applied to emergency services personnel, wherein the Critical Incident Stress Debriefing (CISD) process was described.

Mitchell stated, "The CISD is an organized approach to the management of stress responses in emergency services. It entails either an individual or group meeting" (p. 37). He went on to describe a multicomponent crisis intervention approach that included a small-group crisis intervention referred to as a formal critical incident stress debriefing (CISD). Considerable semantic confusion resulted from Mitchell's use of the term CISD to denote more than one thing: (1) the overarching framework for his crisis intervention system (CISD), (2) a specific, six-phase small-group discussion process ("formal" CISD), and (3) the optional follow-up intervention (follow-up CISD). As a result, the current literature is plagued with references to "individual debriefings" and the perpetuated, but erroneous, notion that the CISD group discussion was intended to be a stand alone, or "one-off" intervention. In an effort to rectify the lexical discord and expand the original formulations, the term Critical Incident Stress Management (CISM) was chosen to denote the overarching, multicomponent approach to crisis intervention, thus replacing the term CISD as it was originally used. CISD is now reserved to describe a seven-stage postincident group discussion.

RESEARCH FINDINGS AND THE EFFECTIVENESS OF CRISIS INTERVENTION

The issue of the effectiveness of crisis intervention first emerged in the clinical literature in the 1960s. Artiss (1963) reported that the psychotherapeutic elements of immediacy, proximity, and expectancy had been employed successfully in military psychiatry to reduce psychiatric morbidity and increase rates of return to combat for American soldiers. Solomon and Benbenishty (1986) confirmed with Israeli soldiers what Artiss had observed with the U.S. military. These authors concluded that early intervention, proximal intervention, and the role of expectation were each associated with positive outcome. Parad and Parad (1968) reviewed 1,656 social work cases and found crisis-oriented intervention to be effective in reducing florid psychiatric complaints and in improving patients' ability to cope with stress. Langsley, Machotka, and Flomenhaft (1971) followed 300 psychiatric patients randomly assigned to inpatient treatment or family crisis intervention groups. The crisis intervention group was found to be superior in reducing the need for subsequent hospital admissions at 6- and 18-month intervals. A similar finding was recorded by Decker and Stubblebine (1972) using a single-group, 2.5-year longitudinal design. Finally, Bordow and Porritt (1979), through randomized experimental design, initially demonstrated that multicomponent crisis intervention was superior to single crisis tactics. Empirical evidence such as this argues for the effectiveness of early intervention and crisis-based psychological support tactics, while at the same time arguing against the attribution of psychotherapeutic exclusivity to traditional individual or group psychotherapy.

Questions concerning the effectiveness of CISM arose in the relevant literature with the publication of two Australian studies. McFarlane (1988) reported on the longitudinal course of posttraumatic morbidity in the wake of bush fires. One aspect of the study found that acute posttraumatic stress was predicted by avoidance of thinking about problems, property loss, and not attending undefined forms of psychological debriefings. The delayed-onset posttraumatic stress group, however, not only had higher premorbid neuroticism scores and greater property loss but also attended the undefined debriefings. Somewhat unexplainably, this study is often cited as a basis for questioning the effectiveness of crisis intervention, especially "debriefing," although the term is not defined.

Another study that has been cited to cast doubt upon crisis intervention is that of Kenardy et al. (1996). This investigation was purported to assess the effectiveness of stress debriefings for 62 "debriefed helpers" compared to 133 helpers who apparently were not debriefed subsequent to an earthquake in New Castle, Australia. This study is often cited as evidence for the ineffectiveness of debriefings, yet the authors state, "We were not able to influence the availability or nature of the debriefing" (p. 39). They continue, "It was assumed that all subjects in this study who reported having been debriefed did in fact receive posttrauma debriefing. However, there was no standardization of debriefing services" (p. 47). These rather remarkable revelations by the authors have failed to deter critics of the "debriefing" process, whatever the term may mean.

Perhaps the greatest contention regarding the utilization of crisis intervention in general, and debriefings specifically, has arisen from reports constructed by Wessely, Rose, and Bisson (1998), sometimes referred to as the Cochrane Review. This review is considered methodologically robust because it employs only investigations using randomization. Of six studies investigating crisis intervention, two found positive outcome, two found negative outcome, and two reported no differences between groups. An analysis of the two "negative" outcome investigations reveals epistemological problems, however.

Bisson, Jenkins, Alexander, and Bannister (1997) randomly assigned 110 patients with severe burns to either a "debriefing" group or a control group. The clinical standard *group* debriefing was abandoned for an *individual* adaptation. The goal of the randomization was not met, in that the "debriefed" individuals had more severe burns, greater pain, and greater previous trauma than the nondebriefed individuals. The debriefed group also suffered greater financial problems, which, in and of itself, could have accounted for the differences in outcome; thus, direct comparison was inappropriate. The preintervention differences, as would be expected, predicted poorer psychological outcome. More specifically, the "debriefed" group had more severe traumatic stress scores at 13-month follow-up. Despite the lack of equivalent groups, a plausible alternative explanation for poorer psychological outcome could be the inappropriate use of the debriefing with medical patients who were either in pain or on analgesic medications, and the failure to follow standard clinical protocols for group debriefings. Nevertheless, these authors contend that the results cast serious doubt upon the utility of debriefings.

Hobbs, Mayou, Harrison, and Warlock (1996) performed a randomized trial of debriefings for 106 (54 debriefed and 52 control subjects) motor vehicle accident victims. Once again, randomization failed to achieve equivalent groups for comparison, in that debriefed individuals had more severe injuries and spent more days in the hospital. Both factors predicted poorer psychological outcome. Similarly, the clinical standard group process was abandoned so as to employ individual debriefings. Not surprisingly, the individuals receiving the debriefings had higher traumatic stress scores at follow-up. Despite nonequivalent groups and the failure to use the clinical standard group-based intervention, these data have been used to argue that debriefing may be injurious. Yet closer scrutiny reveals that the actual traumatic stress scores were not in a clinical range at any time; furthermore, the overall change went from 15.13 to 15.97 (clinical ranges begin around 26). Such a change has no clinical significance whatsoever. In a 4-year, longitudinal follow-up investigation, Mayou, Ehlers, and Hobbs (2000) found that the intervention group (individualized debriefings) remained symptomatic. Once again, however, the *group* debriefing process was not utilized, and the debriefing was used in a stand alone manner (contrary to a multicomponent prescription including follow-up). It seems a nonsequitur to conclude that psychological debriefing is ineffective, and to further conclude that it is inappropriate for trauma patients when the debriefing process was individualized, as opposed to a group format, and when the debriefing was taken out of its prescribed multicomponent context.

The results of these often-cited reviews appear self-evident. Their lack of precise refinement of the independent variables makes any pursuit of external validity difficult, at best, and would seem to restrict the utility of their findings to the idiosyncratic nature of their unique interventions. Therefore, rather than support the notion that crisis intervention in general, or group debriefings specifically, are ineffectual and may be harmful, these data would appear to support a very different set of conclusions.

First, these studies would appear to support the conclusion that clinicians should avoid attempting to implement a group crisis intervention protocol with individuals (Busuttil & Busuttil, 1995). Obviously, none of the therapeutic elements of group process (Yalom, 1970) are available to be utilized when a group protocol is employed one patient at a time. This would appear similar to attempting group psychotherapy protocols with individual psychotherapy patients.

Second, these findings would suggest caution in the use of individualized (nonstandardized) psychological crisis intervention tactics with primary medical patients who have minimal temporal distance from their medical stressors, or with primary medical patients who are in physical distress. Turnbull, Busuttil, and Pittman (1997) argue that such applications are inappropriate due to the timing of the intervention and the nature of the patients' crisis event or trauma. As a crisis intervention tactic, group debriefing is best suited for acute situational crisis responses. Debriefings are certainly not a substitute for psychotherapy, psychotropic medication, analgesics, reconstructive surgery, or psychological rehabilitation.

Third, the studies that used debriefing absent a positive outcome appeared to use the debriefing as a stand alone intervention, outside the prescribed multifaceted CISM-like context (Everly & Mitchell, 1999). Kraus (1997), in agreement with Everly and Mitchell (1999) and the British Psychological Society (1990), argues that debriefing should not be a stand alone intervention.

To paraphrase the philosopher/psychologist William James, "To disprove the assertion that all crows are black, one need only find one crow that is white!" Therefore, to disprove the assertion that all forms of crisis intervention are ineffective, or that all debriefings are ineffectual, one need only find some evidence that crisis intervention is indeed effective, or find that one model of debriefing that is effective!

The effectiveness of integrated multicomponent CISM programs has now been suggested through thoughtful qualitative analyses (Dyregrov, 1997, 1998, 1999; Everly, Flannery, & Mitchell, 2000; Everly & Mitchell, 1999; Miller, 1999; Mitchell & Everly, 1997), as well as through empirical investigations (Corrigan, Flannery, & Penk, 1999; Flannery et al., 1995, 1998, 2000; Mitchell, Schiller, Eyler, & Everly, 1999; Western Management Consultants, 1996) and even meta-analytical statistical reviews (Everly, Flannery, Eyler, & Mitchell, 2001; Flannery et al., 2000). Flannery's (ASAP) program is an exemplary CISM crisis intervention approach (Flannery, 1998, 1999a,b,c) used in hospitals, clinics, and schools. Research has consistently shown the ASAP program to be an effective crisis intervention. The ASAP model of CISM was chosen one of the 10 best mental health programs in 1996 by the American Psychiatric Association. A recent meta-analysis of five ASAP studies found Cohen's d meta-analytic coefficient to be in excess of 1.00, showing a highly significant clinical effect (Flannery et al., 2000). The latest and largest of the meta-analytic studies conducted on CISM coalesced eight investigations. Results of the combined analysis of a wide variety of subjects across diverse settings revealed a Cohen's *d* in excess of 1.00. As would be predicted (Everly, Flannery, & Eyler, in press; Richards, 1999), studies have demonstrated the relative superiority of the multicomponent CISM compared to the singular CISD, consistent with expectations and prescription.

Clearly, randomized research designs that can assess the effectiveness of crisis intervention are certainly welcomed, if they can be instituted without sacrificing internal content validity. We noted earlier that CISM has been submitted to meta-analytical scrutiny and initially found to be effective on the basis of empirical investigations (Everly et al., 2001; Flannery et al., 2000). Although the component investigations were quasi-experimental, they are not without epistemological value for several reasons. First, the use of such designs, even single-case designs, can be useful in contributing meaningful data to the inquiry (Blampied, 2000; Hersen & Barlow, 1976). Second, faithful adherence to the standardized protocols (specifically CISD or CISM) serves as the foundation of internal validity and enhances specified external validity. Third, the use of meta-analysis serves to diminish the likelihood of systematic error across the participant investigations and compensate for specific threats to internal validity.

SUMMARY

Swanson and Carbon (1989), writing for the American Psychiatric Association Task Force Report on Treatment of Psychiatric Disorders state, "Crisis intervention is a proven approach to helping in the pain of an emotional crisis" (p. 2520). While there is a compelling logic to support the notion of early psychological intervention subsequent to a critical incident and empirical evidence to support the utilization of a multifaceted crisis intervention system, continued empirical validation and clinical refinement are worthy pursuits for the future. Clearly, crisis intervention technologies are best directed toward acute situational adversity, well circumscribed stressors, and acute, adult-onset traumatic reactions (Dyregrov, 1997, 1998, 1999; Everly & Mitchell, 1999; Richards, 1999). Crisis intervention is neither a form of therapy per se nor a substitute for treatment. Crisis intervention is designed to complement more traditional psychotherapeutic services. This is readily apparent if we understand that one of the expressed goals of the crisis intervention, as defined in this chapter, is to assess the need for continued care and to facilitate access to a higher level of care, if required or desired. To do nothing other than identify care seems a worthwhile goal in and of itself, and justification for studying and implementing this form of acute stress management.

22

Hans Selye and the Birth of the Stress Concept

Paul J. Rosch

This volume has been dedicated to assist the reader in developing greater proficiency in the treatment of the human stress response. Such a proficiency must be based upon a foundation of increased phenomenological understanding; more specifically, clinical proficiency is based upon an understanding of the phenomenology of the human stress response. Chapters 1–6 have provided the reader with a scientifically accurate yet clinically relevant introduction to the phenomenology of the stress response and its clinical implications and manifestations. But no review of phenomenology would be complete without a historical review. Virtually every chapter of this volume is replete with important historical references. Yet the authors decided to offer a final, rather unique contribution to this volume. Most of what we know about stress is attributable to one man—Hans Selye. While not always correct, Selye is nevertheless the father of the science of human stress. What drove the scientific investigations of human stress was not only the personality of the man but also his brilliance. We offer this chapter as a means of understanding the "background" of the nature and treatment of the human stress response.

For those who knew him intimately, Hans Selye would easily qualify for the *Reader's Digest*'s "Most Unforgettable Character I Ever Met" designation. However, few individuals, especially those in the scientific community, ever

Paul J. Rosch • President, The American Institute of Stress, Clinical Professor of Medicine and Psychiatry, New York Medical College, American Institute of Stress, Yonkers, New York, 10703. This chapter has been published in previous forms in *Stress Medicine* and the *International Journal of Emergency Mental Health*. Used with permission.

enjoyed that privilege because of his apparently aloof attitude. His father Hugo was a surgeon in the Imperial Austro-Hungarian Army, and it was possibly his early upbringing that resulted in his stiff, authoritarian, Prussian demeanor, which many interpreted as an air of arrogance. Born in 1907 in Komarom, a small town that at the time was in the Hungarian part of the Empire, midway between Vienna and Budapest, he attended school at a Benedictine monastery. Since his family had produced four generations of physicians, Selye entered the German Medical School in Prague at the age of 17 and later earned a doctorate in organic chemistry.

In medical school, Selye noted that patients suffering from very different diseases often exhibited identical signs and symptoms in the very early stages of their illness. All had low grade fevers, feelings of malaise, fatigue, generalized aching, and "they just looked sick." Excited about the possibility of studying the biochemical changes and mechanisms that might be responsible for these common findings and possibly lead to some treatment or form of relief, Selye made an appointment to speak to the Chairman of the Department of Physiology to ask if he could study in the laboratory on weekends or in his free time after school. This individual's full name, including titles, was Hofrat Professor Doktor Armin Tschermak Edler (Nobleman) vonSysenegg. Since that was quite a mouthful, it was agreed that his highest title should be used; he, therefore expected to be addressed as "Herr Hofrat" (Counsel to the Imperial Court). Selye, who was 19 at the time and unaware of this, innocently called him "Herr Professor." Apparently, that was the only part of his enthusiastic presentation that sank in, because when he had finished, the only response was "Well, if you are that chummy, why don't you just call me by my first name, Armin." Even after his profuse apologies, Selye's request was rejected as being so childish that it was not worth discussing. He was told that obviously, if a person is sick, he looks sick, just as if he is fat, he looks fat. He was warned not to bring the subject up again, and to concentrate on studying for his exams. Selye obeyed this edict and graduated first in his class.

Because of his obvious talent, Selye received a Rockefeller scholarship to study at Johns Hopkins University. He arrived in Baltimore in 1931, rented a cheap room with a kitchenette near the university, and learned how to cook for himself, so that he could save some of his $150 per month stipend. Selye subsisted on mostly canned foods and often referred to this as his "sardine period," since a large tin was a bargain at 10 cents, and he ate sardines daily for months. He was warmly accepted by the other postdoctoral students, and well-meaning faculty wives, who were sorry for "the poor lonely foreign students," constantly arranged parties and social events so that the students could meet people. Although he spoke English fairly well, Selye quickly realized that Americans had their own lingo. On one occasion at a party, when he met a very attractive daughter of a prominent Professor, Selye asked if they could meet again to go to a movie or dinner, and he offered to walk her home. Her response was "Yes, but would you give me a ring first?" Selye was petrified, thinking that she meant an engagement ring; he had heard many stories of the strict enforcement of "breach of promise" laws in the United States. When he congratulated another girl on her beautiful complexion by saying that her "hide" was of the finest quality, she did not take the remark as a compliment. Unfortunately, there was no distinction between *hide* and *skin* in any of the several languages Selye spoke.

He also had difficulties adapting to faculty life at Johns Hopkins, having been reared in a formal, academic European environment, where the rigid class distinctions were much like the military. Full professors were respected and obeyed as if they were Generals in the Army, and Department Heads were demigods. Selye was appalled at the sight of such distinguished middle-aged and older individuals playing charades and acting in an undignified fashion at faculty parties to which underlings and even medical students were invited. Jackets and ties were discarded, and often everyone seemed to be on a first-name basis. Unable to conceive of Professor Hofrat or his other teachers acting in such a degrading way, Selye suffered from a severe case of culture shock. He was confused, and even considered returning home, but was told by friends that Canada was more European, traditional, and sedate. After making inquiries, Selye found that he could transfer the second half of his fellowship to McGill University in Montreal, to work under the renowned biochemist, J. B. Collip. Although fluent in Parisian French, Selye quickly found out that the language spoken by the Quebeçois was quite different. He quickly adapted and ultimately joined the McGill Faculty, became a Canadian citizen, and, in 1945, moved to his own Institute of Experimental Medicine and Surgery at the University of Montreal.

Selye once told me that he never felt he really had any nationality of his own. He spoke fluent German, Hungarian, Czech, Slovak, French, and English, since each had been his national language at one time or another. Based on personal experience, I can confirm that he was also comfortably conversant in Russian, Spanish, Italian, and Portuguese, and could understand Swedish and a few other languages, if they were spoken slowly. Whereas his first name was Austrian, his surname was Hungarian. He was looked down on and considered an Austrian when he was in Hungary, and vice versa. When the Empire collapsed in 1918, Selye became Czechoslovakian without ever moving out of his house. The Czechs and the Slovaks had many disagreements with one another, but they both detested the Austrians and Hungarians. After Selye became an international celebrity, Czechoslovakia, Austria, and Canada, all wanted to claim him as their own. He readily accepted these accolades but confided in me that he was most proud of his Magyar Hungarian heritage. He was particularly fond of Hungarian Bull's Blood, and on several occasions when I visited his home, we consumed liberal amounts of this red wine, along with the superb Hungarian goulash he loved to make.

As instructed, he had not thought anymore about the "just being sick" syndrome that intrigued him in medical school, but by a strange twist of fate, the idea resurfaced a decade later at McGill. At the time, only two types of female hormones had been identified, but Professor Collip thought there was a third, and he assigned Selye to this research. Selye was sent to the slaughterhouses with a large bucket and told to retrieve as many cow ovaries as possible, which Collip then reduced to various extracts for Selye to inject into female rats for several days or weeks. The animals would later be autopsied to look for any changes in their sex organs or other tissues that could be attributed to this new ovarian hormone. However, no such effects could be demonstrated, and to add injury to insult, many of the rats became quite sick, and some died. Although there were no changes in the ovaries of breasts, all of the rats showed enlargement of the adrenals, shrinkage of the thymus and lymphoid tissues, and ulcerations in the stomach. This did not make any sense at all, and Selye searched for some explanation. One possibility was that the changes were due to some contaminant in his chemical concoction. One day, with a bottle of formaldehyde, a toxic substance used to fix tissues for microscopic study, right in front of him, he injected liberal amounts of formaldehyde into several rats on a whim, and was amazed to find that it produced identical results.

He began to wonder if other, or all, noxious substances or stimuli could also produce these same three effects, and what ensued is now history. He exposed rats not only to powerful chemicals but also to the frigid Canadian winter, by leaving them exposed on the windswept roof of the McGill medical building. He put others in a revolving, barrel-like treadmill contraption driven by an electric motor, so that they had to constantly run to stay upright. Sure enough, all who survived developed the same pathology in the adrenals, lymphoid tissues, and stomach. Selye viewed this syndrome as a nonspecific response to what he referred to as "biologic stress." He published these findings in the form of a 74-line letter to the editor of the British journal *Nature* in 1936, entitled "A Syndrome Produced by Diverse Nocuous Agents." He avoided using the word *stress* because of previous criticisms that, in everyday English, it implied nervous strain, and he did not want to create any confusion. However, Selye did suggest the term *alarm reaction* to describe this response, since he viewed it as a generalized mobilization of the body's defensive mechanisms.

In subsequent studies, he found that the same changes could be produced by other noxious challenges and stimuli. Animal activists were not as vocal at the time, and many of these experiments could never be performed today, including exposing rats to brilliant lights after their eyelids had been sewn back, bombarding them with constant deafening noise, making them continuously swim to the point of exhaustion to avoid drowning, and subjecting them to intense psychological frustration that bordered on torture. He also showed that the pathological changes characteristics of the "Alarm Reaction" occurred not only in rats, but also in mice, rabbits, dogs, cats, and all other animals subjected to such acute insults.

Selye then studied the effects of animals' longer exposure to noxious but not lethal stimuli, noting that this resulted in a "Stage of Resistance" during which the body's defense mechanisms were maximized to adapt to these threatening challenges. However, if they persisted, a final "Stage of Exhaustion" ensued, with deterioration and death. He termed this three-stage response the "General Adaptation Syndrome." He performed numerous, detailed autopsies during the various stages of this syndrome, and observed, on gross and microscopic examination, changes identical to those seen in patients with arthritis, kidney disease, hypertension, coronary heart disease, and gastrointestinal ulcers. He suspected that perhaps "stress" might also cause these disorders in humans as well, and therefore considered them to be "Diseases of Adaptation." Actually, "Diseases of Maladaptation" would have been more appropriate. After thousands of additional experiments, Selye found that he could produce many of these disorders selectively, by sensitizing or conditioning the animals through certain dietary or hormonal manipulations, and subjecting them to different types of distressful insults.

He subsequently traced the pathways and mechanisms responsible for the changes seen in the "Alarm Reaction" and demonstrated that they were due to increased pituitary stimulation of the adrenal cortex to produce steroids that would reduce inflammation. This explained why the adrenals were enlarged. Similarly, the stomach ulcers and lymphoid tissue shrinkage were due to the increased amounts of cortisone-like hormones. If he removed the pituitary and repeated the experiments, these manifestations of damage in different organs and structures did not occur. He reasoned that if he could show how such injuries were caused, then perhaps he could also find a way to prevent them, or to treat the resultant diseases more effectively. These were entirely new and very radical concepts.

As a result of Pasteur's research and Koch's postulates, physicians had always been taught that each disease had its own, very specific cause. Tuberculosis was caused by the tubercle bacillus; pneumonia by the pneumococcus; rabies, anthrax, and cholera by other specific microorganisms, and so on. What Selye proposed was actually the complete reverse of this. He had demonstrated that very different, and even opposite physical challenges such as extremes of heat and cold, as well as severe emotional threats, could indeed produce identical pathological findings. While each of these might also have their own specific hallmarks, such as a burn, or frostbite, all nevertheless caused the same nonspecific changes in the adrenal, stomach, and lymphoid tissue he had first seen following the injection of his new ovarian hormone extract. Perhaps this also explained the curious and very common syndrome of "just being sick" that he had observed as a medical student, in the early stage of illness in patients who later went on to develop very different diseases.

He chose the word *stress* to describe this phenomenon, defining it as "the nonspecific response of the body to any demand for change." It turned out to be an unhappy decision that would haunt him the rest of his life. The term had evolved from the Latin *strictus* (tight, narrow) and *stringere* (to draw tight). This became *strece* (narrowness, oppression) in Old French, and *stresse* (hardship, oppression) in Middle English. In vernacular speech, and in Selye's opinion, stress represented a contraction or variant of distress, which would have been appropriate.

Unfortunately, he was not aware that the word *stress* had been used for centuries in physics to explain elasticity, the property of a material that allows it to resume its original size and shape after having been compressed or stretched by an external force. As expressed in Hooke's Law of 1658, the magnitude of an external force, or *stress*, produces a proportional amount of deformation, or *strain*, in a malleable metal. The maximum amount of stress a material can withstand before becoming permanently deformed is referred to as its elastic limit. This ratio of stress to strain, a characteristic property of each material, is called the modulus of elasticity. Its value is high for rigid materials, such as steel, and much lower for flexible metals, such as tin. Selye complained several times to me that had his knowledge of English been more precise, he would have gone down in history as the father of the "strain" concept.

This created considerable confusion when his research had to be translated into foreign languages. There was no suitable word or phrase that could convey what he meant, since he was really describing strain. In 1946, when he was asked to give an address at the prestigious College de France, the academicians responsible for maintaining the purity of the French language struggled with this problem for several days and subsequently decided that a new word would have to be created. Apparently, the male chauvinists prevailed, and *le stress* was born, quickly followed by *el stress, il stress, lo stress,* and *der stress* in other European languages, and similar neologisms in Russian, Japanese, Chinese and Arabic. Stress is one of the very few words you will see preserved in English form among these latter languages. Twenty-four centuries previously, Hippocrates had written that disease was not only *pathos* (suffering) but also *ponos* (toil) as the body fought to restore normalcy. While *ponos* might have sufficed, the Greeks also settled on stress. Selye's concept of stress and its relationship to illness quickly spread from the research laboratory to all branches of medicine, and *stress* ultimately became a "buzz" word in vernacular speech. However, the term was used interchangeably to describe both physical and emotional challenges, the body's response to such stimuli, as well as the ultimate result of this interaction. Thus, an unreasonable and overdemanding boss might give you heartburn or stomach pain, which eventually resulted in an ulcer. For some people, stress was the bad boss, while others used stress to describe either their "agita" or their ulcer.

Because it was clear that most people viewed stress as some unpleasant threat, Selye had to create a new word, *stressor*, in order to distinguish between stimulus and response. Even Selye had difficulties when he tried to extrapolate his laboratory research to apply to humans. In helping to prepare the *First Annual Report on Stress* in 1951, I included the comments of one critic, who, using verbatim citations from Selye's own writings, concluded that "stress, in addition to being itself, was also the cause of itself, and the result of itself."

I first met Selye in 1949, when he was writing his monumental tome, *Stress*. He was already regarded internationally as one of the world's leading authorities on endocrinology, steroid chemistry, experimental surgery, and pathology. He had singly authored one of the first textbooks of endocrinology, as well as a 27-volume *Encyclopedia of Endocrinology*, covering every aspect of this subject. Selye did everything on a grandiose scale. *Stress*, which was published in 1950, was a huge book of over 1,000 pages, containing more than 5,000 references. However, it paled in comparison to his *Encyclopedia of Endocrinology*, where each of the proposed 27 volumes was the size of a metropolitan telephone directory.

A voracious reader, he consumed everything from the most technical and esoteric journals, in eight languages, to popular magazines and pulp fiction, and he did this with lightning speed. He read as fast as most people could skim, and he could skim a book in almost the time it took to turn pages. However, he seemed to retain as much from skimming a page as most of us would from reading it, because of an amazing photographic memory. He could sometimes quote almost verbatim part of an article he had seemingly only glanced at months before. His favorite lay publications were *The New Yorker Magazine*, with its cartoons by Price and Arno, and some obscure Hungarian publication similar to *The Police Gazette*, the forerunner of *The National Enquirer*. He almost compulsively retained copies of every article in any scientific or lay publication remotely dealing with stress, but it did not stop there. He would write away for reprints of all the pertinent citations listed in an article, retrieve the relevant references from those articles when they were received, and then send away for these reprints, repeating this process over and over, which resulted in a never-ending chain of requests for reprints in different languages from all over the world.

The problem lay in deciding where and how to file this mountain of material. If it had to do with cold stress in hypophysectomized and adrenalectomized rats on a high sodium diet to determine the development of hypertension and/or cardiac enlargement, should he make seven copies to store separately under cold stress, hypophysectomy, adrenalectomy, combined hypophysectomy–adrenalectomy, high sodium diet, hypertension, and cardiac hypertrophy? To overcome this problem, he devised his own "Symbolic Shorthand System for Medicine and Physiology," using mnemonic symbols and arrows that transcended language barriers. It was generally acknowledged to be a vast improvement over the conventional Cutter and Dewey decimal systems, since it provided instant retrieval of pertinent information on any stress-related subject from any publications. Subsequently published for others to use, it went through several editions, until the advent of the computer made it obsolete. Selye eventually amassed a monstrous collection of reprints and books in a library that became world renowned. Unfortunately, it was virtually destroyed by a fire in 1962, but since his classification system allowed him to identify each item, Selye immediately set about completely restoring it by writing to everyone he knew, asking them to send copies of all the reprints on stress in their collections—many of which they had originally obtained from him during the course of their research!

Few people were aware of Selye's superb skills as an experimental surgeon. In order to trace the pathways of the response to stress, it was necessary to demonstrate the role of the pituitary and adrenal glands by studying the effects of removal of these organs. Taking out the adrenals required only an abdominal incision and a rudimentary knowledge of anatomy, but the pituitary posed a formidable problem. In humans, removal of pituitary tumors at the time required opening the skull at a very specific site, followed by 5 hours of painstaking surgery to go deep into the brain without damaging other important structures. Outside of Harvey Cushing and a few others, few neurosurgeons were experienced in this transcranial operative procedure, and morbidity and mortality rates were high. Removing a rat's pituitary without harming the animal was not much easier, and to obtain the dozen or more hypophysectomized but otherwise healthy animals required for each experiment would have taken weeks. Selye found a way to remove the pituitary within 2 minutes, and it was so simple and safe that we all quickly learned to do it on an assembly-line basis. It consisted of a rectangular block of wood with a 1-inch staple partially embedded in it at the top, and a very heavy rubber band encircling the bottom. To the right, we had a beaker filled with ether-soaked balls of cotton, next to which was a cage of rats to be operated on. We would put a rat in the beaker, and after it was anesthetized, which took a minute or two, we placed its upper teeth under the staple and pulled down on the body until the mouth was fully open, maintaining this position by snapping the rubber band over the lower portion of the body or tail. We wore flashlights on our foreheads and used magnifying spectacles, which allowed us to see clearly into the open mouth. Once we had identified where the soft palate met the hard palate, we used a dentist's drill to make a small hole in the center of this junction, which clearly revealed the pituitary and its stalk, and much like a little cherry on a stem, it could easily be removed. The comatose rat was then put in an empty cage on the left to wake up, a new anesthetized rat was taken from the beaker and laid out the same way, then replaced by another to be anesthetized. We hardly ever lost an animal, and with a little practice, most of us could obtain two dozen specimens in a half hour. Selye told me he was visited by Harvey Cushing, who had heard about this remarkable achievement, and also taught him how to perform the procedure.

In later experiments, it was necessary to study the effects of removal of part of the liver on the metabolism of hormones and responses to stress, but this had to be done in some standardized fashion, and without damaging other structures. Selye discovered a way to also accomplish this in less than 2 minutes. Since the lobes of the liver are well differentiated and readily apparent on opening the abdomen, it was simply necessary to tie a suture completely around two of them, which allowed their bloodless removal, resulting in a two-thirds partial hepatectomy. Selye also devised a unique technique for studying the inflammatory response in order to prove that ACTH and glucocorticoids reduced inflammation, while STH (growth hormone) and mineralocorticoids promoted it. This was much more complicated, since it required the ability to quantify the irritant and the body's response to allow accurate measurements and to ensure consistency. There was also the need to separate the two major components of inflammation, the cellular reaction, with its resultant tissue proliferation, and the production of inflammatory fluid. He solved this in an ingenious fashion by shaving the skin on the back of a rat and then injecting air, so that a transparent sac resulted. Various irritants could then be injected and the amount of inflammatory fluid that was produced could be visualized and quantified on a daily basis by transilluminating the sac with a flashlight. The effects of stress or of injecting various steroids were easily demonstrated, and the tissue response could be measured by studying the thickness of the wall of the sac under the microscope. This granuloma pouch technique was so simple and useful that we could only wonder why no one had thought of it before.

When I was at the Institute, Selye's average work day was 10 to 14 hours, including weekends and holidays. He habitually rose around 5:30 A.M., took a dip in the small pool in the basement of his house, which was across from the McGill campus, and then rode his bike several miles to work. He was usually the first to arrive and the last to leave. On sunny days, he often put aside an hour or so after lunch to "take a nap in Miami." This was not Florida, but rather a solarium on the roof, where he had had the glass ceiling replaced with quartz, so that he could work on his tan during the winter. As a result of his research on the experimental production of myocardial necrosis and the benefits achieved by Sodi Pallares's polarizing solution containing potassium in acute heart attacks, he filled all his salt shakers with potassium chloride. It tasted horrible, but he was convinced it would protect his heart and reduce risk for hypertension and stroke. Recent research findings have shown that he was absolutely correct. He regularly took garlic pills, he told me, not only because of their health benefits but also because his breath discouraged prolonged, close conversations, especially with strangers who frequently cornered him during his travels, and he used this effectively.

Selye's office was a real inner sanctum, guarded by an anteroom of protective secretaries and librarians. We had to make an appointment with these watchdogs if we wished to speak with him. There was a prominent green and a red light over both sides of his entry door. When the red light was on, which was not infrequently, he was absolutely not to be disturbed by anyone, including these wardens. A green light indicated that he could now be approached with messages that had accumulated, or important incoming telephone calls. For some reason, I enjoyed a somewhat special relationship with him right from the start, possibly because he knew that I had been an English teacher before entering medical school. Although his command of the language was superb, he was still struggling with the confusion surrounding what "stress" really signified, and was concerned about the possible connotations of other words or expressions that might have escaped him. Since most of his publications were now in English, he wanted to make absolutely certain that they were letter perfect, and that he had not overlooked anything.

He was extremely generous, inviting me to coauthor the lead Chapter "Integration of Endocrinology" for the American Medical Association's *Textbook of Glandular Physiology and Therapy*, which included contributions from 32 leading authorities on various hormonal disorders. He had given a presentation to the New York Academy of Medicine in 1951, which they wanted to publish. However, it had been an extemporaneous speech, so he asked me to write something up from his notes and to add anything that I deemed appropriate, or that he might have neglected. When a preprint was submitted for his approval, he again insisted that I be listed as a full coauthor, explaining to the Academy that a major portion of this final version had been my contribution.

Selye was not well received by his peers, who considered him arrogant and aloof. Many also resented that they could not evaluate much of his research without purchasing expensive publications from Acta Inc., which Selye owned completely. Selye explained to me that he had established this company in self-defense to speed up publication of *Stress* and subsequent works, rather than for any financial gain. Conventional medical publishing houses often took up to a year to get a book into circulation, and it was difficult to make any changes once the galleys had been set. However, since he had complete control of Acta, located a few miles away, he could readily insert any late-breaking research to ensure accuracy and timeliness. He had quarrels and feuds with prominent endocrinologists such as Dwight Ingle and George Engel, and although he was not liked, he was respected. Even many of his adversaries felt that he should have shared in the Nobel Prize given to Kendall and Hench. I had arranged for him to give a talk at Johns Hopkins when I was involved in the Endocrine Clinic with giants such as John Eager Howard, Lawson Wilkins, Harry Klinefelter, and Sam Asper. Although he was well received, I was surprised at the somewhat antagonistic attitude of these good friends, who also viewed him as somewhat pompous.

We continued to keep in close contact while I was at Johns Hopkins, and later, when I headed the Endocrine Section at Walter Reed Army Medical Center. He periodically commissioned me to write articles or review his own, even after I entered private practice. Over the next two decades, he became an international celebrity. Because of several books written for the public, which were high on the best-seller lists for months, he was in wide demand as a speaker all over the world, attracting large audiences and commanding huge fees. He had numerous requests for consultations but, to the best of my knowledge, never saw a patient. After I entered private practice, he regularly referred many patients to me, including several very famous individuals. He later developed a rare and usually fatal malignancy, and attributed his recovery to his strong desire to continue his research. He asked me to contribute a presentation on Stress and Cancer to a Symposium that his Institute conducted with Sloan-Kettering in 1978, which led to my present interest in this subject. He was adamant about my helping him establish the American Institute of Stress, and later assuming its Presidency, as well as serving on the Board of his International Institute of Stress.

In the final analysis, much of what he believed and proposed was not correct. However, his real legacy can be summed up by what he often reminded me, namely, that theories do not have to be correct—only facts do. He pointed out that many theories are of value simply because of their heuristic benefit, in that they encourage others to discover new facts that then lead to better theories. Hans Selye's propaedeutic contributions to our understanding of stress and its relationship to health and illness vividly illustrate this maxim.

23

Summation and Conclusions

With all its sham, drudgery and broken dreams, it is still a beautiful world.
Be cheerful. Strive to be happy.

MAX EHRMANN

"First study the science. Then practice the art which is born of that science." These words of Leonardo da Vinci have served as the guiding spirit of this volume. Perhaps more than any other pathological process, stress arousal represents the epitome of mind–body interaction. We suggested earlier in this volume that proper clinical understanding and treatment of such conditions that so intimately intertwine psychology and physiology demand that the clinician's attention be directed toward the "science" of physiology (and pathophysiology) as well as the art/science of behavior change. Thus, to be consistent with this stated bias, this volume has first introduced the reader to a rather detailed exploration of the physiological nature and foundations of the human stress response. This, as a preface to the subsequent chapters that directly addressed the treatment of excessive stress arousal and its pathological consequences.

A TREATMENT MODEL

In order to assist the reader in seeing the phenomenology of pathogenic stress arousal in its larger context, this volume has introduced an epiphenomenological model of the human stress response, from stressor to target-organ effect. This model was first introduced in Chapter 2 as Figure 2.6. It represents the larger "overview" of not just stress arousal but its antecedent and consequent constituents. This basic figure was employed again in

365

Chapter 6 (Figure 6.1) but this time with measurement technologies super-imposed. The same basic model was again employed in the introduction to Part II, to demonstrate how treatment interventions might be conceptual-ized in a coherent and cogent manner via a unifying model. Finally, that same figure is replicated once again to assist in the summary of the text (see Figure 23.1).

The stress response is predicated upon an event called a *stressor*. The stressor, which can be real or imagined, is typically then perceived and some *cognitive interpretation* is rendered by the individual. The obvious exception would be sympathomimetic and vasoactive stressors, which bypass interpre-tation (see Appendixes C and D). On the basis of the interpretation, the individual will experience some *affect* emerging from the limbic circuitry. Intimately intertwined with the creation of this affect is the activation of a *neurological triggering mechanism* that transduces psychological events into somatic realities, the most important of which is the initiation of the stress response itself: a psychophysiological mechanism of mediation character-ized by arousal and possessing three basic efferent limbs: the neural, the neuroendocrine, and the endocrine. These stress arousal mechanisms then exert some *target-organ effect*, that is, signs and symptoms. If *coping* mecha-nisms employed by the person are not successful, continued arousal and a *psychosomatic disease* is the likely consequence (refer to Figure 23.1).

Given an understanding of this oversimplified process, we can more appropriately select and implement treatment interventions.

Listed in Table 23.1 are the major treatment interventions discussed within this volume and summarized in Figure 23.1.

Having used a treatment model to summarize this volume, let us turn to a clinical protocol to see how it all fits together.

A TREATMENT PROTOCOL

In Chapter 1, the reader may recall that on the basis of a review by Girdano et al. (2001), we suggested that the treatment of excessive stress arousal may be categorized into three therapeutic genres, or "dimensions":

1. Strategies to avoid/minimize/modify stressors
2. Strategies to reduce excessive arousal and target-organ reactivity/ dysfunction
3. Strategies to ventilate, or express, the stress response

The use of such a summative schema facilitates the creation of a generic, multidimensional treatment protocol. This protocol, compared

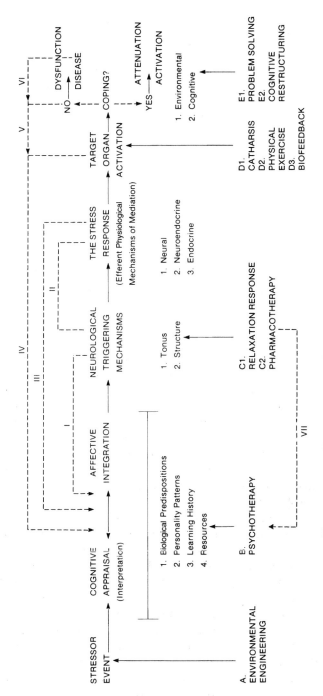

Figure 23.1. A Multidimensional treatment model for the human stress response.

Table 23.1. Treatment Interventions

Treatment options	Chapter discussions	Purpose
Environmental engineering	Chapters 8, 9 Appendices C and D	To allow the patient to avoid or minimize exposure to stressors
Psychotherapy	Chapters 7–9 See also Chapters 11–15	To avoid stressors; to reinterpret stressors; to increase perception of self-efficacy
Relaxation response	Chapters 10–16 Appendix B	To reduce pathogenic arousal; to increase perception of self-efficacy
Psychopharmacotherapy	Chapter 17	To reduce arousal
Reduction of target-organ arousal	Chapters 9, 14–16	To ventilate the stress response in a health-promoting manner; to reduce target-organ arousal or dysfunction
Problem solving and cognitive restructuring	Chapters 8, 9	To attenuate excessive arousal

with Figure 23.1 and Table 23.1, more readily translates into a step-by-step guide for clinical practice and is summarized in Table 23.2.

Having the patient undergo a physical examination is desirable, especially if target-organ disease or dysfunction is manifest. The stress response is the epitome of mind–body interaction. For this reason, it is sometimes difficult to distinguish psychologically induced problems from those problems that possess little or no psychogenic etiology. In some cases, what appear to be stress-related signs and symptoms may in reality be indicative of some neurological pathology or neoplastic phenomenon.

As previously indicated, psychological assessment, especially personologic assessment, can play an important role in treatment planning. The concept of personologic diathesis, when operationalized, provides insight into not only diagnosis but also treatment (see Chapter 7). Broad-spectrum psychological assessments such as the Minnesota Multiphasic Personality Inventory (MMPI) or the Millon Clinical Multiaxial Inventory (MCMI) are useful and efficient assessment tools, especially the latter, which integrates personality assessment (refer also to Chapter 6).

The general protocol described in Table 23.2 is not designed to be "blindly" adhered to by the practicing clinician; rather it is provided as a general guide to allow the clinician to formulate a multidimensional, individualized treatment protocol which is far superior to a unidimensional one. Furthermore, aided by the psychological assessment, the treatment

Table 23.2. A General Treatment Protocol

Physical examination

Psychological assessment (especially personality assessment, see Chapters 6 and 7)

Interventions (three dimensions):

1. Helping the patient develop and implement strategies for the avoidance/minimization/modification of stressors

   A. Patient education (see Chapter 8 for a rationale)
   B. Environmental engineering (see Chapter 9; Appendices C and D)
   C. Psychotherapy (Chapter 9)

2. Helping the patient develop and implement skills that reduce excessive stress arousal and target-organ reactivity/dysfunction

   A. Meditation (Chapter 11)
   B. Neuromuscular relaxation (Chapter 13; Appendix B)
   C. Respiratory control (Chapter 12)
   D. Hypnosis (Chapter 14)
   E. Biofeedback (Chapter 15)
   F. Psychopharmacotherapy (Chapter 17)

3. Helping the patient develop and implement techniques for the healthful ventilation/expression of the stress response

   A. Catharsis (Chapter 9)
   B. Physical exercise (Chapter 16)
   C. Religious beliefs (Chapter 18)

plan can be tailored to the specific needs of the patient. Bhalla (1980) found that multidimensional, individualized treatment protocols were generally superior to unidimensional or otherwise "boilerplate" protocols (see also Meichenbaum & Turk, 1987).

To reiterate the approach taken in this book, effective treatment emerges from accurate and specific diagnosis. To assess the notion of a personologic diathesis, to actively involve the patient in his or her own therapy, and to recognize the therapeutic value of patient education (see Chapter 8) seems a useful and humanistic approach to the treatment of the human stress response and its target-organ consequences.

A WORD ABOUT TREATMENT ADHERENCE

It would be naive to believe or expect that if all of the guidelines in this text are followed, treatment adherence would approach 100%. This is simply not the case. Patient adherence to lifestyle management programs designed to reduce health-related risk factors (e.g., stress management programs) reportedly ranges from a high of 80% to a low of 20%. It has been suggested that adherence to daily home relaxation sessions is as low as 40%. Even adherence to antihypertensive drug regimens may be as low as 60%. See Meichenbaum and Turk (1987) and Blackwell (1997) for a review of these and other treatment adherence issues.

Nevertheless, we hope that our review of the phenomenology and measurement of stress arousal will render clinical success superior to those treatment conditions where such has not been the case. We also highly recommended that the reader review a manual on facilitating treatment adherence before designing any treatment protocols (e.g., Blackwell, 1997; Meichenbaum & Turk, 1987).

SUMMARY

In conclusion, within this chapter, we have seen two forms of summary: the first, a treatment model, provided a more conceptual summary; the second, a treatment protocol, provided a more clinically practical summary. We hope that, by providing both, we convey not only a sense of clinical practicality but also a conceptual understanding that will allow the reader to move beyond the limits of this volume.

Appendixes

Special Considerations in Clinical Practice

A. Self-Report Relaxation Training Form

When we teach the relaxation response, the typical protocol requires the patient to visit the office between one and three times per week. This limited frequency would make it difficult to realize the desired therapeutic effect of a cultivated lower arousal status. Therefore, patients commonly receive relaxation training "homework." This usually consists of asking the patient to employ the relaxation response once or twice a day. In order to provide a useful forum for communications, and to improve compliance, it is highly desirable to have patients complete a relaxation training report form each time they practice the relaxation response. They are then asked to return the completed forms to the therapist at the beginning of each office session. The therapist then uses these forms as a means of reviewing patients' progress.

Following this introduction is a sample relaxation report form that may be used for reporting on the progress made in home relaxation training.

Relaxation Report Form

Name: _____   Time Started _____

Date: _____   Time Finished _____

Beginning SURS* _____   (before the relaxation exercise begins)

Ending SURS   _____   (after the relaxation exercise has ended)

Were you able to relax?   YES   NO   (Circle one)
    If "No", why not? _____
_____

Did your mind wander?   YES   NO
    If "Yes", what were you distracted by? _____
_____

Did you experience anything unusual?   YES   NO
    If "Yes", what? _____
_____

Is there anything else you would like to report? _____
_____
_____
_____
_____
_____

*The SURS (Subjective Units of Relaxation) indication is a method by which you may indicate your subjective levels of relaxation. A SURS of 10 will be indicative of a dreamlike state of profound relaxation; a SURS of 5 is indicative of how you believe the "average" person feels on an "average" day; and a SURS of 1 is indicative of a panic attack. Choose any number between 1 and 10, inclusive, to indicate your beginning and ending SURS levels.

B. Physically Passive Neuromuscular Relaxation

Earlier in this text, we stated that "neuromuscular relaxation" is the term usually reserved for isotonic and isometric contractions of the striated musculature designed to teach the client to relax. The entire discussion on neuromuscular relaxation has addressed that type of physically active procedure. By far the greater part of the literature has been generated on this active form of neuromuscular relaxation—hence our emphasis on reviewing that form. There does exist, however, what may be considered a physically passive form of neuromuscular relaxation. Here, we address that form of relaxation.

Physically passive neuromuscular relaxation fundamentally consists of having the patient focus sensory awareness on a series of individual striated muscle groups and then relax those muscles through a process of direct concentration. In the passive neuromuscular relaxation procedure described here, there is no actual muscular contraction initiated as part of the relaxation cycle—hence "passive" neuromuscular relaxation.

The physically passive neuromuscular relaxation procedure may be considered a form of mental imagery and directed sensory awareness. Mental imagery as a therapeutic intervention has a long and effective history for a wide range of clinical problems (see Leuner, 1969; Sheehan, 1972). When applied to the reduction of muscle tension, the basic mechanism involved in passive neuromuscular relaxation appears to be useful in tension reduction. In a review of investigations into the role of neuromuscular relaxation in general tension reduction, Borkovec et al. (1978) conclude: "Apparently, frequent attempts to relax while focusing on internal sensations are sufficient to promote tension reduction" (p. 527). In our own clinical experience, we have found passive neuromuscular relaxation to be quite effective in reducing subjective as well as electromyographically measured muscle tension.

There do appear to be several distinct advantages and disadvantages when comparing passive neuromuscular relaxation with a physically active form of neuromuscular relaxation. Passive neuromuscular relaxation has the advantage of having no potential limitations based on physical handicaps, as compared with neuromuscular relaxation that involves actual muscle tensing. Another advantage is the fact that the patient can execute a passive protocol without distracting others or drawing attention to him- or herself. Such is obviously not the case with a protocol that involves actual muscle contraction. A final advantage is that a passive protocol generally takes much less time to complete (usually half the time). The major disadvantage in using a passive form of neuromuscular relaxation is that, like meditation or other forms of mental images, it leaves the patient more vulnerable to distracting thoughts. This may be a significant drawback when using a passive protocol with obsessive-type patients or those who have a tendency to get bored easily.

Let us now examine one sample passive protocol (written as if being spoken directly to the patient). The "preparation for implementation" phase will be fundamentally the same as for the physically active form of neuromuscular relaxation, except for few alterations (refer to Chapter 13). In Step 1 of the preparation for implementation (precautions), the precautions are the same as those described for general relaxation. However, the special precautions for meditation prevail here, as opposed to those for the physically active neuromuscular relaxation. The physically passive component here dictates this alteration. Steps 2 through 4 may remain the same. Steps 5 through 8 may be omitted because of their reference to the actual tensing of muscles. The patient is instructed to breathe normally, in a relaxed manner.

BACKGROUND INFORMATION

It has long been known that muscle tension can lead to stress and anxiety—thus, if you can learn to reduce excessive muscle tension, you will reduce excessive stress and anxiety.

What you are about to do is relax the major muscle groups in your body. You can do this by simply focusing your attention on each set of muscles that I describe. Research has shown that with *patience* and *practice*, you can learn to achieve a deeply relaxed state by simply concentrating on relaxing any of the various muscle groups in your body.

First, you should find a quiet place, without interruptions or glaring lights, and a comfortable chair or bed to support your weight. Feel free to loosen restrictive clothing and remove glasses and contact lens if you desire.

ACTUAL INSTRUCTIONS

OK, let's begin. I'd like you to close your eyes and get as comfortable as you can. Let the chair or bed support all your weight. Remember, your job is to concentrate on allowing the muscles that I describe to relax completely.

CHEST AND STOMACH

I'd like you to begin by taking a deep breath. Ready? Begin ... (*pause three seconds*) and now exhale as you feel the tension leave your chest and stomach. Let's do that one more time. Ready? Begin ... (*pause three seconds*) and now relax and exhale as the tension continues to leave and your chest and stomach are relaxed.

HEAD

I'd like you to focus your attention on the muscles in your head. Now begin to feel those muscles relax as a warm wave of relaxation begins to descend from the top of your head. Concentrate on the muscles in your forehead. Now begin to allow those muscles to become heavy and relaxed. Concentrate as your forehead becomes heavy and relaxed (*pause 10 seconds*). Now switch your focus to the muscles in your eyes and cheeks and begin to allow them to become heavy and relaxed. Concentrate as your eyes and cheeks become heavy and relaxed (*pause 10 seconds*). Now switch your focus to the muscles in your mouth and jaw. Allow those muscles to become heavy and relaxed. Concentrate as your mouth and jaw become heavy and relaxed (*pause 10 seconds*).

NECK

Now you can begin to feel that wave of relaxation descend into the muscles of your neck. Your head will remain relaxed as you now shift your attention to your neck muscles. Allow your neck muscles to become heavy and relaxed. Concentrate as your neck becomes heavy and relaxed (*pause 10 seconds*).

SHOULDERS

Now you can begin to feel that wave of relaxation descend into your shoulder muscles. Your head and neck muscles will remain relaxed as you now shift your attention to your shoulder muscles. Allow your shoulder muscles to become heavy and relaxed. Concentrate as your shoulders become heavy and relaxed (*pause 10 seconds*).

ARMS

Now you can begin to feel that wave of relaxation descend into your arms. Your head, your neck, and your shoulders will remain relaxed as you now shift your attention to the muscles in both your arms. Allow both your arms to become heavy and relaxed. Concentrate as your arms become heavy and relaxed (*pause 10 seconds*).

HANDS

Now you can begin to feel that wave of relaxation descend into your hands. Your head, your neck, your shoulders, and your arms will remain relaxed as you now shift your attention to the muscles in both your hands. Allow both your hands to become heavy and relaxed. Concentrate as your hands become heavy and relaxed (*pause 10 seconds*).

THIGHS

Now you can begin to feel that wave of relaxation descend into your thighs. Your head, your neck, your shoulders, your arms, and your hands will remain relaxed as you now shift your attention to the muscles in both your thighs. Allow both your thighs to become heavy and relaxed. Concentrate as your thighs become heavy and relaxed (*pause 10 seconds*).

CALVES

Now you can begin to feel that wave of relaxation descend into your calves. Your head, your neck, your shoulders, your arms, your hands, and your thighs will remain relaxed as you now shift your attention to the muscles in both your calves. Allow both your calves to become heavy and relaxed. Concentrate as your calves become heavy and relaxed (*pause 10 seconds*).

FEET

Now you can begin to feel that wave of relaxation finally descend into your feet. The entire rest of your body will remain relaxed as you now shift your attention to the muscles in both your feet. Allow both your feet to become heavy and relaxed. Concentrate as your feet become heavy and relaxed (*pause 10 seconds*).

CLOSURE

All the major muscles in your body are now relaxed. To help you remain relaxed, simply repeat to yourself each time you exhale, "I am relaxed." Take the next few minutes and continue to relax as you repeat to yourself, "I am relaxed"… "I am relaxed" (*pause about 5 minutes*).

REAWAKEN

Now I want to bring your attention back to yourself and the world around you. I shall count from 1 to 10. With each count, you will feel your mind become more and more awake, and your body become more and more responsive and refreshed. When I reach 10, open your eyes, and you will feel the *best* you've felt all day—you will feel alert, refreshed, full of energy, and eager to resume your activities. Let's begin: 1–2 You are beginning to feel more alert, 3–4–5 you are more and more awake, 6–7 now begin to stretch your hands and feet, 8– now begin to stretch your arms and legs, 9–10 open your eyes, *now!* You feel alert, awake, your mind is clear and your body refreshed.

On concluding the initial passive neuromuscular procedure, inform the patient that he or she can use this procedure to relax once or, preferably, twice a day—before lunch and before dinner. Other times can also be useful as well, particularly as an aid for sleeping.

In summary, Appendix B has presented the clinician with a physically passive alternative form of neuromuscular relaxation, not as a prescription, but as an example of how such a protocol might be created. This option is designed simply to expand the clinician's arsenal of stress-reduction interventions to meet the idiosyncratic needs of individual patients. The ultimate assessment of clinical suitability remains with the clinician, and should be made on an individual, case-by-case basis.

C. Stress-Inducing Sympathomimetic Chemicals

Sympathomimetics are chemical substances that initiate a stress response via biochemical stimulation of the sympathetic branch of the autonomic nervous system. They are also known to stimulate noradrenergic CNS tracts as well. In the psychological domain, sympathomimetics are known to act as psychotropic stimulants causing a sense of stimulation and well-being. The primary mechanism of action for sympathomimetics is the augmentation of norepinephrine and epinephrine release.

Some of the more common sources for sympathomimetics include the following:

1. Coffee (*Coffee arabica*) contains the sympathomimetic substance caffeine. The standard clinical adult dosage of caffeine is 200 mg. The lethal dose is thought to range between 2,000 and 10,000 mg. A 5-ounce cup of drip brewed coffee contains about 150 mg, the same quantity percolated contains about 100 mg, and the same quantity if instant and freeze-dried contains about 65 mg.

2. Tea (*Camelia theca*) contains caffeine as well. Five ounces of tea allowed to brew for 5 minutes contains about 50 mg; if allowed to brew for only 1 minute it contains about 25 mg.

3. Cocoa (5 ounces) contains about 15 mg of caffeine.

4. "Soft drinks" (12 ounces) range from 30 to 65 mg.

5. A 1-ounce chocolate bar contains about 40 mg of caffeine or similar substances.

6. Caffeine is also found in many over-the-counter and prescription medications:

Cafergot—100 mg	Fiorinal—40 mg
Ergocaf—100 mg	Norgesic—30 mg
Fioricet—40 mg	Wigraine—100 mg

Anacin—32 mg   NoDoz—100 mg
Acqua Ban—100 mg   Prolamine—140 mg
Acqua Ban Plus—200 mg   Stay-Alert—250 mg
Dietac—200 mg   Stay Awake—200 mg
Enerjets—65 mg   Slim Plan Plus—200 mg
Excedrin Extra—65 mg   Triaminicin—30 mg
Midol—32 mg   Vivarin—200 mg

The "half-life" of caffeine is about 3 hours. Thus, this chemical can accumulate quite easily over the course of an entire day.

It is generally believed that quantities greater than 350 mg/day can lead to a physical dependence upon caffeine.

7. Other sympathomimetic chemicals include theobromine, theophylline, and amphetamine. Cocaine and nicotine exert sympathomimetic effects as well, yet appear to be far more addicting for some individuals.

8. Within recent years, herbs have gained great popularity as alternatives to traditional therapeutics, as noted in numerous popular and trade magazines. It is sometimes forgotten that herbs and other natural "remedies" may possess powerful stimulant effects. There exist natural stimulants that may induce anxiety or excessive stress reactions in the soma if injested in high quantities. These natural stimulants are reviewed in Appendix K.

The pharmacological information contained within this appendix derived from Schwartz (1987), Katzung (1992), the 2000 volume of the *Physician's Desk Reference*, the *PDR for Herbal Medicines* (1998), and Stephenson (1977); while believed to be accurate at the time of writing, the information cannot be guaranteed.

D. Vascular Headaches and Vasoactive Substances

Many vascular headaches, including the classical migraine, can be induced by vasoactive stimuli. These stimuli interact with what may be a biogenic predisposition for vascular spasticity so as to set the stage for a vascular headache. More specifically, vasoactive stimuli are factors that have the ability to stimulate the sympathetic neural constituency of thusly innervated blood vessels. Through what may be either a vasospastic or a singular vascular rebound phenomenon, these stimuli are believed to have the capability to induce a vascular headache syndrome, including the classical migraine syndrome.

The primary vasoactive substances include the following:

1. Tyramine (a pressor amine)
2. Monosodium glutamate
3. Sodium nitrate
4. Histamine
5. Bright light that creates glare
6. Changes in barometric pressure, especially rapid declines
7. Strenuous physical exercise
8. Loud noise
9. Some sympathomimetics (Despite the fact that sympathomimetic pharmaceuticals are prescribed to treat vascular headaches, the initial ingestion of some "hidden" or naturally occurring sympathomimetics may be sufficient to induce a vasospasm.)

Foods that are relatively high in vasopressor action include the following:

1. Liver
2. Most cheeses

  3. Caviar
  4. Sausages
  5. Coffee (depending upon quantity)
  6. Tea (depending upon quantity)
  7. Chocolate (depending upon quantity)
  8. Marinated herring
  9. Hot dogs (if containing nitrates)
 10. Chianti and other red wines
 11. Many foods that contain brewer's yeast
 12. Fava beans
 13. Many fermented or overripened foods

These lists are provided as general information for the practicing clinician. They should not be used to prescribe medication or to alter the dietary regimen of patients. Rather, the information contained herein is designed to serve as a general guide to assist in formulating diagnostic and/or treatment impressions for appropriate medical and nutritional consultation.

E. The Etiology of Panic Attacks
Nonpsychological Factors

Panic attacks represent a very specific form of pathological stress response. Shader (1984) has suggested prevalence in the United States to be 2.0–4.7%. Any clinician who treats stress- and anxiety-related disorders will invariably be confronted with patients presenting some form of panic disorder and its predictable pattern of subsequent behavioral avoidance.

Panic attacks are characterized by paroxymal episodes of ANS hyper-function usually combined with cognitive–affective symptoms that include dissociation, depersonalization, a generalized morbid fear, fear of dying, fear of losing control, and/or intense emotional manifestation. Proprioception is often interrupted, thus leaving the patient neuromuscularly unstable. Panic attacks typically may last but several minutes, although some attacks could last more than an hour, depending upon etiology.

Although it is widely known that panic attacks can be initiated by psychological factors, it is less widely known that panic attacks are sometimes secondary to variant medical/physiological conditions. Before treating a patient with panic-like symptomatology via psychotherapeutic or psychopharmacological interventions, the clinician should first attempt to determine to what degree medical or physiological factors serve as the etiological basis for the attacks.

Listed below are the most common primary medical/physiological factors that may give rise to secondary panic attacks; clinicians should be sensitive to these factors when constructing a medical history for the patient with some form of panic syndrome.

1. Acute hypoglycemia may serve as a panicogenic stimulus. It is well-established that the arcuate and ventromedial hypothalamic nuclei contain receptors responsible for the neurological monitoring of glucose. Buckley (1985) has argued that acute hypoglycemic inhibition of the hypothalamic

glucoreceptor mechanisms prevents the release of the neurotransmitter beta endorphin and its inhibitory effect upon the panic-related neural networks of the locus ceruleus. When this inhibitory effect is removed, the locus ceruleus becomes far more likely to be massively depolarized. If such depolarization were to occur, a noradrenergically mediated panic attack would most likely result.

2. It has been suggested that some women will suffer panic-like symptoms at the point in their menstrual cycle when progesterone reaches its zenith. This point is usually within 7 days of the onset of menses. This conclusion is based upon the hypothesis that, for some, high levels of progesterone can act as a panicogenic substance (see Carr & Sheehan, 1984).

3. Vigorous anaerobic exercise is believed to be able to induce panic in those patients biologically inclined to suffer from panic disorders. One of the by-products of anaerobic exercise is lactic acid. Pitts and McClure (1967) found that some individuals manifest a biogenic hypersensitivity to lactate (a relative to lactic acid) and this hypersensitivity is manifest in the form of panic attacks. Thus, factors that lead to a rise in lactic acid may be associated with panic.

4. According to Gorman, Liebowitz, and Klein (1984), there exist several medical disorders that either mimic or induce panic attacks. They include:

- Hyperthyroidism
- Hypothyroidism
- Mitral valve prolapse
- Cardiac arrhythmias
- Pheochromocytoma
- Drug or alcohol withdrawal
- Coronary insufficiency
- Amphetamine overdose
- Caffeine overdose

In summary, the assessment of any medical or physiological factors known to serve in the primary etiology of the panic syndrome seems a reasonable course of action prior to treating a patient with a history of panic-like symptoms.

F. Biochemical Bases of Arousal

Throughout this volume, we have emphasized that pathogenic stress represents a disorder of "arousal." Arousal within the human body is mediated through a series of complex neurological networks. Nevertheless, the basis for the activation of these neurological networks resides in the biochemistry of their respective neurotransmitters (refer to Chapter 2). Here we provide a brief summary of the major neurotransmitters that mediate arousal. Also provided is a description of the drugs that affect these neurotransmitters.

There are three major arousal-mediating neurotransmitters: dopamine, norepinephrine, and serotonin.

DOPAMINE

Dopamine is one of the monoaminergic catecholamines. Its synthesis, which is primarily in the neuronal terminals, is described below:

Phenylalanine
 ↓ Phenylalanine hydroxylase
Tyrosine
 ↓ Tyrosine hydroxylase
Dopa
 ↓ Dopa carboxylase
Dopamine (DA)

Dopamine is inactivated by monoamine oxidase (MAO) and catechol-O-methyltransferase (COMT).

Drugs that affect dopamine:

Synthesis inhibitor—alpha-methyl-p-tyrosine
Depletor—reserpine

Reuptake inhibitor—cocaine
Releaser—amphetamine
Receptor blockers—chlorpromazine, haloperidol
Catabolic inhibitor—pargyline
Receptor agonist—apomorphine

NOREPINEPHRINE

Norepinephrine (noradrenalin) is the primary excitatory neurotransmitter. Its synthesis, which occurs primarily in the synaptic vesicles, is described below:

Phenylalanine
  ↓ Phenylalanine hydroxylase
Tyrosine
  ↓ Tyrosine hydroxylase
Dopa
  ↓ Dopa decarboxylase
Dopamine
  ↓ Dopamine-beta-hydroxylase
Norepinephrine (NE)

Norepinephrine is inactivated by MAO and COMT.
Drugs that affect norepinephrine:

Synthesis inhibitor—disulfiram
Depletor—reserpine
Reuptake Inhibitor—cocaine
Releaser—amphetamine
Receptor blocker—phentolamine
Catabolism inhibitor—iproniazid
Receptor agonists—ephedrine, clonidine (alpha-2 agonist)

SEROTONIN

The synthesis of serotonin (5-hydroxytryptamine; 5-HT) is described below:

Tryptophan
  ↓ Tryptophan hydroxylase
5-Hydroxytryptophan
  ↓ 5-HTP decarboxylase
5-Hydroxytryptamine

Serotonin is inactivated primarily by MAO.
    Drugs that affect serotonin:

      Synthesis inhibitor—alpha-methyl-5-HTP
      Depletor—reserpine
      Reuptake inhibitor—nortryptyline
      Releaser—p-chloramphetamine
      Receptor blocker—methysergide
      Catabolic inhibitor—iproniazid
      Receptor agonist—LSD, psilocin

G. Professional Journals for Stress Research

American Journal of Health Promotion
Annals of Behavioral Medicine
Archives of General Psychiatry
Behavioral Medicine (formerly *Journal of Human Stress*)
Biofeedback and Self-Regulation
Crisis Intervention
Health Education
Health Psychology
International Journal of Emergency Mental Health
Journal of Clinical and Consulting Psychology
Journal of Psychosomatic Research
Journal of Traumatic Stress
Psychology and Health
Psychophysiology
Psychosomatic Medicine
Psychosomatics

H. How Do You Cope with Stress?
A Self-Report Checklist Designed for Health Education Purposes

DIRECTIONS: There are many ways to cope with the stress in your life. Some coping techniques are more effective than others. The purpose of this checklist is to help you, the reader, assess how effectively you cope with the stress in your life. Upon completing this checklist, you will have identified many of the ways you choose to cope with stress, while at the same time, through a point system, ascertaining the relative desirability of the coping techniques that you now employ. This is a health education survey, not a clinical assessment instrument. Its sole purpose is to inform you of how you cope with the stress in your life.

In order to complete the checklist, simply follow the instructions given for each of the items listed below. When you have completed all of the 14 items, place your total score in the space provided.

——— 1. Give yourself 10 points if you feel that you have a supportive family.

——— 2. Give yourself 10 points if you actively pursue a hobby.

——— 3. Give yourself 10 points if you belong to some social or activity group that meets at least once a month (other than your family).

——— 4. Give yourself 15 points if you are within 5 pounds of your "ideal" bodyweight, considering your height and bone structure.

——— 5. Give yourself 15 points if you practice some form of "deep relaxation" at least three times a week. Deep relaxation exercises include meditation, imagery, yoga, etc.

—— 6. Give yourself 5 points for each time you exercise 30 minutes or longer during the course of an average week.

—— 7. Give yourself 5 points for each nutritionally balanced and wholesome meal you consume during the course of an average day.

—— 8. Give yourself 5 points for each time you do something that you really enjoy, "just for yourself," during the course of an average week.

—— 9. Give yourself 10 points if you have some place in your home that you can go to in order to relax and/or be by yourself.

—— 10. Give yourself 10 points if you practice time-management techniques in your daily life.

—— 11. Subtract 10 points for each pack of cigarettes you smoke during the course of an average day.

—— 12. Subtract 5 points for each evening during the course of an average week that you take any form of medication or chemical substance (including alcohol) to help you sleep.

—— 13. Subtract 10 points for each day during the course of an average week that you consume any form of medication or chemical substance (including alcohol) to reduce your anxiety or just calm you down.

—— 14. Subtract 5 points for each evening during the course of an average week that you bring work home; work that was meant to be done at your place of employment.

—— Total Score

Now that you've calculated your score, consider that the higher your score, the greater your health-promoting coping practices. A "perfect" score would be around 115. Scores in the 50–60 range are probably adequate to cope with most common sources of stress.

Also keep in mind that items 1–10 represent adaptive, health-promoting coping strategies, and items 11–14 represent maladaptive, health-eroding coping strategies. These maladaptive strategies are self-sustaining because they do provide at least some temporary relief from stress. In the long run, however, their utilization serves to erode one's health. Ideally, health-promoting coping strategies (items 1–10) are the best to integrate into your lifestyle and will ultimately prove to be an effective preventive program against excessive stress.

I. Crisis Management Briefing (CMB)
Large-Group Crisis Intervention in Response to Terrorism, Disasters, and Violence

There can be little doubt that disasters, violence, and acts of terrorism engender a large-scale psychological morbidity. In fact, the explicit goal of any true act of terrorism is to create a condition of fear, uncertainty, demoralization, and helplessness (i.e., "terror"). The direct target or victims of the terrorist act are not the real targets; rather they are but the means to an end. In terrorism, mass disasters, and acts of violence, the "psychological casualties" virtually always outnumber the "physical casualties." Any effective response to such crises must mandate both psychological intervention and physical crisis intervention. For example, the Defense Against Weapons of Mass Destruction Act of 1996 (Nunn, Lugar, & Domenici) mandates the enhancement of domestic preparedness and response capabilities in the wake of attacks against the United States using weapons of mass destruction (WMD). Although a small component, provisions are made for psychological crisis intervention with both emergency responders and primary civilian victim populations. Here we describe a group psychological crisis intervention designed to mitigate against the levels of felt crisis and traumatic stress in the wake of terrorism, mass disasters, violence, and other "large-scale" crises. The intervention, referred to as the "crisis management briefing" (CMB; Everly, 2000a), is designed for use with "large groups" of primary civilian victims, which may range in size from 10 to 300 individuals at one time. This highly efficient intervention takes between 45 and 75 minutes to implement. The CBM may be implemented in school, corporate, and community settings. It is but one component of the comprehensive crisis intervention system.

PHASE 1: ASSEMBLY

The first phase of the CMB consists of bringing together a group of individuals who have experienced a common crisis event. In response to a school crisis, for example, an assembly might be held in the auditorium. Depending upon the number of students, one grade could be addressed at a time, or other divisions of the student body could be utilized. In response to a workplace crisis, a company meeting room or a rented room at a local hotel or commercial meeting facility might be used. In response to mass disasters, large-scale violence, or terrorism, local school auditoriums might be used to address civilian populations within the respective school districts. Announcements to this effect might be made via radio, television, and Internet sites. Obviously, the CMB would be repeated until all constituents have been addressed within the given circumscribed area/population. This act of assembly is the first step in re-establishing the sense of community that is so imperative to the recovery and rebuilding process (Ayalon, 1993).

PHASE 2: FACTS

Once the group has been assembled, the next intervention component is to have the most appropriate and credible sources/authorities explain the *facts* of the crisis event. Objective information serves to (1) control destructive rumors, (2) reduce anticipatory anxiety, and (3) return a sense of control to victims. Without breaching issues of confidentiality, the assembled group should receive factual information concerning what is known and not known regarding the crisis event.

PHASE 3: REACTIONS

The next step is to have credible health care professionals (if available) discuss the most common *reactions* (signs, symptoms, and psychological themes) relevant to the particular crisis event. For example, in the case of a suicide, the psychological theme of suicide should be addressed. In the case of terrorism, the dynamics of terrorism should be discussed. Common signs and symptoms of grief, anger, stress, survivor guilt, and even responsibility guilt among survivors, friends, and others should also be addressed.

PHASE 4: RESOURCES

The final component of the CMB is to address personal coping and self-care strategies that may be of value in mitigating against the distressing reactions to the crisis event. Simple and practical *stress management* strategies should be discussed. Available community and organizational *resources* to facilitate recovery should also be introduced. Questions should be actively entertained, as appropriate.

Each group participant should leave the CMB with a reference sheet that briefly describes common signs and symptoms, stress management techniques, and local professional resources (with contact names and telephone numbers) available to facilitate recovery.

Timing for the CMB is highly situation-specific and flexible. The CMB can be repeated as long as it proves to be useful.

J. Critical Incident Stress Debriefing (CISD)
Small-Group Crisis Intervention

The genre of psychological debriefing interventions has emerged as an innovation in the development of crisis intervention technologies. Psychological debriefings represent group discussions of a crisis or traumatic event designed to mitigate against acute symptoms of distress, to provide a forum for triaging victims, and, if possible, to provide a foundation for psychological closure to the traumatic event. Debriefings have been used with emergency response personnel after acute traumas, with rescue workers after mass disasters, and, most recently, in business and industrial organizations, as well as schools, in the wake of violence and other workplace crises.

The oldest of the formalized psychological debriefing models is Critical Incident Stress Debriefing (CISD), which represents the group crisis intervention technique originally developed by Mitchell (1983). A guided and structured group discussion of a crisis or traumatic event, CISD employs the active mechanisms of early intervention, verbal expression, cathartic ventilation, group support, health education, and assessment for follow-up.

As noted in Chapter 21, CISD was designed as but one component of a comprehensive, multicomponent crisis intervention program referred to as Critical Incident Stress Management (CISM; Everly & Mitchell, 1999). Since its initial development, the CISD technology has enjoyed remarkable popularity because of its perceived efficiency and effectiveness. Although the CISD was never designed to be implemented as a "one-shot" intervention outside of the multicomponent CISM program (Everly & Mitchell, 1999; Mitchell & Everly, 2001), crisis workers have, indeed, found it necessary upon occasion to implement the CISD either outside the CISM framework or with little contextual support.

In the various narrative reviews of the genre of psychological debriefing (Bisson & Deahl, 1994; Dyregrov, 1997, 1998; Everly & Mitchell, 2000; Everly & Mitchell, 1999; Raphael, Meldrum, & McFarlane, 1995; Raphael, Wilson, Meldrum, & McFarlane, 1997; Robinson & Mitchell, 1995; Rose & Bisson, 1998; Watts, 1994), conclusions have been mixed with regard the question of overall effectiveness. Unfortunately, the practical utility of several of these reviews (Bisson & Deahl, 1994; Raphael et al., 1995; Rose & Bisson, 1998) has been compromised because of their failure to clearly define and distinguish the operational nature of the independent variable under scrutiny (i.e., the specific form, or model, of psychological debriefing utilized). A clear and restrictive definition of the independent and dependent variables is an *essential* feature of any review process (Mullen, 1989). Koss and Shiang (1994) emphasize the need for standardization and reliability across interventions as a necessary aspect of any exercise in outcome research. Reviews on effectiveness too often aggregate the debriefing interventions on the basis of terminology alone, without any apparent regard for differences in formal implementation protocols that serve to distinguish various debriefing models, variations in prescribed recipient constituencies, or any other operational factors that might serve functionally to differentiate between the numerous models of psychological debriefing.

In an attempt to clarify the conflicting conclusions surrounding the effectiveness of psychological debriefings, Everly and his colleagues focused solely upon the CISD model of psychological debriefing and offered narrative reviews of the effectiveness of CISD specifically (Everly & Mitchell, 1999; Mitchell & Everly, 1997, 2001). Deahl, et al. (2000), in a randomized controlled trial of CISD with British soldiers, found it associated with decreased alcohol use. See also Campfield & Hills (2001) for a randomized trial of CISD. As Mullen (1989) cogently points out, however, even well-focused narrative reviews are subject to divergent interpretation. He offers, therefore, empirical meta-analysis as a more precise, objective, and compelling exercise in the conduct of inquiry. In a meta-analysis of five quasiexperimental investigations, CISD was found to be associated with decreased stress symptoms (Everly & Boyle, 1999). Let us more closely examine the CISD group crisis intervention by reviewing the seven-phase process itself.

THE CISD PROGRESSION

The CISD contains seven phases. Here, we present one possible set of prompts, or questions, that may be used to initiate each phase of the model:

1. *Introduction:* The CISD intervention team members introduce themselves, define expectations, set limits, and address confidentiality.

2. *Fact Phase*.   This phase is directed toward obtaining the relevant facts concerning the crisis or traumatic event. Prompt (ask each person): "Tell us who you are and what happened" or "Describe the event from your perspective."

3. *Thought Phase*.   This phase is designed to solicit the first cognitive appraisals concerning the crisis event. Prompt (ask each person): "What was your first thought during or just after the crisis?" or "When you had a chance 'think' about the incident, what were your first thoughts?"

4. *Reaction Phase*.   This phase is designed to elicit emotional reactions. Prompts: "What was the worst part of this incident for you?" or "Is there any one specific part that you wish you could erase?" (For this and the remaining phases, ask prompts to the group as a whole, without directly asking any specific individual.)

5. *Symptom Phase*.   Prompts: "How are you different now because of the incident?" and/or "What physical or behavioral changes have you experienced?" or "What has life been like since this event?"

6. *Teaching Phase*.   After soliciting input from the group members, CISD team members teach basic concepts of trauma and stress management. The goal is to normalize most reactions and give helpful hints to aid recompensation or recovery.

7. *Reentry Phase*.   In this phase, CISD team members facilitate a sense of psychological closure concerning the crisis event by emphasizing normalization and answering questions, but the most valuable component of this phase is the summarization to achieve a sense of closure to the event. "Cognitive refraining" should be encouraged (e.g., the identification of positive aspects of the incident, lessons learned, silver lining, etc.).

The CISD group crisis intervention is designed to be used subsequent to a critical incident. Ideal group sizes range from 5 to 15 individuals. The process is designed to last between 1.5 and 3 hours. The CISD is typically implemented between 1 and 10 days postincident. In the case of mass disasters, the CISD should not be implemented until 3 to 4 weeks postdisaster. In the interim, the large-group crisis intervention technique known as the Crisis Management Briefing (CMB; Everly, 2000a) may be utilized.

The CISD intervention requires specialized training for effective implementation (see Mitchell & Everly, 2001, for a recent description of the CISD).

K. Herbal Stimulants

Within recent years, there has been a virtual explosion of interest in non-traditional remedies, including herbs.* One cannot walk into a health food store without finding numerous products, even entire sections, dedicated to herbal agents. While described as "natural," some of these herbs are powerful anxiogenic, even panicogenic, stimulants. The purpose here is to alert the clinician to the most common herbs that may be found as dietary supplements thought to be benign.

There is evidence that the following herbs may have psychotropic and/or somatotropic effects that are consistent with increased arousal of the stress response. Symptoms of excessive utilization of these substances may include irritability, insomnia, anxiety, panic, affective lability, increased libido, and somatic signs and symptoms of increased SNS arousal. These seven herbs should be considered as potential biogenic stressors. They are commercially popular and are often found in "designer" herbal drinks and "natural energy" preparations, and are often sold individually. The following herbs should be the subject of a specific query in the history and interview conducted by the clinician:

Cola (*Cola acuminata*)
Ginkgo biloba
Ginseng
Gotu kola (*Centella asiatica*)
Guarana (*Paullinia cupana*)
Ma huang (*Ephedra sinica*)
Yohimbine (*Pausinystalia yohimbe*)

*SOURCE: *PDR for Herbal Medicines*, 1998.

L. Herbs with Putative Antianxiety Properties

As the popularity of alternative medicine increases, so does that of herbal remedies.* While the well-controlled evidence for the anxiolytic properties of the following herbs is sparse or nonexistent, these herbs have been otherwise reported to possess some relaxing, calming, or otherwise antistress properties:

Kava kava (*Piper methysticum*)
Lavender (*Lavandula angustifolia*)
Primrose (*Primula elatior*)
St. John's wort (*Hypericum perforatum*)
Valerian (*Valeriana officinalis*)

The preceding herbs are listed for the edification of the clinician, but *are not* presented as a recommendation for alternative therapeutics.

*SOURCE: *PDR for Herbal Medicines*, 1998.

References

Abramson, L. Y., Metalsky, G. I., & Alloy, L. B. (1989). Hopelessness depression: A theory-based subtype of depression. *Psychological Review, 96*(2), 358–372.

Abramson, L. Y., Seligman, M. E. P., & Teasdale, J. D. (1978). Learned helplessness in humans: Critique and reformulation. *Journal of Abnormal Psychology, 87*(1), 49–74.

Ackerman, R., & DeRubeis, R. J. (1991). Is depressive realism real? *Clinical Psychology Review, 11*, 565–584.

Ader, R. (1981). *Psychoneuroimmunology*. New York: Academic Press.

Ader, R. (1985). Conditioned immunopharmacologic effects in animals: Implications for a conditioning model of pharmacotherapy. In L. White, B. Tursky, & G. Schwartz (Eds.), *Placebo: Theory, research, and mechanisms* (pp. 306–323). New York: Guilford.

Ader, R., & Cohen, N. (1975). Behaviorally conditioned immunosuppression. *Psychosomatic Medicine, 37*, 333–340.

Ader, R., & Cohen, N. (1982). Behaviorally conditioned immunosuppression and murine systemic lupus erythematosus. *Science, 214*, 1534–1536.

Ader, R., & Cohen, N. (1993). Psychoneuroimmunology: Conditioning and stress. *Annual Review of Psychology, 44*, 53–85.

Ader, R., Felten, D. L., & Cohen, N. (Eds.). (1991). *Psychoneuroimmunology* (2nd ed.). New York: Academic Press.

Adler, A. (1929). *The science of living*. New York: Greenberg.

Adler, C., & Morrissey-Adler, S. (1983). Strategies in general psychiatry. In J. Basmajian (Ed.), *Biofeedback* (pp. 239–254). Baltimore: Williams & Wilkins.

Affleck, G., Tennen, H., Croog, S., & Levine, S. (1987). Causal attribution, perceived control, and recovery from a heart attack. *Journal of Social and Clinical Psychology, 5*(3), 339–355.

Affleck, G., Tennen, H., Pfeiffer, C., & Fifield, J. (1987). Appraisals of control and predictability in adapting to chronic disease. *Journal of Personality and Social Psychology, 53*, 273–279.

Aggleton, J. P. (Ed.). (1992). The Amygdala. New York: Wiley-Liss.

Alcoholics Anonymous World Services. (1990). *Alcoholics Anonymous 1989 membership survey*. New York: Author.

Alexander, A. B. (1975). An experimental test of the assumptions relating to the use of EMG: Biofeedback as a general relaxation training technique. *Psychophysiology, 12*, 656–662.

Alexander, C. N., Langer, E. J., Newman, R. I., Chandler, H. M., & Davies, J. (1989). Transcendental meditation, mindfulness, and longevity: An experimental study with the elderly. *Journal of Personality and Social Psychology, 57*(6), 950–964.

Alexander, F. (1950). *Psychosomatic medium.* New York: Norton.

Alhambra, M. A., Fowler, T. P., & Alhambra, A. A. (1995). EEG biofeedback: A new treatment option for ADD/ADHD. *Journal of Neurotherapy, 1*(2), 39–43.

Allen, K. D., & Shriver, M. D. (1997). Enhanced performance feedback to strengthen biofeedback treatment outcome with childhood migraine. *Headache, 37*(3), 169–173.

Allen, R. (1981). Controlling stress and tension. *Journal of School Health, 17*, 360–364.

Alloy, L. B., & Clements, C. M. (1992). Illusion of control: Invulnerability to negative affect and depressive symptoms after laboratory and natural stressors. *Journal of Abnormal Psychology, 101*(2), 234–245.

Alloy, L. B., Just, N., & Panzarella, C. (1997). Attributional style, daily life events, and hopeless-ness depression: Subtype validation by prospective variability and specificity of symptoms. *Cognitive Therapy and Research, 21*(3), 321–344.

Alloy, L. B., Kelly, K. A., Mineka, S., & Clements, C. M. (1990). Comorbidity in anxiety and depressive disorders: A helplessness–hopelessness perspective. In J. D. Maser & C. R. Cloninger (Eds.), *Comorbidity in anxiety and mood disorders* (pp. 499–543). Washington, DC: American Psychiatric Press.

Almy, T. P., Kern, F., & Tulin, M. (1949). Alterations in colonic function in man under stress. *Gastroenterology, 12*, 425–436.

American College of Sports Medicine. (1995). *Guidelines for graded exercise testing and exercise prescription.* Baltimore: Williams & Wilkins.

American Psychiatric Association. (1968). *Diagnostic and statistical manual of mental disorders* (2nd ed.). Washington, DC: Author.

American Psychiatric Association. (1980). *Diagnostic and statistical manual of mental disorders* (3rd ed.). Washington, DC: Author.

American Psychiatric Association. (1987). *Diagnostic and statistical manual of mental disorders* (3rd ed., rev.). Washington, DC: Author.

American Psychiatric Association. (1994). *Diagnostic and statistical manual of mental disorders* (4th ed.). Washington, DC: Author.

American Psychiatric Association. (2000). *Diagnostic and statistical manual of mental disorders,* 4th Edition, Text revision. Washington, DC: Author.

American Psychological Association. (1976). Contributions of psychology to health research. *American Psychologist, 31*, 263–273.

American Society of Clinical Hypnosis. (1973). *A syllabus on hypnosis and a handbook of therapeutic suggestions.* Des Plaines, IL: American Society of Clinical Hypnosis Education and Research Foundation.

American Society of Hospital Pharmacists. (2000). *American Hospital Formulary Services Drug Information,* 2000. Bethesda, MD: American Society of Health-System Pharmacists.

Ames, B. N., Gold, L. S., & Willett, W. C. (1995). The causes and prevention of cancer. *Proceedings of the National Academy of Science USA, 92*, 5258–5265.

Ametz, B., Fjeliner, B., Eneroth, P., & Kaliner, A. (1986). Neuroendocrine response selectivity to standardized psychological stressors. *International Journal of Psychosomatics, 33*, 19–27.

Amkraut, A., & Solomon, G. (1974). From symbolic stimulus to the pathophysiologic response: Immune mechanisms. *International Journal of Psychiatry in Medicine, 5*, 541–563.

Anderson, B., Hovmoller, S., Karlsson, C., & Svensson, S. (1974). Analysis of urinary catecholamines. *Clinica Chimica Acta, 51*, 13–28.

Andreassi, J. (1980). *Psychophysiology.* New York: Oxford University Press.

Antoni, M. H., Schneiderman, N., Fletcher M. A., Goldstein, D. A., Ironson, G., & Laperriere, A. (1990). Psychoneuroimmunology and HIV-1. *Journal of Consulting and Clinical Psychology, 58*(1), 38–49.

Arena, J. G., Bruno, G. M., Hannah, S. L, & Meador, K. J. (1995). A comparison of frontal electromyographic biofeedback training, trapezius electromyographic biofeedback training, and progressive muscle relaxation therapy in the treatment of tension headache. *Headache, 35*(7), 411–419.

Argas, W. S., Taylor, C. B., Kraemer, H. C., Southam, M. A., & Schneider, J. A. (1987). Relaxation training for essential hypertension at the worksite: II. The poorly controlled hypertensive. *Psychosomatic Medicine, 49*, 264–273.

Arnarson, E., & Sheffield, B. (1980, March). *The generalization of the effects of EMG and temperature biofeedback.* Paper presented at the Annual Meeting of the Biofeedback Society of America, Colorado Springs, CO.

Arnkoff, D. B., & Glass, C. R. (1992). Cognitive therapy and psychotherapy integration. In D. Freedheim (Ed.), *History of psychotherapy: A century of change* (pp. 657–694). Washington, DC: American Psychological Association.

Arnold, M. (1970). *Feelings and emotions.* New York: Academic Press.

Arnold, M. (1984). *Memory and the brain.* Hillsdale, NJ: Erlbaum.

Arnold, M. B. (1960). *Emotion and personality* (2 vols.). New York: Columbia University Press.

Artiss, K. (1963). Human behavior under stress: From combat to social psychiatry. *Military Medicine, 128*, 1011–1015.

Astin, J. A. (1997). Stress reduction through mindfulness meditation: Effects on psychological symptomatology, sense of control, and spiritual experiences. *Psychotherapy and Psychosomatics, 66*(2), 97–106.

Austin, J. H. (1998). *Zen and the brain: Toward an understanding of meditation and consciousness.* Cambridge, MA: MIT Press.

Avants, S. K., Margolin, A., & Salovey, P. (1990). Stress management techniques: Anxiety reduction, appeal, and individual differences. *Imagination, Cognition and Personality, 10*, 3–23.

Averill, J. (1973). Personal control over aversive stimuli and its relationship to stress. *Psychological Bulletin, 80*, 286–307.

Avorn, J., & Langer, E. J. (1982). Induced disability in nursing home patients. *Journal of the American Geriatrics Society, 30*(6), 379–400.

Axelrod, J., & Reisine, T. (1984). Stress hormones. *Science 224*, 452–459.

Ayalon, O. (1993). Posttraumatic stress recovery of terrorist survivors. In J. Wilson & B. Raphael (Eds.), *International handbook of traumatic stress syndromes* (pp. 855–866). New York: Plenum.

Bachman, R. (1994, July 6). Violence and theft in the workplace. In *Crime data brief: National crime victimization survey.* Washington, DC: U.S. Department of Justice.

Backus, F., & Dudley, D. (1977). Observations of psychosocial factors and their relationship to organic disease. In Z. J. Lipowski, D. Lipsitt, & P. Whybrow (Eds.), *Psychosomatic medicine* (pp. 187–205). New York: Oxford University Press.

Baehr, E., Rosenfeld, J. P., & Baehr, R. (1997). The clinical use of an alpha asymmetry protocol in the neurofeedback treatment of depression: Two case studies. *Journal of Neurotherapy, 2*(3), 10–23.

Ballentine, R. (1976). *Science of breath.* Glenview, IL: Himalayan International Institute.

Ballieux, R. E. (1994). The mind and the immune system. *Theoretical Medicine, 15*, 387–395.

Ballieux, R. E., & Heijnen, C. J. (1989). Stress and immune response. In H. Weiner, I. Florin, R. Mursion, & D. Hellhammer (Eds.), *Frontiers of stress research* (pp. 51–55). Stuttgart: Hans Huber.

Balog, L. F. (1978). *The effects of exercise on muscle tension and subsequent muscle relaxation.* Unpublished doctoral dissertation, University of Maryland, College Park.

Bandura, A. (1977). Self-efficacy: Toward a unifying theory of behavioral change. *Psychological Review, 84*, 191–215.

Bandura, A. (1982a). Self-efficacy mechanism in human agency. *American Psychologist, 37*, 122–147.

Bandura, A. (1982b). The self and mechanisms of agency. In J. Suls (Ed.), *Psychological perspectives on the self* (pp. 3–39). Hillsdale, NJ: Erlbaum.

Bandura, A. (1997). *Self-efficacy: The exercise of control.* New York: Freeman.

Bandura, A., Taylor, C. B., Williams, S. L., Mefford, I. N., & Barchas, J. D. (1985). Catecholamine secretion as a function of perceived coping self-efficacy. *Journal of Consulting and Clinical Psychology, 5*(3), 406–414.

Banwell, B., & Ziebell, B. (1985). Psychological and sexual health in rheumatic diseases. In W. Kelly, E. Harris, S. Ruddy, & C. Sledge (Eds.), *Textbook of rheumatology* (pp. 497–510). Philadelphia: Saunders.

Barabasz, M., & Spiegel, D. (1989). Hypnotizability and weight loss in obese subjects. *International Journal of Eating Disorders, 8,* 335–341.

Barber, T. X. (1969). *Hypnosis: A scientific approach.* New York: Van Nostrand Reinhold.

Barber, T. X. (1977). Rapid induction analgesia: A clinical report. *American Journal of Clinical Hypnosis, 19,* 138–147.

Barlow, D. H., & Craske, M. G. (1989). *Mastery of your anxiety and panic.* Albany, New York: Graywind.

Barlow, D., & Beck, J. (1984). The psychosocial treatment of anxiety disorders. In J. B. Williams & R. Spitzer (Eds.), *Psychotherapy research* (pp. 29–69). New York: Guilford.

Barnes, V., Schneider, R., Alexander, C., & Staggers, F. (1997). Stress, stress reduction, and hypertension in African Americans: An update and review. *Journal of the National Medical Association, 7,* 464–476.

Barrett, E. (1996). Primary care for women: Assessment and management of headache. *Journal of Nurse Midwifery, 41*(2), 117–124.

Bartrop, R. W., Luckhurst, E., Lazarus, L., Kiloh, L. G., & Penny, R. (1977). Depressed lymphocyte function after bereavement. *Lancet, 1,* 834–836.

Basmajian, J. V. (1963). Control and training of individual motor units. *Science, 141,* 440–441.

Basmajian, J. V. (1989). *Biofeedback: Principles and practice for clinicians* (3rd ed.). Baltimore, Maryland: Williams & Wilkins.

Basmajian, J. V. (1999). The third therapeutic revolution: Behavioral medicine. *Applied Psychophysiological Biofeedback, 24*(2), 107–116.

Basmajian, J. V. (Ed.). (1983). *Biofeedback.* Baltimore: Williams & Wilkins.

Batieha, A. M., Armenian, H. K., Norkus, E. P., Morris, J. S., Spate, V. E., & Comstock, G. W. (1993). Serum micronutrients and the subsequent risk of cervical cancer in a population-based nested case–control study. *Cancer Epidemiology, Biomarkers, and Prevention, 2*(4), 335–339.

Baum, A., & Posluszny, D. M. (1999). Health psychology: Mapping biobehavioral contributions to health and illness. *Annual Review of Psychology, 50,* 137–163.

Baumgaertel, A. (1999). Alternative and controversial treatments for attention-deficit/hyperactivity disorder. *Pediatric Clinics of North America, 46*(5), 977–992.

Beaton, R., Murphy, S., & Corneil, W. (1996, September). *Prevalence of posttraumatic stress disorder symptomatology in professional urban fire fighters in two countries.* Paper presented to the International Congress of Occupational Health, Stockholm, Sweden.

Beck, A. T. (1993). Cognitive approaches to stress. In P. M. Lehrer & R. L. Woolfolk (Eds.), *Principles and practices of stress management* (2nd ed., pp. 333–372). New York: Guilford.

Beck, A. T. (1995). Foreword. In J. S. Beck (author), *Cognitive therapy: Basics and beyond* (pp. vii). New York: Guilford.

Beck, A., & Emery, G. (1985). *Anxiety disorders and phobias: A cognitive perspective.* New York: Basic Books.

Ben-Sira, Z., & Eliezer, R. (1990). The structure of readjustment after heart attack. *Social Science and Medicine, 30,* 523–536.

Benjamin, L. (1963). Statistical treatment of the law of the initial values in autonomic research. *Psychosomatic Medicine, 25,* 556–566.

Benson, H. (1969). Yoga for drug abuse. *New England Journal of Medicine, 281,* 1133.

Benson, H. (1975). *The relaxation response.* New York: Morrow.

Benson, H. (1979). *The mind body effect.* New York: Simon and Schuster.

Benson, H. (1983). The relaxation response: Its subjective and objective historical precedents and physiology. *Trends in Neuroscience, 6,* 281–284.

Benson, H. (1987). *Your maximum mind.* New York: Times Books.

Benson, H. (1996). *Timeless healing.* New York: Scribner.

Benson, H. (1996). *Timeless healing: The power and biology of belief.* New York: Scribner.

Benson, H., & Friedman, R. (1985). A rebuttal to the conclusions of David S. Holme's article: Meditation and somatic arousal reduction. *American Psychologist, 40,* 725–728.

Benson, H., & Stuart, E. (1993). *The Wellness Book.* New York: Fireside.

Benson, H., Beary, J., & Carol, M. (1974). The relaxation response. *Psychiatry, 37,* 37–46.

Benson, H., Frankel, F. H., Apfel, R., Daniels, M. D., Schniewind, H. E., Nemiah, J. C., Sifneos, P. E., Crassweller, K. D., Greenwood, M., Kotch, J. B., Arns, P. A., & Rosner, B. (1978). Treatment of anxiety: A comparison of the usefulness of self-hypnosis and a meditational relaxation technique: An overview. *Psychotherapy and Psychosomatics, 30,* 229–242.

Berczi, I., & Nagy, E. (1991). Effect of hypophysectomy on immune function. In R. Ader, D. L. Felten, & N. Cohen (Eds.), *Psychoneuroimmunology* (2nd ed., pp. 339–375). New York: Academic Press.

Bergin, A. E., & Payne, I. R. (1993). Proposed agenda for a spiritual strategy in personality and psychotherapy. In E. L. Worthington, Jr. (Ed.), *Psychotherapy and religious values* (pp. 243–260). Grand Rapids, MI: Baker.

Berk, L. (1989a). Eustress of mirthful laughter modifies natural killer cell activity. *Clinical Research, 37,* 115.

Berk, L. (1989b). Neuroendocrine and stress hormone changes during mirthful laughter. *American Journal of Medical Science, 298,* 390–396.

Berkun, M. (1962). Experimental studies of psychological stress in man. *Psychological Monographs, 76* (Whole No. 534).

Berne, R. M., Levy, M. N., Koeppen, B. M., & Stanton, B. A. (1998). *Physiology* (4th ed.). St. Louis: Mosby.

Berstein, D., & Borkovec, T. (1973). *Progressive relaxation training.* Champaign, IL: Research Press.

Besedovsky, H. O., Sorkin, E., Keller, M., & Muller, J. (1975). Changes in blood hormone levels during immune response. *Proceedings of the Society for Experimental Biology and Medicine, 150,* 466–470.

Bevan, A. J. W. (1980). Endocrine changes in transcendental meditation. *Clinical and Experimental Pharmacology and Physiology, 7*(1), 75–76.

Bhalla, V. (1980). *Neuroendocrine, cardiovascular, and musculoskeletal analyses of a holistic approach to stress reduction.* Unpublished doctoral dissertation, University of Maryland, College Park.

Biondi, M., & Picardi, A. (1998). Temporomandibular joint pain–dysfunction syndrome and bruxism: Etiopathogenesis and treatment from a psychosomatic integrative viewpoint. In G. A. Fava & H. Freyberger (Eds.), *Handbook of psychosomatic medicine* (pp. 469–490). Madision, CT: International Universities Press.

Bisson, J. I., & Deahl, M. (1994). Psychological debriefing and the prevention of posttraumatic stress: More research is needed. *British Journal of Psychiatry, 165,* 717–720.

Bisson, J. I., Jenkins, P., Alexander, J., & Bannister, C. (1997). Randomized controlled trial of psychological debriefings for victims of acute burn trauma. *British Journal of Psychiatry, 171,* 78–81.

Bisson, J. I., McFarlane, A., & Rose, S. (2000). Psychological debriefing. In E. Foa, A. McFarlane, & M. Friedman (Eds.), *Effective treatments for PTSD* (pp. 39–59). New York: Guilford.

Black, I., Adler, J., Dreyfus, C., Friedman, W., Laganuna, E., & Roach, A. (1987). Biochemistry of information storage in the nervous system. *Science, 236,* 1263–1268.

Black, P. H. (1994). Central nervous system–immune system interactions: Psychoneuroendocrinology of stress and its immune consequences. *Antimicrobial Agents and Chemotherapy, 38*(1), 1–6.

Blackwell, B. (Ed.) (1997). *Treatment compliance and the therapeutic alliance.* Australia: Harwood Academic Publishers.

Blair, S. N., Kampert, J. B., Kohl, H. W., Barlow, C. E., Macera, C. A., Paffenberger, R. S., & Gibbons, L. W. (1996). Influences of cardiorespiratory fitness and other precursors on cardiovascular disease and all-cause mortality in men and women. *Journal of the American Medical Association, 276*(3), 205–210.

Blampied, N. M. (2000). Single-case research designs: A neglected alternative. *American Psychologist, 55*(8), 960.

Blanchard, E. B. (1999). The definition of "applied psychophysiology": A dangerous exercise in exclusivity. *Applied Psychophysiology and Biofeedback, 24*(1), 23–25.

Blanchard, E. B., & Epstein, L. H. (1978). *A biofeedback primer.* Reading, MA: Addison-Wesley.

Blanchard, E. B., Applebaum, K. A., Guarnieri, P., Neff, D. F., Andrasik, F., Jaccard, J., & Barron, K. D. (1988). Two studies of the long-term follow-up of minimal therapist contact treatments of vascular and tension headaches. *Journal of Consulting and Clinical Psychology, 56,* 427–432.

Blanchard, E. B., Eisele, G., Vollmer, A., Payne, A., Gordon, M., Cornish, P., & Gilmore, L. (1996). Controlled evaluation of thermal biofeedback in treatment of elevated blood pressure in unmedicated mild hypertension. *Biofeedback and Self-Regulation, 21*(2), 167–190.

Blanchard, E. B., Nicholson, N. L., Taylor, A. E., Steffeck, B. D., Radnitz, C. L., & Applebaum, K. A. (1991). The role of regular home practice in the relaxation treatment of tension headache. *Journal of Consulting and Clinical Psychology, 59,* 467–470.

Bland, B. (1995). Psychoneuro-nutritional medicine: An advanced paradigm. *Alternative Therapies in Health and Medicine, 1*(2), 22–27.

Bohus, B., & Koolhaas, J. M. (1991). Psychoimmunology of social factors in rodents and other subprimate vertebrates. In R. Ader, D. L. Felten, & N. Cohen (Eds.), *Psychoneuroimmunology* (2nd ed., pp. 807–830). New York: Academic Press.

Bombardier, C. H., D'Amico, C., & Jordan, J. S. (1990). The relationship of appraisal and coping to chronic illness adjustment. *Behaviour Research and Therapy, 28*(4), 297–304.

Bordow, S., & Porritt, D. (1979). An experimental evaluation of crisis intervention. *Social Science and Medicine, 13,* 251–256.

Borkovec, T., Grayson, J., & Cooper, K. (1978). Treatment of general tension: Subjective and physiological effects of progressive relaxation. *Journal of Consulting and Clinical Psychology, 46,* 518–526.

Borysenko, M. (1987). The immune system. *Annals of Behavioral Medicine, 9,* 3–10.

Boutin, G. E., & Tosi, D. J. (1983). Modification of irrational ideas and test anxiety through rational stage directed hypnotherapy (RSDH). *Journal of Clinical Psychology, 39,* 382–391.

Bovbjerg, D. H., Redd, W. H., Maier, L. A., Holland, J. C., Lesko, L. M., Niedzwiecki, D., Rubin, S. C., & Hakes, T. B. (1990). Anticipatory immune suppression and nausea in women receiving cyclic chemotherapy for ovarian cancer. *Journal of Consulting and Clinical Psychology, 58*(2), 153–157.

Bowers, K. S., & Kelly, P. (1979). Stress, disease, psychotherapy, and hypnosis. *Journal of Abnormal Psychology, 88,* 490–505.

Boyd, W. D., & Campbell, S. E. (1998). EEG biofeedback in the schools: The use of EEG biofeedback to treat ADHD in a school setting. *Journal of Neurotherapy, 2*(4), 65–71.

Brandtstadter, J., & Baltes-Gotz, B. (1990). Personal control over development. In M. M. Baltes & P. B. Baltes (Eds.), *Successful aging: Perspectives from the behavioral sciences* (pp. 197–224). Cambridge, UK: Cambridge University Press.

Brehm, B. A. (1998). *Stress management: Increasing your stress resistance.* New York: Longman.

Brenman, M., & Gill, M. M. (1947). *Hypnotherapy.* New York: Wiley.

Brennan, D., & Stevens, J. (1998). A grounded theory approach towards understanding the self perceived effects of meditation on people being treated for cancer. *Australian Journal of Holistic Nursing, 5*(2), 20–26.

Breslau, N., Kessler, R., Chilcoat, H., Schultz, L., Davis, G., & Andreski, P. (1998). Trauma and posttraumatic stress disorder in the community. *Archives of General Psychiatry, 55,* 626–633.

Brett, E., & Ostroff, R. (1985). Imagery and PTSD. *American Journal of Psychiatry, 142,* 417–424.

British Psychological Society. (1990). *Psychological aspects of disaster.* Leicester, UK: Author.

Broocks, A., Bandelow, B., Pekrun, G., George, A., Meyer, T., Bartmann, U., Hillmer-Vogel, U., & Ruther, E. (1998). Comparison of aerobic exercise, chlomipramine, and placebo in the treatment of panic disorder. *American Journal of Psychiatry, 155,* 603–609.

Brooks, J. (1994). The application of Maharishi Ayur-Veda to mental health and substance abuse treatment. *Alcoholism Treatment Quarterly, 11*(3–4), 395–411.

Brooks, W. H., Cross, R. J., Roszman, T. L., & Markesbery, W. R. (1982). Neuroimmunomodulation: Neural anatomical basis of impairment and facilitation. *Annals of Neurology, 12,* 56–61.

Brown, B. (1977). *Stress and the art of biofeedback.* New York: Harper & Row.

Brown, C., Rakel, R., Wells, B., Downs, J., & Akiskal H. (1993). A practical update on anxiety disorders and their pharmacologic treatment. *Archives of Internal Medicine, 151,* 873–884.

Brown, G. W. (1972). Life events and psychiatric illness. *Journal of Psychosomatic Research, 16,* 311–320.

Buckley, R. (1985, November). *Post-prandial hypoglycemic anxiety.* Paper presented to the 32nd Annual Meeting of Psychosomatic Medicine, San Francisco, CA.

Budzynski, T. (1979, November). *Biofeedback and stress management.* Paper presented at the Johns Hopkins Conference on Clinical Biofeedback, Baltimore, MD.

Budzynski, T., & Stoyva, J. (1969). An instrument for producing deep muscle relaxation by means of analog information feedback. *Journal of Applied Behavioral Analysis, 2,* 231–237.

Budzynsky, T. H., Stoyva, J. M., & Adler, C. S. (1976, September). *The use of feedback-induced muscle relaxation in tension headache: A controlled study.* Paper presented at the annual meeting of the American Psychological Association, Miami Beach, FL.

Bureau of Justice Statistics. (1997). *Criminal victimization 1996.* Washington, DC: U.S. Department of Justice.

Bureau of Justice Statistics. (1997). *National crime victimization survey.* Washington, DC: U.S. Department of Justice.

Burgio, K. L., & Goode, P. S. (1997). Behavioral interventions for incontinence in ambulatory geriatric patients. *American Journal of the Medical Sciences, 314*(4), 257–261.

Buselli, E. F., & Stuart, E. M. (1999). Influence of psychosocial factors and biopsychosocial interventions on outcomes after myocardial infarction. *Journal of Cariovascular Nursing, 13*(3), 60–72.

Busuttil, A., & Busuttil, W. (1995). Psychological debriefing. *British Journal of Psychiatry, 166,* 676–677.

Busuttil, W., Turnbull, G., Neal, L., Rollins, J., West, A., Blanch, N., & Herepath, R. (1995). Incorporating psychological debriefing techniques within a brief group psychotherapy programme for the treatment of post-traumatic stress disorder. *British Journal of Psychiatry, 167,* 495–502.

Butler, R. N., Maby, J. I., Montela, J. M., & Young, G. P. (1999). Urinary incontinence: Primary care therapies for the older woman. *Geriatrics, 54*(11), 31–34, 39–40, 43–44.

Byrd, R. B. (1988). Positive therapeutic effects of intercessory prayer in a coronary care unit population. *Southern Medical Journal, 81,* 826–829.

Cain, D. P. (1992). Kindling and the amygdala. In J. P. Aggleton (Ed.), *The amygdala* (pp. 539–560). New York: Wiley-Liss.

Caldwell, M. F. (1992). Incidence of PTSD among staff victims of patient violence. *Hospital and Community Psychiatry, 8,* 838–839.

Caldwell, R. A., Pearson, J. L., & Chin, R. J. (1987). Stress-moderating effects: Context of gender and locus of control. *Personality and Social Psychology Bulletin, 13,* 5–17.

Campernolle, T., Kees, H., & Leen, J. (1979). Diagnosis and treatment of the hyperventilation syndrome. *Psychosomatics, 20,* 612–625.

Campfield, K. & Hills, A. (2001). Effect of timing of Critical Incident Stress Debriefing on posttraumatic symptoms. *Journal of Traumatic Stress, 14,* 327–340.

Cannon, W. B. (1914). The emergency function of the adrenal medulla in pain and in the major emotions. *American Journal of Physiology, 33,* 356–372.

Cannon, W. B. (1929). *Bodily changes in pain, fear, hunger, and rage.* New York: Appleton.

Cannon, W. B. (1942). "Voodoo" death. *American Anthropologist, 44*(2), 169–181.

Cannon, W. B. (1953). *Bodily changes in pain, hunger, fear, and rage.* Boston: Branford.

Cannon, W. B., & Paz, D. (1911). Emotional stimulation of adrenal secretion. *American Journal of Physiology, 28,* 64–70.

Caplan, G. (1961). *An approach to community mental health.* New York: Grune & Stratton.

Caplan, G. (1964). *Principles of preventive psychiatry.* New York: Basic Books.

Capra, F. (1975). *The tao of physics.* Boulder, CO: Shambala.

Cardena, E., & Spiegel, D. (1993). Dissociative reactions to the Bay Area Earthquake. *American Journal of Psychiatry, 150,* 474–478.

Carey, M. P., & Burish, T. G. (1987). Providing relaxation training to cancer chemotherapy patients: A comparison of three delivery techniques. *Journal of Consulting and Clinical Psychology, 55,* 732–737.

Carey, M. P., & Burish, T. G. (1988). Etiology and treatment of the psychological side effects associated with cancer chemotherapy: A critical review and discussion. *Psychological Bulletin, 104,* 307–325.

Carr, D., & Sheehan, D. (1984). Panic anxiety: A new biological model. *Journal of Clinical Psychiatry, 45,* 323–330.

Carrington, P. (1993). Modern forms of meditation. In P. Lehrer & R. Woolfolk (Eds.). *Principles and practice of stress management* (pp. 139–168). New York: Guilford.

Carruthers, M., & Taggart, P. (1973). Vagotonicity of violence. *British Medical Journal, 3,* 384–389.

Caspersen, C. J., Merritt, R. K., & Stephens, T. (1994). International physical activity patterns: A methodological perspective. In R. K. Dishman (Ed.), *Advances in exercise adherence* (pp. 73–110). Champaign, IL: Human Kinetics.

Cassel, J. (1974). *Psychosocial Processes and "Stress.": The Behavioral Sciences and Preventive Medicine.* Washington, DC: Public Health Service.

Cattell, R. B. (1972). *The sixteen personality factor.* Champaign, IL: Institute for Personality and Ability Testing.

Cattell, R. B., & Scheier, I. (1961). *The meaning and measurement of neuroticism and anxiety.* New York: Ronald Press.

Caudill, M. (1994). *Managing pain before it manages you.* New York: Guilford.

Caudill, M., Schnable, R., Zuttermeister, P., Benson, H., & Friedman, R. (1991). Decreased clinic utilization by chronic pain patients. *Clinical Journal of Pain, 7,* 305–310.

Cella, D. F., Pratt, A., & Holland, J. C. (1986). Persistent anticipatory nausea, vomiting, and anxiety in cured Hodgkin's disease patients after completion of chemotherapy. *American Journal of Psychiatry, 143,* 641–643.

Chang, E. C. (1998). Dispositional optimism and primary and secondary appraisal of a stressor: Controlling for confounding influences and relations to coping and psychological and physical adjustment. *Journal of Personality and Social Psychology, 74,* 1109–1120.

Chanowitz, B., & Langer, E. J. (1981). Premature cognitive commitment. *Journal of Personality and Social Psychology, 41,* 1051–1063.

Chaouloff, F., Berton, O., & Mormède, P. (1999). Serotonin and stress. *Neuropsychopharmacology, 21,* 28S–32S.

Charney, D. S., Deutch, A., Krystal, J., Southwick, S., & Davis, M. (1993). Psychobiologic mechanisms of posttraumatic stress disorder. *Archives of General Psychiatry, 50,* 294–299.

Chavat, J., Dell, P., & Folkow, B. (1964). Mental factors and cardiovascular disorders. *Cardiologia, 44,* 124–141.

Chen, W. W., & Sun, W. Y. (1997). Tai chi chuan, an alternative form of exercise for health promotion and disease prevention for older adults in the community. *International Quarterly of Community Health Education, 16*(4), 333–339.

Chrousos, G. P., & Gold, P. W. (1992). The concepts of stress and stress system disorders. *Journal of the American Medical Association, 267,* 1244–1252.

Cluss, P. A., & Epstein, L. H. (1985). The measurement of medical compliance in the treatment of disease. In P. Karoly (Ed.), *Measurement strategies in health psychology* (pp. 403–432). New York: Wiley.

Cohen, F., & Lazarus, R. S. (1979). Coping with the stresses of illness. In G. Stone, F. Cohen, & N. Adler (Eds.), *Health psychology* (pp. 217–254). San Francisco: Jossey-Bass.

Cohen, J. (1977). *Statistical power analysis for the sciences* (2nd ed.). New York: Academic Press.

Cohen, J. (1984). The benefits of meta-analysis. In J. Williams & R. Spitzer (Eds.), *Psychotherapy research* (pp. 332–339). New York: Guilford.

Cohen, S., & Herbert, T. B. (1996). Health psychology: Psychological factors and physical disease from the perspective of human psychoneuroimmunology. *Annual Review of Psychology, 47,* 113–142.

Cohen, S., & Herbert, T. B. (1996). Health psychology: Psychological factors and physical disease from the perspective of human psychoneuroimmunology. *Annual Review of Psychology, 47,* 113–142.

Cohen, S., Evans, G. W., Stokols, D., & Krantz, D. S. (Eds.). (1986). *Behavior, health, and environmental stress.* New York: Plenum Press.

Cooper, J. R., Bloom, F., & Roth, R. (1982). *The biochemical basis of neuropharmacology.* New York: Oxford University Press.

Cooper, K. H. (1977). *The aerobics way: New data on the world's most popular exercise program.* New York: M. Evans.

Corley, K. (1985). Psychopathology of stress. In S. Burchfield (Ed.), *Stress* (pp. 185–206). New York: Hemisphere.

Corneil, D. W. (1993). *Prevalence of post-traumatic stress disorders in a metropolitan fire department.* Dissertation, School of Hygiene and Public Health, Johns Hopkins University, Baltimore, MD.

Corson, S., & Corson, E. (1971). Psychosocial influences on renal function: Implications for human pathophysiology. In L. Levi (Ed.), *Society, stress, and disease* (Vol. 1, pp. 338–351). New York: Oxford University Press.

Cortright, B. (1997). *Psychotherapy and spirit: Theory and practice in transpersonal psychotherapy.* Albany, NY: State University of New York Press.

Coyne, J. C., & Holroyd, K. (1982). Stress, coping, and illness. In T. Millon, C. Green, & R. Meagher (Eds.), *Handbook of clinical health psychology* (pp. 103–128). New York: Plenum Press.

Craft, L. L., & Landers, D. M. (1998). The effect of exercise on clinical depression and depression resulting from mental illness: A meta-analysis. *Journal of Sport and Exercise Psychology, 20*(4), 339–357.

Crasilneck, H. B., & Hall, J. A. (1975). *Clinical hypnosis: Principles and applications.* New York: Grune & Stratton.

Crider, A. B., & Glaros, A. G. (1999). A meta-analysis of EMG biofeedback treatment of temporomandibular disorders. *Journal of Orofacial Pain, 13*(1), 29–37.

Cromwell, R. L., Butterfield, E. C., Brayfield, F. M., & Curry, J. J. (1977). *Acute myocardial infarction: Reaction and recovery.* St. Louis: Mosby.

Crook, T. H., & Miller, N. E. (1985). The challenge of Alzheimer's disease. *American Psychologist, 40*(11), 1245–1250.

Cross, R. J., Brooks, W. H., Roszman, T. L., & Markesbery, W. R. (1982). Hypothalamic–immune interactions: Effect of hypophysectomy on neuroimmunomodulation. *Journal of the Neurological Sciences, 53,* 557–566.

Cullinan, W., Herman, J. P., Helmreich, D., & Watson, S. (1995). A neuroanatomy of stress. In M. J. Friedman, D. Charney, & A. Deutch (Eds.), *Neurobiological and clinical consequences of stress* (pp. 3–26). Philadelphia: Lippincott-Raven.

Cunnick, J. E., Lysle, D. T., Armfield, A., & Rabin, B. S. (1988). Shock induced modulation of lymphocyte responsiveness and natural killer cell activity: Differential mechanisms of induction. *Brain, Behavior, and Immunity, 2,* 102–112.

Damon Corporation. (1981). *Evaluation of adrenocortical function.* Needham Heights, MA: Author.

Dann, J. A., Wachtel, S. S., & Rubin, A. L. (1979). Possible involvement of the central nervous system in graft rejection. *Transplantation, 27,* 223–226.

Dantzer, R., & Kelley, K. W. (1989). Stress and immunity: An integrated view of relationships between the brain and immune system. *Life Sciences, 44,* 1995–2008.

Davidson, J. (1976). The physiology of meditation and mystical states of consciousness. *Perspectives in Biology and Medicine, 19,* 345–379.

Davis, M., Eshelman, E. R., & McKay, M. (1988). *Relaxation and stress reduction workbook* (3rd ed.). Oakland, CA: New Harbinger.

De la Torre, B. (1994). Psychoendocrinologic mechanisms of life stress. *Stress Medicine, 10,* 107–114.

Deadwyler, S., Gribkoff, V., Cotman, D., & Lynch, G. (1976). Long-lasting chances in the spontaneous activity of hippocampal neurons following stimulation of the entorhinal cortex. *Brain Research Bulletin, 169,* 1–7.

Deahl, M., Srinivasan, M., Jones, N., Thomas, J., Neblett, C., & Jolly, A. (2000). Preventing psychological trauma in soldiers: The role of operational stress training and psychological debriefing. *British Journal of Medical Psychology, 73,* 77–85.

Debenham, G., Sargent, W., Hill, D., & Slater, E. (1941). Treatment of war neurosis. *Lancet, 3,* 107–110.

Decker, J., & Stubblebine, J. (1972). Crisis intervention and prevention of psychiatric disability: A follow-up. *American Journal of Psychiatry, 129,* 725–729.

Dekker, E., Pelser, H. E., & Groen, J. (1957). Conditioning as a cause of asthamatic attacks. *Journal of Psychosomatic Research, 2,* 97–108.

Delanoy, R., Tucci, D., & Gold, P. (1983). Amphetamine effects on LTP in dendate granule cells. *Pharmacology, Biochemistry, and Behavior, 18,* 137–139.

Delmonte, M. (1984). Physiological concomitants of meditation practice. *International Journal of Psychosomatics, 31,* 23–36.

Dembroski, T., & Costa, P. (1988). Assessment of coronary-prone behavior. *Annals of Behavioral Medicine, 10,* 60–63.

Der, D., & Lewington, P. (1990). Rational self-directed hypnotherapy: A treatment for panic attacks. *American Journal of Clinical Hypnosis, 32,* 160–167.

Derogatis, L. (1977). *The SCL-90-R: Administration, scoring and procedures manual 1.* Baltimore: Clinical Psychometric Research.

Derogatis, L. (1980). *The Derogatis stress profile.* Baltimore: Clinical Psychometric Research.

deVries, H. (1966). *Physiology of exercise.* Dubuque, IA: Brown.

deVries, H. (1968). Immediate and long-term effects of exercise upon resting muscle action potential level. *Journal of Sports Medicine and Physical Fitness, 8,* 1–11.

deVries, H. (1981). Tranquilizer effect of exercise. *America's Journal of Physical Medicine, 60,* 57–66.

Dewe, P. J. (1992). The appraisal process: Exploring the role of meaning, importance, control, and coping in work stress. *Anxiety, Stress, and Coping, 5,* 95–109.

DiCara, L. V., & Miller, N. E. (1968a). Changes in heart rate instrumentally learned by curarized rats as avoidance responses. *Journal of Comparative Physiology and Psychology, 65,* 8–12.

DiCara, L. V., & Miller, N. E. (1968b). Instrumental learning of systolic blood pressure responses by curarized rats: Dissociation of cardiac and vascular changes. *Psychosomatic Medicine, 30,* 489–494.

DiCara, L. V., & Miller, N. E. (1968c). Instrumental learning of vasomotor responses by rats: Learning to respond differently in the two ears. *Science, 159,* 1485.

DiFilippo, J. M., & Overholser, J. C. (1999). Cognitive-behavioral treatment of panic disorder: Confronting situational precipitants. *Journal of Contemporary Psychotherapy, 29*(2), 99–113.

Dillon, K., & Baker, K. (1985). Positive emotional states and enhancement of the immune system. *International Journal of Psychiatric Medicine, 5,* 13–18.

DiLorenzo, T. M., Bargman, E. P., Stucky-Ropp, R., Brassington G. S., Frensch, P. A., & LaFontaine, T. (1999). Long-term effects of aerobic exercise on psychological outcomes. *Preventive Medicine, 28,* 75–85.

Dimsdale, J. E., & Moss, J. (1980). Plasma catecholamines in stress and exercise. *Journal of the American Medical Association, 243,* 340–342.

Dishman, R. K. (1994). *Advances in exercise adherence.* Champaign, IL: Human Kinetics.

Dishman, R. K., & Buckworth, J. (1997). Adherence to physical exercise. In W. Morgan (Ed.), *Physical activity and mental health* (pp. 63–80). Washington, DC: Taylor & Francis.

Doane, B. (1986). Clinical psychiatry and the physiodynamics of the limbic system. In B. Doane & K. Livingston (Eds.), *The limbic system* (pp. 285–315). New York: Raven Press.

Dobson, K. S., & Shaw, B. F. (1995). Cognitive therapies in practice. In B. Bongar & L. E. Bentler (Eds.), *Comprehensive textbook of psychotherapies: Theory and practice* (pp. 159–172). New York: Oxford University Press.

Domar, A., Seidel, M., & Benson, H. (1990). The mind body program for infertility. *Infertility and Sterility, 53,* 246–249.

Domar, A., Zuttermeister, P., Seibel, M., & Benson, H. (1992). Psychological improvement in infertile women after behavioral treatment. *Infertility and Sterility, 55,* 144–147.

Donahue, M. J. (1985). Intrinsic and extrinsic religiousness: Review and meta-analysis. *Journal of Personality and Social Psychology, 48,* 400–419.

Donoghue, S. (1977). The correlation between physical fitness, absenteeism, and work performance. *Canadian Journal of Public Health, 68,* 201–203.

Dorpat, T. L., & Holmes, T. H. (1955). Mechanisms of skeletal muscle pain and fatigue. *Archives of Neurology and Psychiatry, 74,* 628–640.

Dotevall, G. (1985). *Stress and the common gastrointestinal disorders.* New York: Praeger.

Duffy, E. (1962). *Activation and behavior.* New York: Wiley.

Duman, R. S., Malberg, J., & Thome, J. (1999). Neural plasticity to stress and antidepressant treatment. *Biolilogical Psychiatry, 46,* 1181–1191.

Dunbar, H. F. (1935). *Emotions and bodily changes.* New York: Columbia University Press.

Dunn, A. J. (1989). Psychoneuroimmunology for the psychoneuroendocrinologist: A review of animal studies of nervous–immune system interactions. *Psychoneuroendocrinology, 14,* 251–274.

Dunn, A. J. (1993). Infection as a stressor: A cytokine mediated activation of the hypothalamo–pituitary–adrenal area. In *Corticotropin releasing factor* (Ciba Foundation Symposium 172, pp. 226–243). West Sussex, UK: Wiley.

Dyregrov, A. (1997). The process of psychological debriefing. *Journal of Traumatic Stress, 10,* 589–604.

Dyregrov, A. (1998). Psychological debriefing: An effective method? *Traumatology, 4*(2), Article 1.

Dyregrov, A. (1999). Helpful and hurtful aspects of psychological debriefing groups. *International Journal of Emergency Mental Health, 1,* 175–181.

Earle, J. B. (1981). Cerebral laterality and meditation: A review of the literature. *Journal of Transpersonal Psychology, 13,* 155–173.

Edelberg, R. (1972). Electrical activity of the skin. In N. Greenfield & R. Sternbach (Eds.), *Handbook of psychophysiology* (pp. 367–418). New York: Holt, Rinehart & Winston.

Edinger, J. (1982). Incidence and significance of relaxation treatment side effects. *Behavior Therapist, 5,* 137–138.

Eisenberg, D. M., Davis, R. B., Ettner, S. L., Appel, S., Wilkey, S., Van Rompay, M., & Kessler, R. C. (1998). Trends in alternative medicine use in the United States, 1990–1997: Results of a follow-up national survey. *Journal of the American Medical Association, 280*(18), 1569–1575.

Eisler, R., & Polak, P. (1971). Social stress and psychiatric disorder. *Journal of Nervous and Mental Disease, 153,* 227–233.

Eizenman, D. R., Nesselroade, J. R., Featherman, D. L., & Rowe, J. W. (1997). Intraindividual variability in perceived control in an older sample: The MacArthur successful aging studies. *Psychology and Aging, 12*(3), 489–502.

Eliot, R. (1979). *Stress and the major cardiovascular diseases.* Mt. Kisco, NY: Futura.

Eller, L. S. (1996). Effects of two cognitive-behavioral interventions on immunity and symptoms in persons with HIV. *Annals of Behavioral Medicine, 17,* 339–348.

Ellis, A. (1962). *Reason and emotion in psychotherapy.* Secaucus, NJ: Lyle Stuart.

Ellis, A. (1971). Emotional disturbance and its treatment in a nutshell. *Canadian Counselor, 5,* 168–171.

Ellis, A. (1973). *Humanistic psychology: The rational-emotive approach.* New York: Julian.

Ellis, A. (1985). The use of hypnosis with rational-emotive therapy. *Journal of Integrative & Eclectic Psychotherapy, 2,* 15–22.

Ellis, A. (1991). The revised ABC's of rational-emotive therapy (RET). *Journal of Rational-Emotive and Cognitive-Behavior Therapy, 9,* 139–177.

Ellis, A. (1995). Reflections on rational-emotive therapy. In M. Mahoney (Ed.), *Cognitive and constructive psychotherapies: Theory, research, and practice* (pp. 69–86). New York: Springer.

Elton, D. (1993). Combined use of hypnosis and EMG biofeedback in the treatment of stress-induced conditions. *Stress Medicine, 9,* 25–35.

Emmons, M. (1978). *The inner source: A guide to meditative therapy.* San Luis Obispo, CA: Impact.

Engel, G. L. (1968). A life setting conducive to illness. *Annals of Internal Medicine, 69,* 293–300.

Engel, G. L. (1971). Sudden and rapid death during psychological stress. *Annals of Internal Medicine, 74,* 771–782.

Engels, W. (1985). Dermatological disorders. In W. Dorftnan & L. Cristofar (Eds.), *Psychosomatic illness review* (pp. 146–161). New York: Macmillan.

English, E., & Baker, T. (1983). Relaxation training and cardiovascular response to experimental stressors. *Health Psychology, 2,* 239–259.

Enqvist, B., Von Konow, L., & Bystedt, H. (1995). Stress reduction, preoperative hypnosis and perioperative suggestion in maxillofacial surgery: Somatic responses and recovery. *Stress Medicine, 11,* 229–233.

Epstein, S., & Coleman, M. (1970). Drive theories of schizophrenia. *Psychosomatic Medicine, 32,* 114–141.

Erdman, L. (1993). Laughter therapy for patients with cancer. *Journal of Psychosocial Oncology, 11*(4), 55–67.

Eschelman, M. M. (1996). *Introductory nutrition and nutrition therapy* (3rd ed.). Philadelphia: Lippincott.

Esterling, B. A., Antoni, M. H., Fletcher, M. A., Marguiles, S., & Schneiderman, N. (1994). Emotional disclosure through writing or speaking modulates latent Epstein–Barr virus reactivation. *Journal of Consulting and Clinical Psychology, 62*, 130–140.

Esterling, B. A., Kiecolt-Glaser, J. K., & Glaser, R. (1996). Psychosocial modulation of cytokine-induced natural killer cell activity in older adults. *Psychosomatic Medicine, 58*, 264–272.

Esterling, B. A., Kiecolt-Glaser, J. K., Bodnar, J. C., & Glaser, R. (1994). Chronic stress, social support, and persistent alterations in the natural killer cell response to cytokines in older adults. *Health Psychology, 13*(4), 291–298.

Euler, U. S. V., & Lishajko, F. (1961). Improved techniques for the fluorimetric estimation of catecholamines. *Acta Physiologica Scandinavia, 51*, 348–355.

Everly, G. S., Jr. (1978). *The Organ Specificity Score as a measure of psychophysiological stress reactivity.* Unpublished doctoral dissertation, University of Maryland, College Park.

Everly, G. S., Jr. (1979a). *Strategies for coping with stress: An assessment scale.* Washington, DC: Office of Health Promotion, Department of Health and Human Services.

Everly, G. S., Jr. (1979b). Technique for the immediate reduction of psychophysiological reactivity. *Health Education, 10*, 44.

Everly, G. S., Jr. (1979c). A psychophysiological technique for the rapid onset of a trophotropic state. *IRCS Journal of Medical Science, 7*, 423.

Everly, G. S., Jr. (1985a). Occupational stress. In G. S. Everly & R. Feldman (Eds.), *Occupational health promotion* (pp. 49–73). New York: Wiley.

Everly, G. S., Jr. (1985b, November). *Biological foundations of psychiatric sequelae in trauma and stress-related "disorders of arousal."* Paper presented to the 8th National Trauma Symposium, Baltimore, MD.

Everly, G. S., Jr. (1986). A "biopsychosocial analysis" of psychosomatic disease. In T. Millon & G. Kierman (Eds.), *Contemporary directions in psychopathology* (pp. 535–551). New York: Guilford.

Everly, G. S., Jr. (1987). The principle of personologic primacy. In C. Green (Ed.), *Proceedings of the conference on the Millon Clinical Inventories* (pp. 3–7). Minneapolis: National Computer Systems.

Everly, G. S., Jr. (1993). Psychotraumatology: A two-factor formulation of posttraumatic stress disorder. *Integrative Physiology and Behavioral Science, 28*, 270–278.

Everly, G. S., Jr. (1994). Brief psychotherapy for posttraumatic stress disorder. *Stress Medicine, 10*, 191–196.

Everly, G. S., Jr. (1995). An integrative model of posttraumatic stress. In G. S. Everly, Jr. & J. M. Lating (Eds.), *Psychotraumatology* (pp. 27–48). New York: Plenum.

Everly, G. S., Jr. (2000a). Crisis management briefings. *International Journal of Emergency Mental Health, 2*, 53–57.

Everly, G. S., Jr. (2000b). Pastoral crisis intervention: Toward a definition. *International Journal of Emergency Mental Health, 2*, 69–71.

Everly, G. S., Jr., & Benson, H. (1989). Disorders of arousal and the relaxation response. *International Journal of Psychosomatics, 36*, 15–21.

Everly, G. S., Jr., & Boyle, S. (1999). Critical Incident Stress Debriefing (CISD): A meta-analysis. *International Journal of Emergency Mental Health, 1*, 165–168.

Everly, G. S., Jr., Boyle, S., & Lating, J. (1999). Effectiveness of psychological debriefing with vicarious trauma: A meta-analysis. *Stress Medicine, 15*, 229–233.

Everly, G. S., Jr., Flannery, R. B., & Mitchell, J. (2000). Critical Incident Stress Management: A review of literature. *Aggression and Violent Behavior: A Review Journal, 5*, 23–40.

Everly, G. S., Jr., Flannery, R. B., Jr., & Eyler, V. (in press). Critical Incident Stress Management (CISM): A statistical review of the literature. *Psychiatric Quarterly.*

Everly, G. S., Jr., Flannery, R. B., Jr., Eyler, V., & Mitchell, J. T. (2001). Sufficiency analysis of an integrated multicomponent approach to crisis intervention: Critical Incident Stress Management. *Advances in Mind-Body Medicine, 17*, 171–183.

Everly, G. S., Jr., & Horton, A. (1989). Neuropsychology of posttraumatic stress disorder, *Perceptual and Motor Skills, 68*, 807–810.

Everly, G. S., Jr., & Lating, J. (Eds.). (1995). *Psychotraumatology.* New York: Plenum.

Everly, G. S., Jr., & Lating, J. (in press). *A personality-guided approach to the treatment of Posttraumatic Stress Disorder.* Washington, DC: American Psychological Association.

Everly, G. S. Jr., & Mitchell, J. T. (1999). *Critical Incident Stress Management: A new era and standard of care in crisis intervention* (2nd ed.). Ellicott City, MD: Chevron.

Everly, G. S., Jr., & Mitchell, J. T. (2001). *Critical Incident Stress Management (CISM). A New Era and Standard of Care in Crisis Intervention* (3rd ed.). Ellicott City, MD: Chevron.

Everly, G. S., Jr., & Piacentini, A. (1999, March). The Effects of CISD on trauma symptoms: A meta-analysis. Paper presented to the *APA-NIOSH Work, Stress and Health '99: Organization of Work in a Global Economy* conference, Baltimore.

Everly, G. S., Jr., & Sobelman, S. H. (1987). *The assessment of the human stress response: Neurological, biochemical, and psychological foundations.* New York: American Management Systems Press.

Everly, G. S., Jr., Spollen, M., Hackman, A., & Kobran, E. (1987). Undesirable side-effects and self-regulatory therapies. *Proceedings of the Eighteenth Annual Meeting of the Biofeedback Society of America* (pp. 166–167).

Everly, G. S., Jr., Welzant, V., Machado, P. & Miller, K. (1989). *The correlation between frontalis muscle tension and sympathetic nervous system activity.* Unpublished research report.

Faggiotto, A., Poli, A., & Catapano, A. L. (1998). Antioxidants and coronary artery disease. *Current Opinion in Lipidology, 9*, 541–549.

Fairbank, J., McCaffery, R., & Keane, T. (1985). Psychometric detection of fabrication symptoms of PTSD. *American Journal of Psychiatry, 142*, 501–503.

Farrow, J. T., & Herbert, R. (1982). Breath suspension during the transcendental meditation technique. *Psychosomatic Medicine, 44*(2), 133–153.

Faymonville, M. E., Mambourg, P. H., Joris, J., Vrijens, B., Fissette, J., Albert, A., & Lamy, M. (1997). Psychological approaches during conscious sedation: Hypnosis versus stress reducing strategies: A prospective randomized study. *Pain, 73*, 361–367.

Felten, D. L., Cohen, N., Ader, R., Felten, S. Y., Carlson, S. L., & Roszman, T. L. (1991). Central neural circuits involved in neural–immune interactions. In R. Ader, D. L. Felten, & N. Cohen (Eds.), *Psychoneuroimmunology* (2nd ed., pp. 3–25). New York: Academic Press.

Felten, S. Y., & Felten, D. L. (1991). Innervation of lymphoid tissue. In R. Ader, D. L. Felten, & N. Cohen (Eds.), *Psychoneuroimmunology* (2nd ed., pp. 27–61). New York: Academic Press.

Feske, U. (1998). Eye movement desensitization and reprocessing treatment for posttraumatic stress disorder. *Clinical Psychology: Science and Practice, 5*(2), 171–181.

Fibiger, W., & Singer, G. (1984). Physiological changes during physical and psychological stress. *Australian Journal of Psychology, 36*, 317–326.

Fiske, D. W. (1983). The meta-analysis revolution in outcome research. *Journal of Consulting and Clinical Psychology, 51*, 65–70.

Fixx, J. F. (1977). *The complete book of running.* New York: Random House.

Flannery, R. B., Jr. (1992). *Posttraumatic Stress Disorder: The victim's guide to healing and recovery.* New York: Continuum.

Flannery, R. B., Jr. (1998). *The Assaulted Staff Action Program.* Ellicott City, MD: Chevron.

Flannery, R. B., Jr. (1999a). Treating family survivors of mass casualties: A CISM family crisis intervention approach. *International Journal of Emergency Mental Health, 1*, 243–250.

Flannery, R. B., Jr. (1999b). Critical Incident Stress Management (CISM): The assaultive psychiatric patient. *International Journal of Emergency Mental Health, 1*, 169–174.

Flannery, R. B., Jr. (1999c). Critical Incident Stress Management and the Assaulted Staff Action Program. *International Journal of Emergency Mental Health, 1*, 103–108.

Flannery, R. B., Jr., Anderson, E., Marks, L., & Uzoma, L. (2000). The Assaulted Staff Action Program (ASAP) and declines in rates of assaults: Mixed replicated findings. *Psychiatric Quarterly, 71*, 165–175.

Flannery, R. B., Jr., Everly, G. S., Jr., & Eyler, V. (2000). The Assaulted Staff Action Program (ASAP) and declines in Assaults: A meta-analysis. *International Journal of Emergency Mental Health, 2*, 143–146.

Flannery, R. B., Jr., Hanson, M. A., Penk, W., Goldfinger, S., Pastva, G., & Navon, M. (1998). Replicated declines in assault rates after the implementation of the Assaulted Staff Action Program. *Psychiatric Services, 49*, 241–243.

Flannery, R. B., Jr., Hanson, M., Penk, W., Flannery, G., & Gallagher, C. (1995). The Assaulted Staff Action Program: An approach to coping with the aftermath of violence in the workplace. In L. Murphy, J. Hurrell, S. Sauter, & G. Keita (Eds.), *Job stress interventions* (pp. 199–212). Washington, DC: American Psychological Association Press.

Flannery, R. B., Penk, W., & Corrigan, M. (1999). Assaulted Staff Action Program (ASAP) and declines in the prevalence of assaults: Community-based replication. *International Journal of Emergency Mental Health, 1*, 19–22.

Fleshner, M., Laudenslager, M. L., Simons, L., & Maier, S. F. (1989). Reduced serum antibodies associated with social defeat in rats. *Physiology and Behavior, 42*, 485–489.

Fletcher, G. F., Balady, G., Blair, S. N., Blumenthal, J., Caspersen, C., Chaitman, B., Epstein, S., Sivarajan-Froelicher, E. S., Froelicher, V. F., Pina, I. L., & Pollock, M. L. (1996). Statement on exercise: Benefits and recommendations for physical activity programs for all Americans: A statement for health professionals by the committee on exercise and cardiac rehabilitation of the Council on Clinical Cardiology, American Heart Association. *Circulation, 94*, 857–862.

Foa, E., Davidson, J., & Frances, A. (1999). *Journal of Clinical Psychiatry*, Entire Supplement 16.

Foa, E., Keane, T., & Friedman, M. (Eds.). (2000). *Effective treatments for PTSD*. New York: Guilford.

Folkow, B., & Neil, E. (1971). *Circulation*. London: Oxford University Press.

Folks, D. G., & Kinney, F. C. (1995). Dermatologic conditions. In A. Stoudemire (Ed.), *Psychological factors affecting medical conditions* (pp. 123–140). Washington, DC: American Psychiatric Press.

Food and Nutrition Board Institute of Medicine. (2000). *Dietary reference intakes for vitamin C, vitamin E, selenium, and carotenoids* (A Report of the Panel on Dietary Antioxidants and Related Compounds, Subcommittees on Upper Reference Levels of Nutrients and Interpretation and Uses of Dietary Reference Intakes, and the Standing Committee on the Scientific Evaluation of Dietary Reference Intakes). Washington, DC: National Academy Press.

Foon, A. E. (1985). Similarity between therapists' and clients' locus of control: Implications for therapeutic expectations and outcome. *Psychotherapy, 22*(4), 711–717.

Foss, M. L., & Keteyian, S. J. (1998). *Fox's physiological basis for exercise and sport* (6th ed.). Boston: McGraw-Hill.

Fowers, B. J. (1994). Perceived control, illness status, stress, and adjustment to cardiac illness. *Journal of Psychology, 128*(5), 567–576.

Foy, D. W. (1992). *Treating PTSD*. New York: Guilford.

Foy, D., Sipprelle, R., Rueger, D., & Carroll, E. (1984). Etiology of PTSD in Vietnam veterans. *Journal of Consulting and Clinical Psychology, 52*, 79–87.

Frances, A. (1982). Categorical and dimensional systems of personality diagnosis. *Comprehensive Psychiatry, 23,* 516–527.

Frances, A., & Hale, R. (1984). Determining how a depressed woman's personality affects the choice of treatment. *Hospital and Community Psychiatry, 35,* 883–884.

Frank, J. D. (1974). The restoration of morale. *American Journal of Psychiatry, 131,* 271–274.

Frankel, F. H. (1976). *Hypnosis: Trance as a coping mechanism.* New York: Plenum Press.

Frankenhaeuser, M. (1980). Psychoneuroendocrine approaches to the study of stressful person-environment transactions. In H. Selye (Ed.), *Selye's guide to stress research* (pp. 46–70). New York: Van Nostrand Reinhold.

Frazier, T. W. (1966). Avoidance conditioning of heart rate in humans. *Psychophysiology, 3,* 188–202.

Freedman, R., & Papsdorf, J. (1976). Generalization of frontal EMG biofeedback training to other muscles. Paper presented to the 7th Annual Meeting of the Biofeedback Society, Colorado Springs.

Freeman, G. L. (1939). Toward a psychiatric Plimsoll Mark. *Journal of Psychology, 8,* 247–252.

Freud, S. (1921). *Forward in psychoanalysis and the war neurosis.* New York: International Psychoanalytic Press.

Fried, R. (1987). *The hyperventilation syndrome: Research and clinical treatment.* Baltimore: Johns Hopkins University Press.

Fried, R. (1993). The role of respiration in stress and stress control: Toward a theory of stress as a hypoxic phenomenon. In P. M. Lehrer & R. L. Woolfolk (Eds.), *Principles and practice of stress management* (2nd ed., pp. 301–331). New York: Guilford.

Friedland, N., Keinan, G., & Regev, Y. (1992). Controlling the uncontrolable: Effects of stress on illusory perceptions of controllability. *Journal of Personality and Social Psychology, 63*(6), 923–931.

Friedlander, Y., Kark, J. D., & Stein, Y. (1986). Religious orthodoxy and myocardial infarction in Jerusalem: A case control study. *International Journal of Cardiology, 10,* 33–41.

Friedman, H., & Booth-Kewley, S. (1987). The "disease-prone personality". *American Psychologist, 42,* 539–555.

Friedman, M. (1969). *Pathogenesis of coronary artery disease.* New York: McGraw-Hill.

Friedman, M. J., & Schnurr, P. P. (1995). The relationship between trauma, postraumatic stress disorder, and physical health. In M. J. Friedman, D. Charney, & A. Deutch (Eds.), *Neurobiological, and clinical consequences of stress* (pp. 507–526). Philadelphia: Lippincott-Raven.

Friedman, M. J., Charney, D., & Deutch, A. (Eds.). (1995). *Neurobiological, and clinical consequences of stress.* Philadelphia: Lippincott-Raven.

Friedman, M., & Rosenman, R. (1974). *Type A behavior and your heart.* New York: Knopf.

Froberg, J., Karlsson, C., Levi, L., & Lidberg, L. (1971). Physiological and biochemical stress reactions induced by psychosocial stimuli. In L. Levi (Ed.), *Society, stress, and disease* (Vol. 1, pp. 280–295). New York: Oxford University Press.

Frysinger, R., & Harper, R. (1989). Cardiac and respiratory correlations with unit discharge in human amygdala and hippocampus. *Electroencephalography and Clinical Neurophysiology, 72,* 463–470.

Fuller, G. (1972). *Biofeedback: Methods and procedures in clinical practice.* San Francisco: Biofeedback Institute.

Ganong, W. F. (1997). *Review of medical physiology* (18th ed.). Stamford, CT: Appleton & Lange.

Ganong, W. F. (1997). *Review of medical physiology.* Stamford, CT: Appleton & Lange.

Gaston, L., Crombez, J. C., & Dupuis, G. (1989). An imagery and meditation technique in the treatment of psoriasis: A case study using an A-B-A design. *Journal of Mental Imagery, 13*(1), 31–38.

Gatchel, R., & Price, K. (1979). Biofeedback: An introduction and historical overview. In R. Gatchel & K. Price (Eds.), *Clinical applications of biofeedback: Appraisal and status.* Elmsford, NY: Pergamon Press.

Gawler, I. (1998). The creative power of imagery: Specific techniques for people affected by cancer. *Australian Journal of Clinical Hypnotherapy and Hypnosis, 19*(1), 17–30.

Gelderloos, P., Walton, K. G., Orme-Johnson, D. W., & Alexander, C. N. (1991). Effectiveness of the transcendental meditation program in preventing a substance misuse: A review. *International Journal of the Addictions, 26*(3), 293–325.

Gellhorn, E. (1957). *Autonomic imbalance and the hypothalamus.* Minneapolis: University of Minnesota Press.

Gellhorn, E. (1958a). The physiological basis of neuromuscular relaxation. *Archives of Internal Medicine, 102,* 392–399.

Gellhorn, E. (1958b). The influence of curare on hypothalamic excitability and the electroencephalogram. *Electroencephalography and Clinical Neurophysiology, 10,* 697–703.

Gellhorn, E. (1964a). Motion and emotion. *Psychological Review, 71,* 457–472.

Gellhorn, E. (1964b). Sympathetic reactivity in hypertension. *Acta Neurovegetative, 26,* 35–44.

Gellhorn, E. (1965). The neurophysiological basis of anxiety. *Perspectives in Biology and Medicine, 8,* 488–515.

Gellhorn, E. (1967). *Principles of autonomic–somatic integrations.* Minneapolis: University of Minnesota Press.

Gellhorn, E. (1968). Central nervous system tuning and its implications for neuropsychiatry. *Journal of Nervous and Mental Disease, 147,* 148–162.

Gellhorn, E. (1969). Further studies on the physiology and pathophysiology of the tuning of the central nervous system. *Psychosomatics, 10,* 94–104.

Gellhorn, E., & Kiely, W. (1972). Mystical states of consciousness. *Journal of Nervous and Mental Disease, 154,* 399–405.

Gellhorn, E., & Loofbourrow, G. (1963). *Emotions and emotional disorders.* New York: Harper & Row.

Gessel, A. H. (1989). Edmund Jacobson, M. D., Ph.D.: The founder of scientific relaxation. *International Journal of Psychosomatics, 36*(1–4), 5–14.

Gevarter, W. (1978). *Psychotherapy and the brain.* Unpublished paper, NASA, Washington, DC.

Gherman, E. M. (1982). *Stress and the bottom line.* New York: AMACOM.

Gifford, S., & Gunderson, J. G. (1970). Cushing's disease as a psychosomatic disorder: A selective review. *Perspectives in Biology and Medicine, 13,* 169–221.

Gillespie, R. D. (1942). *Psychological effects of war on citizen and soldier.* New York: Norton.

Girdano, D. A., & Everly, G. S., Jr. (1986). *Controlling stress and tension* (2nd ed.). Englewood Cliffs, NJ: Prentice-Hall.

Girdano, D. A., Dusek, D. E., & Everly, G. S., Jr. (2001). *Controlling stress and tension* (6th ed.). Boston: Allyn & Bacon.

Girdano, D. A., Everly, G. S., Jr., & Dusek, D. E. (1997). *Controlling stress and tension* (5th ed.). Boston: Allyn & Bacon.

Glaser, R., Kiecolt-Glaser, J. K., Bonneau, R. H., Malarkey, W., Kennedy, S., & Hughes, J. (1992). Stress-induced modulation of the immune response to recombinant hepatitis B vaccine. *Psychosomatic Medicine, 54,* 22–29.

Glaus, K., & Kotses, H. (1977). Generalization of conditioned frontalis tension. Paper presented to the 8th Annual Meeting of the Biofeeback Society. Orlando, FL.

Glaus, K., & Kotses, H. (1978). Generalization of conditioned frontalis tension: a closer look. Paper presented to the 9th Annual Meeting of the Biofeeback Society. Albuquerque, NM.

Gloor, P. (1986). Role of the human limbic system in perception, memory, and affect. In B. Doane & K. Livingston (Eds.), *The limbic system* (pp. 159–169). New York: Raven Press.

Gloor, P. (1992). Role of the amygdala in temporal lobe epiepsy. In J. P. Aggleton (Ed.), *The amygdala* (pp. 561–574). New York: Wiley-Liss.

Glueck, B., & Stroebel, C. (1978). Psychophysiological correlates of relaxation. In A. Sugerman & R. Tarter (Eds.), *Expanding dimensions of consciousness* (pp. 99–129). New York: Springer.

Glueck, G., & Stroebel, C. (1975). Biofeedback and meditation in the treatment of psychiatric illness. *Comprehensive Psychiatry, 16,* 309.

Goddard, G., & Douglas, R. (1976). Does the engram of kindling model the engram of normal long-term memory? In J. Wads (Ed.), *Kindling* (pp. 1–18). New York: Raven Press.

Goddard, G., McIntyre, D., & Leech, C. (1969). A permanent change in brain function resulting from daily electrical stimulation. *Experimental Neurology, 25,* 295–330.

Goldberg, J., Flowerdew, G., Smith, E., Brody, J. A., & Tso, M. O. (1988). Factors associated with age-related macular degeneration. *American Journal of Epidemiology, 128,* 700–710.

Goldsby, R. A., Kindt, T. J., & Osborne, B. A. (2000). *Kuby immunology.* New York: W. H. Freeman.

Goleman, D., & Schwartz, G. (1976). Meditation as an intervention in stress reactivity. *Journal of Consulting and Clinical Psychology, 15,* 110–111.

Gorman, J., Dillon, D., Fyer, A., Liebowitz, M., & Klein, D. (1985). The lactate infusion model. *Psychopharmacology Bulletin, 21,* 428–433.

Gorman, J., Liebowitz, M., & Klein, D. (1984). *Panic disorder and agoraphobia.* Kalamazoo, MI: Upjohn.

Grace, W., Seton, P., Wolf, S., & Wolff, H. G. (1949). Studies of the human colon: 1. *American Journal of Medical Science, 217,* 241–251.

Graham, C., Cook, M. R., Cohen, H. D., Gerkovich, M. M., Phelps, J. W., & Fotopoulous, S. S. (1986). Effects of variation in physical effort on frontalis EMG activity. *Biofeedback and Self-Regulation, 11*(2), 135–141.

Gravitz, M. A. (1991). Early theories of hypnosis: A clinical perspective. In S. J. Lynn & J. W. Rhue (Eds.), *Theories of hypnosis: Current models and perspectives* (pp. 19–42). New York: Guilford.

Gravitz, M. A. (1995). Hypnosis in the treatment of functional infertility. *American Journal of Clinical Hypnosis, 38,* 22–26.

Gravitz, M. A. (1997). First uses of "hypnotism" nomenclature: A historical record. *Hypnos, 24,* 42–46.

Gray, J. (1982). *The neuropsychology of anxiety.* New York: Oxford University Press.

Gray, J. (1985). Issues in the neuropsychology of anxiety. In A. Tuma & J. Maser (Eds.), *Anxiety and anxiety disorders* (pp. 5–26). Hillsdale, NJ: Erlbaum.

Greden, J. F. (1974). Anxiety or caffeinism: A diagnostic dilemma. *American Journal of Psychiatry, 131,* 1089–1092.

Green, E., & Green, A. (1977). *Beyond biofeedback.* San Francisco: Delta.

Green, E., & Green, A. (1983). General and specific applications of thermal biofeedback. In J. V. Basmajian (Ed.), *Biofeedback* (pp. 211–797). Baltimore: Williams & Wilkins.

Green, E., & Green, A. (1989). General and specific applications of thermal biofeedback. In J. V. Basmajian (Ed.), *Biofeedback* (3rd ed., pp. 209–221). Baltimore: Williams & Wilkins.

Green, H. (1986). *Fit for America: Health, fitness, sport, and American society.* New York: Pantheon Books.

Greenberg, J. S., Dintiman, G. B., & Myers-Oakes, B. (1998). *Physical fitness and wellness* (2nd ed.). Boston: Allyn & Bacon.

Greenfield, N., & Sternbach, R. (1972). *Handbook of psychophysiology.* New York: Holt, Rinehart & Winston.

Greengard, P. (1978). Phosphorylated proteins and physiological affectors. *Science, 199,* 146–152.

Grimsley, S. R. (1995). Anxiety disorders. In L. Y. Young, M. A. Koda-Kimble, W. A. Kradjan, & B. J. Guglielmo (Eds.), *Applied therapeutics: The clinical use of drugs* (6th ed., pp. 73-1–73-31). Vancouver, WA: Applied Therapeutics.

Grinker, R. R., & Spiegel, J. P. (1945). War neuroses in flying personnel overseas and after return to the U.S.A. *American Journal of Psychiatry, 101,* 619–624.

Groff, J., Gropper, S., & Hunt, S. M. (1995). *Advanced nutrition and human metabolism* (2nd ed.). Minneapolis, St. Paul: West.

Grossman, P., & DeSwart, J. C. G. (1984). Diagnosis of hyperventilation syndrome on the basis of reported complaints. *Journal of Psychosomatic Research, 28,* 97–104.

Gruzelier, J. H. (2000). Redefining hypnosis: Theory, methods, and integration. *Contemporary Hypnosis, 17,* 51–70.

Gullette, E. C., Blumenthal, J. A., Babyak, M., Jiang, W., Waugh, R. A., Frid, D. J., O'Connor, C. M., Morris, J. J., & Krantz, D. S. (1997). Effects of mental stress on myocardial ischemia during daily life. *Journal of the American Medical Association, 277*(19), 1521–1526.

Guyton, A. C. (1982). *Textbook of medical physiology.* Philadelphia: Saunders.

Guyton, A. C. (1987). *Human physiology and mechanisms of disease* (4th ed.). Philadelphia: Saunders.

Guyton, A. C. (1996). *Textbook of medical physiology* (9th ed.). Philadelphia: Saunders.

Guyton, A. C., & Hall, J. E. (1996). *Textbook of medical physiology.* Philadelphia: Saunders.

Gwynne, P. H., Tosi, D. J., & Howard, L. (1978). Treatment of nonassertion through rational stage directed hypnotherapy (RSDH) and behavioral rehearsal. *American Journal of Clinical Hypnosis, 20,* 263–271.

Hall, N. R. S., & O'Grady, M. P. (1991). Psychosocial interventions and immune function. In R. Ader, D. L. Felten, & N. Cohen (Eds.), *Psychoneuroimmunology* (2nd ed., pp. 1067–1080). New York: Academic Press.

Hall, N. R. S., Anderson, J. A., & O'Grady, M. P. (1994). Stress and immunity in humans: Modifying variables. In R. Glaser & J. K. Kiecolt-Glaser (Eds.), *Handbook of human stress and immunity* (pp. 183–215). San Diego: Academic Press.

Halliwell, B. (1998). Can oxidative DNA damage be used as a biomarker for cancer risk in humans? Problems, resolutions and preliminary results from nutritional supplement studies. *Free Radical Research, 29,* 469–486.

Hamberger, L., & Lohr, I. (1984). *Stress and stress management.* New York: Springer.

Hammarberg, M. (1992). Penn Inventory for posttraumatic stress disorder: Psychometric properties. *Psychological Assessment, 4,* 67–76.

Hammond, D. C. (1990). *Handbook of hypnotic suggestions and metaphors.* New York: Norton.

Han, J. N., Stegen, K., de Valck, C., & Clement, J. (1996). Influence of breathing therapy on complaints, anxiety and breathing pattern in patients with hyperventilation syndrome and anxiety disorders. *Journal of Psychosomatic Research, 41*(5), 481–493.

Hardonk, H. J., & Beumer, H. M. (1979). Hyperventilation syndrome. In P. J. Vinken & G. W. Bruyn (Eds.), *Handbook of clinical neurology* (Vol. 38, pp. 309–360). Amsterdam: North-Holland.

Harper, H. A. (1975). *Review of physiological chemistry.* Los Altos, CA: Lange.

Harris, A. H. S., Thoresen, C. E., McCullough, M. E., & Larson, D. B. (1999). Spirituality and religiously oriented health interventions. *Journal of Health Psychology, 4*(3), 413–433.

Harris, T. (1991). Life stress and illness: The question of specificity. *Annals of Behavioral Medicine, 13,* 211–219.

Harvey, J. (1978). Diaphragmatic breathing: A practical technique for breath control. *Behavior Therapist, 1,* 13–14.

Haskell, W. L. (1995). Physical activity in the prevention and management of coronary heart disease. *Physical Activity and Fitness Research Digest, 2,* 1–8.

Hatch, M. C., Wallenstein, S., Beyea, J., Nieves, J. W., & Susser, M. (1991). Cancer raters after the Three Mile Island nuclear accident and proximity of residence to the plant. *American Journal of Public Health, 81*(6), 719–724.

Hegel, M. T., Abel, G. G., Etscheidt, M., Cohen-Cole, S., & Wilmer, C. I. (1989). Behavioral treatment of angina-like chest pain in patients with hyperventilation syndrome. *Journal of Behavior Therapy and Experimental Psychiatry, 20*(1), 31–39.

Hegel, M. T., & Ahles, T. A. (1992). Behavioral analysis and treatment of reflexive vomiting associated with visceral sensations: A case study of interoceptive conditioning? *Journal of Behavior Therapy and Experimental Psychiatry, 23*(3), 237–242.

Hegstrand, L. R., & Eichelman, B. (1981). Determination of rat brain tissue catecholamines using liquid chromatography with electrochemical detection. *Journal of Chromatography, 22*, 107–111.

Heide, F., & Borkovec, T. (1983). Relaxation induced anxiety. *Journal of Consulting and Clinical Psychology, 51*, 171–182.

Heisel, J. S. (1972). Life changes as etiologic factors in juvenile rheumatoid arthritis. *Journal of Psychosomatic Research, 17*, 411–420.

Helgeson, V. S. (1992). Moderators of the relation between perceived control and adjustment to chronic illness. *Journal of Personality and Social Psychology, 63*(4), 656–666.

Hellman, C. (1990). Overview of behavioral medicine. *Practical Reviews in Psychiatry*, Audiocassette volume 14.

Hellman, C. J., Budd, M., Borysenko, J., McClelland, D. C., & Benson, H. (1990). A study of the effectiveness of two group behavioral medicine interventions for patients with psychosomatic complaints. *Behavioral Medicine, 16*, 165–173.

Hemenover, S. H., & Dienstbier, R. A. (1996). The effects of an appraisal manipulation: Affect, intrusive cognitions, and performance for two cognitive tasks. *Motivation and Emotion, 20*, 319–340.

Heninger, G. R. (1995). Neuroimmunology of stress. In M. J. Friedman, D. Charney, & A. Deutch (Eds.), *Neurobiological, and clinical consequences of stress*, (pp. 381–402). Philadelphia: Lippincott-Raven.

Henke, P. G. (1992). Stomach pathology and the amygdala. In J. P. Aggleton (Ed.). *The amygdala* (pp. 323–338). New York: Wiley-Liss.

Hennekens, C. H., Buring, J. E., Manson, J. E., Stampfer, M., Rosner, B., Cook, N. R., Belanger, C., LaMotte, F., Gaziano, J. M., Ridker, P. M., Willett, W., & Peto, R. (1996). Lack of effect of long-term supplementation with beta carotene on the incidence of malignant neoplasms and cardiovascular disease. *New England Journal of Medicine, 334*(18), 1145–1149.

Henry, J. L., Wilson, P. H., Bruce, D. G., Chisholm, D. J., & Rawling, P. J. (1997). Cognitive-behavioural stress management for patients with non-insulin dependent diabetes mellitus. *Psychology, Health and Medicine, 2*(2), 109–118.

Henry, J. P., & Ely, D. (1976). Biologic correlates of psychosomatic illness. In R. Grenen & S. Galay (Eds.), *Biological foundations of psychiatry* (pp. 945–986). New York: Raven Press.

Henry, J. P., & Stephens, P. (1977). *Stress, health, and the social environment*. New York: Springer-Verlag.

Herbert, R., & Lehmann, D. (1977). Theta bursts: An EEG pattern in normal subjects practicing the transcendental meditation technique. *Electroencephalography and Clinical Neurophysiology, 42*, 245–252.

Herbert, T. B., & Cohen, S. (1993). Stress and immunity in humans: A meta-analytic review. *Psychosomatic Medicine, 55*, 364–379.

Herman, C., Blanchard, E. B., & Flor, H. (1997). Biofeedback treatment for pediatric migraine: Prediction of treatment outcome. *Journal of Consulting and Clinical Psychology, 65*(4), 611–616.

Hersen, M., & Barlow, D. (1976). *Single-case experimental designs*. Oxford, UK: Pergamon Press.

Hess, W. (1957). *The functional organization of the diencephalon*. New York: Grune & Stratton.

Hewitt, J. (1977). *The complete yoga book*. New York: Schocken.

Hill, L. E. (1930). *Philosophy of a biologist*. London: Arnold.

Hiroto, D. S. (1974). Locus of control and learned helplessness. *Journal of Experimental Psychology, 102*(2), 187–193.

Ho, D. D., Neumann, A. U., Perelson, A. S., Chen, W., Leonard, J. M., & Markowitz, M. (1995). Rapid turnover of plasma virions and CD4 lymphocytes in HIV-1 infection. *Nature, 373*, 123–126.

Hobbs, M., Mayou, R., Harrison, B., & Worlock, P. (1996). A randomized controlled trial of psychological debriefing for victims of road traffic accidents. *British Medical Journal, 313*, 1438–1439.

Hoch, F., Werle, E., & Weicker, H. (1988). Sympathoadrenergic regulation in elite fencers in training and competition. *International Journal of Sports Medicine, 9*, 141–145.

Hodis, H. N., Mack, W. J., LaBree, L., Cashin-Hemphill, L., Sevanian, A., Johnson, R., & Azen, S. P. (1995). Serial coronary angiographic evidence that antioxidant vitamin intake reduces progression of coronary artery atherosclerosis. *Journal of the American Medical Association, 273*(23), 1849–1854.

Hoffman, J., Benson, H., Arns, P., Stainbrook, G., Landsberg, L., Young, J., & Gill, A. (1982). Reduced sympathetic relaxation response. *Science, 215*, 190–192.

Holland, J. C., & Tross, S. (1987). Psychosocial considerations in the therapy of epidemic Kaposi's sarcoma. *Seminars in Oncology, 14*, 48–53.

Holloway, E. A. (1994). The role of the physiotherapist in the treatment of hyperventilation. In B. H. Timmons & R. Ley (Eds.), *Behavioral and psychological approaches to breathing disorders* (pp. 157–175). New York: Plenum Press.

Holmes, T. H., & Rahe, R. (1967). The social readjustment rating scale. *Journal of Psychosomatic Research, 11*, 213–218.

Holmes, T. H., & Wolff, H. G. (1952). Lift situations, emotions and backache. *Psychosomatic Medicine, 14*, 18–33.

Holmes, T. H., Trenting, T., & Wolff, H. (1951). Lift situations, emotions, and nasal disease. *Psychosomatic Medicine, 13*, 71–82.

Holroyd, J. (1987). How hypnosis may potentiate psychotherapy. *American Journal of Clinical Hypnosis, 29*, 194–200.

Holroyd, K. A., & Penzien, D. B. (1994). Psychosocial interventions in the management of recurrent headache disorders: I. Overview and effectiveness. *Behavioral Medicine, 20*(2), 53–63.

Horowitz, M. (1974). Stress response syndrome. *Archives of General Psychiatry, 31*, 768–781.

Horowitz, M., Wilner, N., Kaltreider, N., & Alvarez, W. (1980). Signs and symptoms to post-traumatic stress disorder. *Archives of General Psychiatry, 37*, 85–92.

Houldin, A. D., Lev, E., Prystowsky, M. B., Redei, E., & Lowery, B. J. (1991). Psychoneuroimmunology: A review of literature. *Holistic Nursing Practice, 5*(4), 10–21.

Humphrey, J., & Everly, G. S., Jr. (1980). Factor dimensions of stress responsiveness in male and female students. *Health Education, 11*, 38–39.

Hymes, A. (1980). Diaphragmatic breath control and post surgical care. *Research Bulletin of the Himalayan International Institute, 1*, 9–10.

Ide, B. A. (1996). Psychometric review of family disruption from Illness Scale. In B. H. Stamm (Ed.), *Measurement of stress trauma, and adaptation*. Lutherville, MD: Sidran Press.

Imboden, B. (1994). T lymphocytes and natural killer cells. In D. Stites, A. I. Terr, & T. G. Parslow (Eds.), *Basic and clinical immunology* (8th ed., pp. 94–104). Norwalk, CT: Appleton & Lange.

Ironson, G., Wynings, C., Schneiderman, N., Baum, A., Rodriguez, M., Greenwood, D., Benight, C., Antoni, M., LaPerriere, A., Huang, H., Klimas, N., & Fletcher, M. A. (1997). Posttraumatic stress symptoms, instrusive thoughts, loss, and immune function after Hurricane Andrew. *Psychosomatic Medicine, 59*, 128–141.

Irwin, M., Daniels, M., Smith, T. L., Bloom, E., & Weiner, H. (1987). Life events, depressive symptoms, and immune function. *American Journal of Psychiatry, 144*, 437–441.

Irwin, M., Lacher, U., & Caldwell, C. (1992). Depression and reduced natural killer cytotoxicity: A longitudinal study of depressed patients and control subjects. *Psychological Medicine, 22,* 1045–1050.

Isaacson, R. L. (1982). *The limbic system.* New York: Plenum Press.

Jacobs, D. S., Demott, W., Finly, P., Horvat, R., Kasten, B., & Tilzer, L. (1994). *Laboratory test handbook* (3rd ed.). Cleveland: Lexi-Comp.

Jacobs, G. D., Benson, H., & Friedman, R. (1996). Topographic EEG mapping of the relaxation response. *Biofeedback and Self-Regulation, 21*(2), 121–129.

Jacobsen, P. B., Bovbjerg, D. H., & Redd, W. H. (1993). Anticipatory anxiety in women receiving chemotherapy for breast cancer. *Health Psychology, 12*(6), 469–475.

Jacobsen, P. B., Bovbjerg, D. H., Schwartz, M. D., Andrykowski, M. A., Futterman, A. D., Gilewski, T., Norton, L., & Redd, W. H. (1993). Formation of food aversions in cancer patients receiving repeated infusions of chemotherapy. *Behaviour Research and Therapy, 31*(8), 739–748.

Jacobsen, P. B., Bovbjerg, D. H., Schwartz, M. D., Hudis, C. A., Gilewski, T. A., & Norton, L. (1995). Conditioned emotional distress in women receiving chemotherapy for breast cancer. *Journal of Consulting and Clinical Psychology, 63*(1), 108–114.

Jacobson, E. (1938). *Progressive relaxation.* Chicago: University of Chicago Press.

Jacobson, E. (1970). *Modern treatment of tense patients.* Springfield, IL: Charles C. Thomas.

Jacobson, E. (1978). *You must relax.* New York: McGraw-Hill.

Jakes, S. C., Hallam, R. S., Rachman, S., & Hinchcliffe, R. (1986). The effects of reassurance, relaxation training and distraction on chronic tinnitus sufferers. *Behavioural Research and Therapy, 24,* 497–507.

James, L. C., & Folen, R. A. (1996). EEG biofeedback as a treatment for chronic fatigue syndrome: A controlled case report. *Behavioral Medicine, 22*(2), 77–81.

Janoff-Bulman, R. (1988). Victims of violence. In S. Fisher & J. Reason (Eds.), *Handbook of life stress, cognition and health* (pp. 101–113). New York: Wiley.

Janoff-Bulman, R. (1992). *Shattered Assumptions.* New York: Free Press.

Jasper, H. (1949). Diffuse projection systems. *Electroencephalography and Clinical Neuropsychology, 1,* 405–420.

Jemmott, J. B., III. (1985). Psychoneuroimmunology: The new frontier [Special Issue, Health psychology: Emerging issues]. *American Behavioral Scientist, 28,* 497–509.

Jencks, B. (1977). *Your body: Biofeedback at its best.* Chicago: Nelson-Hall.

Jevning, R., Wallace, R. K., & Beidebach, M. (1992). The physiology of meditation: A review. A wakeful hypometabolic integrated response. *Neuroscience and Biobehavioral Reviews, 16,* 415–424.

Johnson, R. H. & Spalding, J. M. (1974). *Disorders of the autonomic nervous system.* Philadelphia: Davis.

Johnson, T. M., & Ouslander, J. G. (1999). Urinary incontinence in the older man. *Medical Clinics of North America, 83*(5), 1247–1266.

Johnson, W. B., DeVries, R., Ridley, C. R., Pettorini, D., & Peterson, D. R. (1994). The comparative efficacy of Christian and secular rational-emotive therapy with Christian clients. *Journal of Psychology and Theology, 22,* 130–140.

Johnston, M., Gilbert, P., Partridge, C., & Collins, J. (1992). Changing perceived control in patients with physical disabilities: An intervention study with patients receiving rehabilitation. *British Journal of Clinical Psychology, 31*(1), 89–94.

Jones, G. E., & Evans, P. A. (1981). Effectiveness of frontalis feedback training in producing general body relaxation. *Biological Psychology, 12*(4), 313–320.

Joseph, M. (1998). The effect of strong religious beliefs on coping with stress. *Stress Medicine, 14,* 219–224.

Joy, R. (1985). The effects of neurotoxicants on kindling and kindled seizures. *Fundamental and Applied Toxicology, 5,* 41–65.

Kabat-Zinn, J. (1993). Mindfulness meditation: Health benefits of an ancient Buddhist practice. In D. Coleman & J. Gurin (Eds.), *Mind–body medicine: How to use your mind for better health* (pp. 259–275). Yonkers, NY: Consumer Reports Books.

Kabat-Zinn, J., Lipworth, L., & Burney, R. (1985). The clinical use of mindfulness meditation for the self-regulation of chronic pain. *Journal of Behavioral Medicine, 8*(2), 163–190.

Kabat-Zinn, J., Massion, A. O., Kristeller, J., Peterson, L. G., Fletcher, K. E., Pbert, L., Lenderking, W. R., & Santorelli, S. F. (1992). Effectiveness of a meditation based stress reduction program in the treatment of anxiety disorders. *American Journal of Psychiatry, 149,* 936–943.

Kabat-Zinn, J., Wheeler, E., Light, T., Skillings, A., Scharf, M. J., Cropley, T. G., Hosmer, D., & Bernhard, J. D. (1998). Influence of a mindfulness meditation-based stress reduction intervention on rates of skin clearing in patients with moderate to severe psoriasis undergoing phototherapy (UVB) and photochemotherapy (PUVA). *Psychosomatic Medicine, 60*(5), 625–632.

Kamiya, J. (1969). Operant control of the EEG alpha rhythm and some of its reported effects on consciousness. In C. T. Tart (Ed.), *Altered states of consciousness* (pp. 507–517). New York: Wiley.

Kang, D. H., Coe, C. L., & McCarthy, D. O. (1996). Academic examinations significantly impact immune responses, but not lung function, in healthy and well-managed asthmatic adolescents. *Brain, Behavior, and Immunity, 10,* 164–181.

Kanner, A. D., Coyne, J. C., Schaefer, C., & Lazarus, R. S. (1981). Comparison of two modes of stress measurement: Daily hassles and uplifts versus major life events. *Journal of Behavioral Medicine, 4,* 1–39.

Kaplan, G. A., & Camacho, T. (1983). Perceived health and mortality: A nine-year follow-up of the Human Population Laboratory cohort. *American Journal of Epidemiology, 117,* 292–304.

Kaplan, K. H., Goldenberg, D. L., & Galvin-Nadeau, M. (1993). The impact of a meditation-based stress reduction program on fibromyalgia. *General Hospital Psychiatry, 15*(5), 284–289.

Kardiner, A. (1941). *The traumatic neuroses of war.* New York: Hoeber.

Kark, J. D., Goldman, S., & Epstein, L. (1995). Iraqi missle attacks on Israel. The association of mortality with a life-threatening stressor. *Journal of the American Medical Association, 273*(15), 1208–1210.

Katayama, M., Kobayashi, S., Kuramoto, N., & Yokoyama, M. M. (1987). Effects of hypothalamic lesions on lymphocyte subsets in mice. *Annals of the New York Academy of Sciences, 496,* 366–376.

Katzung, B. G. (1992). *Basic and clinical Pharmacology* (5th ed.). Norwalk, CT: Lange.

Kayser, A., Robinson, D., Nies, A., & Howard, D. (1985). Response to phenelzine among depressed patients with features of hysteroid dysphoria. *American Journal of Psychiatry, 142,* 486–488.

Keane, T., Malloy, P., & Fairbank, J. (1984). Empirical development of an MMPI scale for combat related PTSD. *Journal of Consulting and Clinical Psychology, 52,* 888–891.

Kelley, K. W. (1989). Growth hormone, lymphocytes and macrophages. *Biochemical Pharmacology, 38,* 705–713.

Kelley, K. W., Johnson, R. W., & Dantzer, R. (1994). Immunology discovers physiology. *Veterinary Immunology and Immunopathology, 43,* 157–165.

Kemeny, M. E. (1994). Psychoneuroimmunology of HIV infection. *Psychiatric Clinics of North America, 17*(1), 55–68.

Kemeny, M. E., Weiner, H., Duran, R., Taylor, S. E., Visscher, B., & Fahey, J. L. (1995). Immune system changes after the death of a partner in HIV-positive gay men. *Psychosomatic Medicine, 57*, 547–554.

Kenardy, J. A., Webster, R. A., Lewin, T. J., Carr, V. J., Hazell, P. L., & Carter, G. L. (1996). Stress debriefing and patterns of recovery following a natural disaster. *Journal of Traumatic Stress, 9*, 37–49.

Kendall, M. D. (1998). *Dying to live: How our bodies fight disease.* Cambridge, UK: Cambridge University Press.

Kent, J. M., Coplan, J. D., & Gorman, J. M. (1998). Clinical utility of the selective serotonin reuptake inhibitors in the spectrum of anxiety. *Biological Psychiatry, 44*, 812–824.

Kent, S., Bluthé, R. M., Dantzer, R., Hardwick, A. J., Kelley, K. W., Rothwell, N. J., & Vannice, J. L. (1992). Different receptor mechanisms mediate the pyrogenic and behavioral effect of interleukin-1. *Proceedings of the National Academy of Sciences, 89*, 9117–9120.

Kent, S., Bluthé, R. M., Kelley, K. W., & Dantzer, R. (1992). Sickness behavior as a new target for drug development. *Trends in Pharmacologic Science, 13*(1), 24–28.

Kesterson, J., & Clinch, N. F. (1989). Metabolic rate, respiratory exchange ratio and apneas during meditation. *American Journal of Physiology, 256*(3, Pt. 2), R632–R638.

Khan, A. U. (1977). Effectiveness of biofeedback and counterconditioning in the treatment of bronchial asthma. *Journal of Psychosomatic Research, 21*, 97–104.

Khansari, D. N., Murgo, A. J., & Faith, R. E. (1990). Effects of stress on the immune system. *Immunology Today, 11*, 170–175.

Kiecolt-Glaser, J. K., Dura, J. R., Speicher, C. E., Trask, O. J., & Glaser, R. (1991). Spousal caregivers of dementia victims: Longitudinal changes in immunity and health. *Psychosomatic Medicine, 53*, 345–362.

Kiecolt-Glaser, J. K., Fisher, L., Ogrocki, P., Stout, J. C., Speicher, C. E., & Glaser, R. (1987). Marital quality, marital disruption, and immune function. *Psychosomatic Medicine, 49*, 13–34.

Kiecolt-Glaser, J. K., Garner, W., Speicher, C., Penn, G. M., Holliday, J., & Glaser, R. (1984). Psychosocial modifiers of immunocompetence in medical students. *Psychosomatic Medicine, 46*, 7–13.

Kiecolt-Glaser, J. K., Kennedy, S., Malkoff, S., Fisher, L., Speicher, C. E., & Glaser, R. (1988). Marital discord and immunity in males. *Psychosomatic Medicine, 50*, 213–229.

Kiecolt-Glaser, J. K., Malarkey, W. B., Chee, M., Newton, T., Cacioppo, J. T., Hsiao-Yin, M. H, & Glaser, R. (1993). Negative behavior during marital conflict is associated with immunological down-regulation. *Psychosomatic Medicine, 55*, 395–409.

Kimble, G. A. (1961). *Hilgard and Marquis' conditioning and learning.* New York: Appleton–Century–Crofts.

Kirsch, I. (1996). Hypnotic enhancement of cognitive-behavioral weight loss treatments— another meta-reanalysis. *Journal of Consulting and Clinical Psychology, 64*, 517–519.

Kirsch, I., Montgomery, G., & Sapirstein, G. (1995). Hypnosis as an adjunct to cognitive-behavioral psychotherapy: A meta-analysis. *Journal of Consulting and Clinical Psychology, 63*, 214–220.

Kirtz, S., & Moos, R. H. (1974). Physiological effects of social environments. *Psychosomatic Medicine, 36*, 96–114.

Klajner, F., Hartman, L., & Sobell, M. (1984). Treatment of substance abuse by relaxation training. *Addictive Behaviors, 9*, 41–55.

Knapp, P. (1982). Pulmonary disorders and psychosocial stress. In W. Farm, I. Karacan, A. Pakorny, & R. Williams (Eds.), *Phenomenology and treatment of psychophysiological disorders* (pp. 15–34). New York: Spectrum.

Knekt, P., Heliovaara, M., Rissanen, A., Aromaa, A., & Aaran, R. K. (1992). Serum antioxidant vitamins and risk of cataracts. *British Medical Journal, 305,* 1392–1394.

Kobasa, S. (1979). Stressful life events, personality, and health. *Journal of Personality and Social Psychology, 37,* 1–11.

Kobasa, S., & Puccetti, M. (1983). Personality and social resources in stress resistance. *Journal of Personality and Social Psychology, 45,* 839–850.

Kocsis, A. (1996). Relaxation. In J. Green & A. McCreaner (Eds.), *Counselling in HIV infection and AIDS* (2nd ed., pp. 270–278). Cambridge, MA: Blackwell Scientific.

Koenig, H. G. (1997). *Is religion good for your health? The effects of religion on physical and mental health.* New York: Hayworth Pastoral Press.

Koenig, H. G., Cohen, J. J., Blazer, D. G., & Krishnan, K. R. R. (1995). Religious coping and cognitive symptoms of depression in elderly medical patients. *Psychosomatics, 36,* 369–375.

Koenig, H. G., Kvale, J. N., & Ferrel, C. (1988). Religion and well-being in later life. *The Gerontologist, 28,* 18–28.

Kolb, L. C. (1984). The post traumatic stress disorders of combat. *Military Medicine, 149,* 237–243.

Kolb, L. C. (1987). A neuropsychological hypothesis explaining post traumatic stress disorders. *American Journal of Psychiatry, 144,* 989–995.

Koltyn, K. F., Raglin, J. S., O'Conner, P. J., & Morgan, W. P. (1995). Influence of weight training on state anxiety, body awareness and blood pressure. *International Journal of Sports Medicine, 16,* 266–269.

Koolhaas, J. M., & Bohus, B. (1989). Social control in relation to neuroendocrine and immunological responses. In A. Steptoe & A. Appels (Eds.), *Stress, personal control and health* (pp. 295–304). Chichester, UK: Wiley.

Koolhaas, J. M., & Bohus, B. (1995). Animal models of stress and immunity. In B. E. Leonard & K. Miller (Eds.), *Stress, the immune system and psychiatry* (pp. 69–83). Chichester, UK: Wiley.

Kopin, L. (1976). Catecholamines, adrenal hormones, and stress. *Hospital Practice, 11,* 49–55.

Koss, M., & Shiang, J. (1994). Research on brief psychotherapy. In A. Bergin & S. Garfield (Eds.), *Handbook of psychotherapy and behavior change* (pp. 664–700). New York: Wiley.

Koss, M., Woodrugg, W. J., & Koss, P. (1991). Criminal victimization among primary care medical patients: Prevalence, incidence, and physician usage. *Behavioral Sciences and the Law, 9*(1), 85–96.

Krantz, D. S. (1980). Cognitive processes and recovery from heart attack: A review and theoretical analysis. *Journal of Human Stress, 6*(3), 27–38.

Krantz, D. S., Baum, A., & Wideman, M. V. (1980). Assessment for preferences for self-treatment and information in health care. *Journal of Personality and Social Psychology, 39,* 977–990.

Kraus, H., & Raab, W. (1961). *Hypokinetic disease.* Springfield, IL: Charles C. Thomas.

Kraus, R. P. (1997). Randomised controlled trial of psychological debriefing for victims of acute burn trauma: Comment. *British Journal of Psychiatry, 171,* 583.

Kristeller, J., & Hallett, B. C. (1999). An exploratory study of a meditation-based intervention for binge eating disorder. *Journal of Health Psychology, 4*(3), 357–363.

Krug, E. G., Kresnow, M., Peddicord, J., Dahlberg, L., Powell, K., Crosby, A., & Annest, J. (1998). Suicide after natural disasters. *New England Journal of Medicine, 338,* 373–378.

Kusnecov, A. V., Husband, A. J., & King, M. G. (1988). Behaviorally conditioned suppression of mitogen-induced proliferation and immunoglobulin production: Effect of time span between conditioning and reexposure to the conditioned stimulus. *Brain, Behavior and Immunity, 2,* 198–211.

Kutz, I., Borysenko, J., & Benson, H. (1985). Meditation and psychotherapy. *American Journal of Psychiatry, 142,* 1–8.

Lacey, J., & Lacey, B. (1958). Verification and extension of the principle of autonomic response-stereotype. *American Journal of Psychology, 71,* 50–73.

Lacey, J., & Lacey, B. (1962). The law of initial value in the longitudinal study of autonomic constitution. *Annals of the New York Academy of Sciences, 98,* 1257–1290.

Lachman, M. E., & Leff, R. (1989). Perceived control and intellectual functioning in the elderly: A 5-year longitudinal study. *Developmental Psychology, 25*(5), 722–728.

Lachman, S. (1972). *Psychosomatic disorders: A behavioristic interpretation.* New York: Wiley.

Lader, M. H. (1969). Psychophysiological aspects of anxiety. In M. H. Lader (Ed.), *Studies of anxiety* (pp. 53–61). Ashford, Kent, UK: Headly Brothers.

Lake, C. R., Ziegler, M., & Kopin, L. (1976). Use of plasma norepinephrine for evaluation of sympathetic neuronal function in man. *Life Sciences, 18,* 1315–1326.

Lang, I. M. (1975). *Limbic involvement in the vagosympathetic arterial pressor response of the rat.* Unpublished master's thesis, Temple University, Philadelphia.

Lang, R., Dehof, K., Meurer, K., & Kaufmann, W. (1979). Sympathetic activity and transcendental meditation. *Journal of Neural Transmission, 44,* 117–135.

Langer, E. J. (1975). The illusion of control. *Journal of Personality and Social Psychology, 32,* 311–328.

Langer, E. J., & Benevento, A. (1978). Self-induced dependence. *Journal of Personality and Social Psychology, 36*(8), 886–893.

Langer, E. J., & Rodin, J. (1976). The effects of choice and enhanced personal responsibility for the aged: A field experiment in an institutional setting. *Journal of Personality and Social Psychology, 34*(2), 191–198.

Langer, E. J., Janis, L. L., & Wolfer, J. A. (1975). Reduction of psychological stress in surgical patients. *Journal of Experimental Social Psychology, 11,* 155–165.

Langer, E. J., Rodin, J., Beck, P., Weinman, C., & Spitzer, L. (1979). Environmental determinants of memory improvement in late adulthood. *Journal of Personality and Social Psychology, 37*(11), 2003–2013.

Langsley, D., Machotka, P., & Flomenhaft, K. (1971). Avoiding mental health admission: A follow-up. *American Journal of Psychiatry, 127,* 1391–1394.

LaPerriere, A. R., Antoni, M. H., Schneiderman, N., Ironson, G., Klimas, N., Caralis, P., & Fletcher, M. A. (1990). Exercise intervention attenuates emotional distress and natural killer cell decrements following notification of positive serologic status for HIV-1. *Biofeedback and Self-Regulation, 15,* 229–242.

LaPerriere, A. R., Fletcher, M. A., Antoni, M. H., Klimas, N. G., Ironson, G., & Schneiderman, N. (1991). Aerobic exercise training in an AIDS risk group. *International Journal of Sports Medicine, 12*(Suppl. 1), S53–S57.

LaPerriere, A., Goldstein, A., Klimas, N., Ironson, G., Majors, P., Maik, G., Talluto, C., Fletcher, M. A., & Schneiderman, N. (1997). Non-compliant exercise decreases CD4+ cells in early symptomatic HIV-1 infection. *Proceedings of the Society of Behavior Medicine's Eighteenth Annual Meeting,* S059, PA 4E.

Larson, D. B., & Larson, S. S. (1994). *The forgotten factor in physical and mental health: What does the research show?* Rockville, MD: National Institute for Healthcare Research.

Latimer, P. (1985). Irritable bowel syndrome. In W. Dorfman & L. Cristofar (Eds.), *Psychosomatic illness review* (pp. 61–75). New York: Macmillan.

Laudenslager, M. L., Fleshner, M., Hofstadter, P., Held, P. E., Simons, L., & Maier, S. F. (1988). Suppression of specific antibody production by inescapable shock: Stability under varying conditions. *Brain, Behavior, and Immunity, 2,* 92–101.

Lavey, R., & Taylor, C. (1985). The nature of relaxation therapy. In S. Burchfield (Ed.), *Stress* (pp. 329–358). New York: Hemisphere.

Lazar, A. (1975). Effects of the TM program on anxiety, drug abuse, cigarette smoking and alcohol consumption. In D. Orme-Johnson, L. Domash, & J. Farrow (Eds.), *Scientific research on the TM program* (pp. 243–250). Geneva: MIV Press.

Lazarus, R. S. (1966). *Psychological stress and the coping process.* New York: McGraw-Hill.

Lazarus, R. S. (1975). A cognitively oriented psychologist looks at biofeedback. *American Psychologist, 30,* 553–561.

Lazarus, R. S. (1982). Thoughts on the relations between emotions and cognition. *American Psychologist, 37,* 1019–1024.

Lazarus, R. S. (1984). On the primacy of cognition. *American Psychologist, 39,* 124–129.

Lazarus, R. S. (1991). *Emotion and adaptation.* New York: Oxford University Press.

Lazarus, R. S. (1996). The role of coping in the emotions and how coping changes over the life course. In C. Magai & S. H. McFadden (Eds.), *Handbook of emotion, adult development, and aging* (pp. 289–306). New York: Academic Press.

Lazarus, R. S. (1999). *Stress and emotion: A new synthesis.* New York: Springer.

Lazarus, R. S., & Folkman, S. (1984). *Stress, appraisal, and coping.* New York: Springer.

Leahy, A., Clayman, C., Mason, I., Lloyd, G., & Epstein, O. (1998). Computerised biofeedback games: A new method for teaching stress management and its use in irritable bowel syndrome. *Journal of the Royal College of Physicians of London, 32*(6), 552–556.

Le Blanc, J. (1976, July). *The role of catecholamines in adaptation to chronic and acute stress.* Paper presented at the proceedings of the International Symposium on Catecholamines and Stress, Bratislava, Czechoslovakia.

LeDoux, J. E. (1992). Emotion and the amygdala. In J. P. Aggleton (Ed.), *The amygdala* (pp. 339–352). New York: Wiley-Liss.

Lee, C., Slade, P., & Lygo, V. (1996). The influence of psychological debriefing on emotional adaptation in women following early miscarriage. *British Journal of Psychiatry, 69,* 47–58.

Lee, I. M. (1994). Physical activity, fitness, and cancer. In C. Bouchard, R. J. Shephard, & T. Stephens (Eds.), *Physical activity, fitness, and health: International proceedings and consensus statement* (pp. 814–831). Champaign, IL: Human Kinetics.

Lee, I. M. (1995). Physical activity and cancer. *Physical Activity and Fitness Research Digest, 2,* 1–8.

Lee, K., Schottler, F., Oliver, M., & Lynch, G. (1980). Brief bursts of high-frequency stimulation produce two types of structural change in rat hippocampus. *Journal of Neurophysiology, 44,* 247–258.

Lehmann, J., Goodale, I., & Benson, H. (1986). Reduced pupillary sensitivity to topical phenylephrine associated with the relaxation response. *Journal of Human Stress, 12,* 101–104.

Lehrer, P. M. (1995). Recent research findings on stress management techniques. *Directions in Clinical Psychology, 5,* whole issue 9.

Lehrer, P. M., & Woolfolk, R. (1984). Are stress reduction techniques interchangable, or do they specific effects? In R. Woolfolk & P. Lehrer (Eds.), *Principles and practice of stress management* (pp. 404–477). New York: Guilford.

Lehrer, P. M., & Woolfolk, R. L. (1993). *Principles and practices of stress management* (2nd ed.). New York: Guilford.

Lehrer, P. M., Carr, R., Sargunaraj, D., & Woolfolk, R. L. (1994). Stress management techniques: Are they all equivalent, or do they have specific effects? *Biofeedback and Self-Regulation, 19*(4), 353–401.

Leor, J., Poole, W. K., & Kloner, R. A. (1996). Sudden cardiac death triggered by an earthquake. *New England Journal of Medicine, 334*(7), 413–419.

Leuner, H. (1969). Guided affective imagery. *American Journal of Psychotherapy, 23,* 4–21.

Levi, L. (1972). Psychosocial stimuli, psychophysiological reactions and disease. *Acta Medica Scandinavica* (entire Suppl. 528).

Levi, L. (1975). *Emotions: Their parameters and measurement.* New York: Raven Press.

Levi, L., & Andersson, L. (1975). *Psychosocial stress.* New York: Wiley.

Levin, P., Lazrove, S., & van der Kolk, B. (1999). What psychological testing and neuroimaging tell us about the treatment of posttraumatic stress disorder by eye movement desensitization and reprocessing. *Journal of Anxiety Disorders, 13*(1–2), 159–172.

Levine, L. J. (1996). The anatomy of disappointment: A natural test of appraisal models of sadness, anger, and hope. *Cognition and Emotion, 10,* 337–359.

Liebowitz, M., Quitkin, F. M., Stewart, J. W., McGrath, P. J., Harrison, W., Rabkin, J. G., Tricamo, E., Markowitz, J. S., & Klein, D. F. (1984). Psychopharmacologic validation of atypical depression. *Journal of Clinical Psychiatry, 45*(7), 22–25.

Lindsley, D. B. (1951). Emotion. In S. S. Stevens (Ed.), *Handbook of experimental psychology.* New York: Wiley.

Lindsley, D. B., & Sassaman, W. (1938). Autonomic activity and brain potentials associated with "voluntary" control of pilomotors. *Journal of Neurophysiology, 1,* 342–349.

Linn, M. W., Linn, B. S., & Jensen, J. (1984). Stressful events, dysphoric mood, and iuume responsiveness. *Psychological Reports, 54,* 219–222.

Lipke, H. (2000). *EMDR and psychotherapy integration: Theoretical and clinical suggestions with focus on traumatic stress.* Boca Raton, FL: CRC Press.

Lipowski, Z. J. (1984). What does the word "psychosomatic" really mean? *Psychosomatic Medicine, 46,* 153–171.

Lorig, K., & Fries, J. F. (1990). *The arthritis helpbook: A tested self-management program for coping with your arthritis.* Reading, MA: Addison-Wesley.

Lown, B., Temte, J. V., Reich, P., Gaughan, C., Regestein, Q., & Hai, H. (1976). Basis for recurring ventricular fibrillation in the absence of coronary heart disease and its management. *New England Journal of Medicine, 294,* 623–629.

Lubar, J. F. (1991). Discourse on the development of EEG diagnostics and biofeedback treatment for attention-deficit/hyperactivity disorders. *Biofeedback and Self-Regulation, 16,* 201–225.

Lubar, J. F. (1995). Neurofeedback for the management of attention-deficit/hyperactivity disorders. In M. Schwartz and Associates (Eds.), *Biofeedback: A practioner's guide* (2nd ed., pp. 493–522). New York: Guilford.

Lubar, J. F., & Deering, W. M. (1981). *Behavioral approaches to neurology.* New York: Academic Press.

Lubar, J. F., & Shouse, M. N. (1976). EEG and behavioral changes in a hyperkinetic child concurrent with training of the sensorimotor rhythm (SMR): A preliminary report. *Biofeedback and Self-Regulation, 3,* 293–306.

Lubar, J. F., Swartwood, M. O., Swartwood, J. N., & O'Donnell, P. H. (1995). Evaluation of the effectiveness of EEG neurofeedback training for ADHD in a clinical setting as measured by changes in T. O. V. A. scores, behavioral ratings, and WISC-R performance. *Biofeedback and Self-Regulation, 20*(1), 83–99.

Lucas, O. (1975). The use of hypnosis in hemophilia dental care. *Annals of the New York Academy of Sciences, 240,* 263–266.

Lum, L. C. (1975). Hyperventilation: The tip of the iceberg. *Journal of Psychosomatic Research, 19,* 375–383.

Lundberg, U., & Forsman, L. (1978). *Adrenal medullary and adrenal cortical responses to understimulation and overstimulation* (Report No. 541). Stockholm: Department of Psychology, University of Stockholm.

Luparello, T. J., Stein, M., & Park, D. E. (1964). A stereotaxic atlas of the hypothalamus of the guinea pig. *Journal of Comparative Neurology, 122,* 201–218.

Luria, A. R. (1958). *The mind of a mnemonist* (L. Solotaroff, trans.). New York: Basic Books.

Luthe, W. (Ed.). (1969). *Autogenic therapy* (Vols. I–VI). New York: Grune & Stratton.

Macht, M. (1996). Effects of high- and low-energy meals on hunger, physiological processes and reactions to emotional stress. *Appetite, 26*(1), 71–88.

Mackenzie, J. N. (1896). The production of the so-called "rose cold" by means of an artificial rose. *American Journal of Medical Science, 91,* 45–57.

MacLean, P. D. (1949). Psychosomatic disease and the "visceral brain." *Psychosomatic Medicine, 11*, 338–353.

MacLean, P. D. (1975). On the evolution of three mentalities. *Man–Environment System, 5*, 213–994.

Madison, D., & Nicoll, R. (1982). Noradrenaline blocks accommodation of pyramidal cell discharge in the hippocampus. *Nature, 299*, 636–638.

Mahl, C. F., & Brody, E. (1954). Chronic anxiety symptomatology, experimental stress and HCL secretion. *Archives of Neurological Psychiatry, 71*, 314–325.

Mahler, H. I., & Kulik, J. A. (1990). Preferences for health care involvement, perceived control, and surgical recovery: A prospective study. *Social Science and Medicine, 31*(7), 743–751.

Maier, S. F., Watkins, L. R., & Fleshner, M. (1994). Psychoneuroimmunology: The interface between behavior, brain, and immunity. *American Psychologist, 49*(12), 1004–1017.

Makara, G., Palkovits, M., & Szentagothal, J. (1980). The endocrine hypothalamus and the hormonal response to stress. In H. Selye (Ed.), *Selye's guide to stress research* (pp. 280–337). New York: Van Nostrand Reinhold.

Malmo, R. B. (1966). Studies of anxiety. In C. Spielberger (Ed.), *Anxiety and behavior* (pp. 157–177). New York: Academic Press.

Malmo, R. B. (1975). *On emotions, needs, and our archaic brain.* New York: Holt, Rinehart & Winston.

Malmo, R. B., & Shagass, C. (1949). Physiologic study of symptom mechanisms in psychiatric patients under stress. *Psychosomatic Medicine, 11*, 25–29.

Malmo, R. B., Shagass, C., & Davis, J. (1950). A method for the investigation of somatic response mechanisms in psychoneurosis. *Science, 112*, 325–328.

Mann, D. M. A. (1992). The neuropathology of the amygdala in ageing and in dementia. In J. P. Aggleton (Ed.), *The amygdala* (pp. 561–574). New York: Wiley-Liss.

Manuck, S. B., Marsland, A. L., Kaplan, J. R., & Williams, J. K. (1995). The pathogenicity of behavior and its neuroendocrine mediation: An example from coronary artery disease. *Psychosomatic Medicine, 57*(3), 275–283.

Manuck, S., & Krantz, D. (1984). Psychophysiologic reactivity in coronary artery disease. *Behavioral Medicine Update, 6*, 11–15.

Maranon, G. (1924). Contribution a l'etude de l'action emotive de l'ademaline. *Revue Francais d'Endrocrinologie, 2*, 301–325.

Marcus, B. H., Eaton, C. A., Rossi, J. S., & Harlow, L. L. (1994). Self-efficacy, decision making, and stages of change: An integrated model to physical exercise. *Journal of Applied Social Psychology, 24*, 489–508.

Marcus, S., Marquis, P., & Sakai, C. (1997). Controlled study of treatment of PTSD using EMDR in HMO setting. *Psychotherapy, 34*, 307–315.

Mariela, S. C., Matt, D. A., & Burish, T. G. (1992). Comparison of frontalis, multiple muscle site, and reactive muscle site feedback in reducing arousal under stressful and nonstressful conditions. *Medical Psychotherapy: An International Journal, 5*, 133–148.

Markus, C., Panhuysen, G., Tuiten, A., Koppeschaar, H., Fekkes, D., & Peters, M. (1998). Does carbohydrate-rich, protein-poor food prevent a deterioration of mood and cognitive performance of stress-prone subjects when subjected to a stressful task? *Appetite, 31*(1), 49–65.

Martinsen, E. G., & Morgan, W. P. (1997). Antidepressant effects of physical activity. In W. Morgan (Ed.), *Physical activity and mental health* (pp. 93–106). Washington, DC: Taylor & Francis.

Maslow, A. H. (1970). *Motivation and personality.* New York: Harper & Row.

Mason, J. B. (1971). A re-evaluation of the concept of non-specificity in stress theory. *Journal of Psychiatric Research, 8*, 323–333.

Mason, J. W. (1968a). A review of psychendocrine research on the sympathetic–adrenal medullary system. *Psychosomatic Medicine, 30,* 631–653.

Mason, J. W. (1968b). Organization of psychoendocrine mechanisms. *Psychosomatic Medicine, 30* (entire P. 2).

Mason, J. W. (1968c). A review of psychoendocrine research on the pituitary–adrenal–cortical system. *Psychosomatic Medicine, 30,* 576–607.

Mason, J. W. (1972). Organization of psychoendocrine mechanisms: A review and reconsideration of research. In N. Greenfield & R. Sternbach (Eds.), *Handbook of psychophysiology* (pp. 3–76). New York: Holt, Rinehart & Winston.

Mason, J. W., Maher, J., Hartley, L., Mougey, E., Perlow, M., & Jones, L. (1976). Selectivity of corticosteroid and catecholamine responses to various natural stimuli. In G. Servan (Ed.), *Psychopathology of human adaptation* (pp. 147–171). New York: Plenum Press.

Mason, J. W., Wang, S., Yehuda, R., Bremner, J. D., Riney, S., Lubin, H., Johnson, D. R., Southwick, S. M., & Charney, D. (1995). Some approaches to the study of clinical implications of thyroid alterations in post-traumatic stress disorder. In M. J. Friedman, D. Charney, & A. Deutch (Eds.), *Neurobiological, and clinical consequences of stress,* (pp. 367–380). Philadelphia: Lippincott-Raven.

Matthews, D. A., Larson, D. B., & Barry, C. P. (1993). *The faith factor: An annotated bibliography of clinical research on spiritual subjects* (Vol. 1). John Templeton Foundation.

Mayne, S. T. (1996). Beta carotene, carotenoids, and disease prevention in humans. *The FASEB Journal, 10,* 690–701.

Mayne, S. T., & Goodwin, W. J. (1993). Chemoprevention of head and neck cancer. *Current Opinion in Otolaryngology, Head and Neck Surgery, 1,* 126–132.

Mayou, R. A., Ehlers, A., & Hobbs, M. (2000). Psychological debriefing for road traffic accident victims: Three-year follow-up of a randomised controlled trial. *British Journal of Psychiatry, 176,* 589–593.

McCabe, P., & Schneiderman, N. (1984). Psychophysiologic reactions to stress. In N. Schneiderman & J. Tapp (Eds.), *Behavioral medicine* (pp. 3–32). Hillsdale, NJ: Erlbaum.

McCain, N. L., & Zeller, J. M. (1996). Psychoneuroimmunological studies in HIV disease. *Annual Review of Nursing Research, 14,* 23–55.

McCaul, K., Solomon, S., & Holmes, D. (1979). The effects of paced respiration and expectations on physiological responses to threat. *Journal of Personality and Social Psychology, 37,* 564–571.

McClelland, D. C., & Cheriff, A. D. (1997). The immunoenhancing effects of humor on secretory IgA and resistance to respiratory infections. *Psychology and Health, 12*(3), 329–344.

McClelland, D. C., Ross, G., & Patel, V. (1985). The effect of an academic examination on salivary norepinephrine and immunoglobulin levels. *Journal of Human Stress, 11,* 52–59.

McClure, C. (1959). Cardiac arrest through volition. *California Medicine, 90,* 440–448.

McDaniel, J. S. (1992). Psychoimmunology: Implications for future research. *Southern Medical Journal, 85*(4), 388–396.

McDermott, W. (1987). The diagnosis of PTSD using the MCMI. In C. Green (Ed.), *Proceedings of the conference on the Millon inventories* (pp. 257–262). Minneapolis: National Computer Systems.

McDonald, D. G., & Hodgdon, J. A. (1991). *The psychological effects of aerobic fitness training: Research and theory.* New York: Springer-Verlag.

McDowell, B. J., Engberg, S., Sereika, S., Donovan, N., Jubeck, M. E., Weber, E., & Engberg, R. (1999). Effectiveness of behavioral therapy to treat incontinence in homebound older adults. *Journal of the American Geriatric Society, 47*(3), 309–318.

McFarlane, A. C. (1988). The longitudinal course of posttraumatic morbidity. *Journal of Nervous and Mental Disease, 176,* 30–39.

McGinnis, J. M., & Foege, W. H. (1993). Actual causes of death in the United States. *Journal of the American Medical Association, 270,* 2207–2212.

McGrady, A., Graham, G., & Bailey, B. (1996). Biofeedback-assisted relaxation in insulin-dependent diabetes: A replication and extension study. *Annals of Behavioral Medicine, 18*(3), 185–189.

McGrath, P. J. (1999). Clinical psychology issues in migraine headaches. *Canadian Journal of the Neurological Sciences, 26*(Suppl. 3), S33–S36.

McGuigan, F. J. (1991). *Calm down: A guide for stress and tension control* (rev. ed.). Dubuque, IA: Kendall/Hunt.

McGuigan, F. J. (1993). Progressive relaxation: Origins, principles, and clinical applications. In P. M. Lehrer & R. L. Woolfolk (Eds.), *Principles and practices of stress management* (2nd ed.), pp. 17–52. New York: Guilford.

McGuire, E. J. (1996). Stress incontinence: New alternatives. *International Journal of Fertility and Menopausal Studies, 41*(2), 142–147.

McKerns, K., & Pantic, V. (1985). *Neuroendocrine correlates of stress.* New York: Plenum Press.

McNair, D., Lorr, M., & Droppleman, L. (1971). *Profile of mood states manual.* San Diego: Educational and Industrial Testing Service.

McNeil, F. (1996). Psychometric review of Common Grief Response Questionnaire. In B. H. Stamm (Ed.). *Measurement of stress trauma, and adaptation.* Lutherville, MD: Sidran Press.

Meany, J., McNamara, M., Burks, V., Berger, T. W., & Sayle, D. M. (1988). Psychological treatment of an asthmatic patient in crisis: Dreams, biofeedback, and pain behavior modification. *Journal of Asthma, 25*(3), 141–151.

Medansky, R. S. (1971). Emotion and the skin. *Psychosomatics, 12,* 326–329.

Medical Economics. (1998). *PDR for herbal medicines.* Montvale, New Jersey: Author.

Meehl, P. (1973). *Psychodiagnosis.* New York: Norton.

Mefferd, R. (1979). The developing biological concept of anxiety. In W. Fann, I. Karacan, A. D. Porkorny, & R. L. Williams (Eds.), *Phenomenology and treatment of anxiety* (pp. 111–124). New York: Spectrum.

Meichenbaum, D. (1977). *Cognitive-behavior modification.* New York: Plenum Press.

Meichenbaum, D. (1985). *Stress innoculation training.* New York: Plenum Press.

Meichenbaum, D. (1993). Stress inoculation training: A 20-year update. In P. M. Lehrer & R. L. Woolfolk (Eds.), *Principles and practice of stress management* (2nd ed., pp. 373–406). New York: Guilford.

Meichenbaum, D. (1994). *A clinical handbook/practical therapist manual for assessing and treating adults with posttraumatic stress disorder.* Waterloo: Institute.

Meichenbaum, D. (1995). Changing conceptions of cognitive behavior modification: Retrospect and prospect. In M. Mahoney (Ed.), *Cognitive and constructive psychotherapies: Theory, research, and practice* (pp. 20–26). New York: Springer.

Meichenbaum, D., & Jaremko, M. (1983). *Stress reduction and prevention.* New York: Plenum Press.

Meichenbaum, D., & Turk, D. (1987). *Facilitating treatment adherence.* New York: Plenum Press.

Meichenbaum, D., & Turk, D. (1987). *Facilitating treatment adherence.* New York: Plenum Press.

Metal'nikov, S., & Chorine, V. (1926). Role des reflexes conditionnels dans l'immunite. *Annales de l'Institute Pasteur, Paris, 40,* 893–900.

Metal'nikov, S., & Chorine, V. (1928). Role des relexes conditionnels dans la formation des anticorps. *Comptes Rendus des Seances de la Societe de Biologie et de Ses Filales, 102,* 133–134.

Metalsky, G. I., & Joiner, Jr., T. E. (1992). Vulnerability to depressive symptomatology: A prospective test of the diathesis–stress and causal mediation components of the hopelessness theory of depression. *Journal of Personality and Social Psychology, 63*(4), 667–675.

Metalsky, G. I., & Joiner, T. E. (1997). The hopelessness depression symptom questionnaire. *Cognitive Therapy and Research, 21*(3), 359–384.

Michaels, R., Haber, M., & McCann, D. (1976). Evaluation of transcendental meditation as a method of reducing stress. *Science, 192*, 1242–1244.

Michaels, R., Parra, J., McCann, D., & Vander, A. (1979). Renin, cortisol, and aldosterone during Transcendental Meditation. *Psychosomatic Medicine, 41*, 49–54.

Miehlke, A. (1973). *Surgery of the facial nerve*. Philadelphia: Saunders.

Miller, D. K., & Allen, T. E. (1995). *Fitness: A lifetime commitment* (5th ed.). Boston: Allyn & Bacon.

Miller, J. J., Fletcher, K., & Kabat-Zinn, J. (1995). Three-year follow-up and clinical implications of a mindfulness meditation-based stress reduction intervention in the treatment of anxiety disorders. *General Hospital Psychiatry, 17*(3), 192–200.

Miller, L. (1999). Critical incident stress debriefing: Clinical applications and new directions. *International Journal of Emergency Mental Health, 1*, 253–265.

Miller, L., & Smith, A. (1982). *The Stress Audit Questionnaire*. Boston: Neuromedical Consultants.

Miller, N. E. (1969). Learning of visceral and glandular responses. *Science, 163*, 434–445.

Miller, N. E. (1978). Biofeedback and visceral learning. *Annual Review of Psychology, 29*, 373–404.

Miller, N. E. (1979). General discussion and a review of recent results with paralyzed patients. In R. Gatchel & K. Price (Eds.), *Clinical applications of biofeedback* (pp. 215–225). Oxford, UK: Pergamon Press.

Miller, N. E., & Dworkin, B. (1977). Critical issues in therapeutic applications of biofeedback. In G. Schwartz & J. Beatty (Eds.), *Biofeedback: Theory and research* (pp. 129–162). Chicago: Aldine.

Miller, N. E., & Dworkin, B. R. (1974). Visceral learning: Recent difficulties with curarized rats and significant problems for human research. In P. A. Obrist, A. H. Black, J. Brener, & L. V. DiCara (Eds.), *Cardiovascular psychophysiology* (pp. 313–331). Chicago: Aldine.

Miller, R. M., & Chang, M. W. (1999). Advances in the management of dysphagia caused by stroke. *Physical Medicine and Rehabilitation Clinics of North America, 10*(4), 925–941.

Millon, T. (1981). *Disorders of personality: DSM-III, Axis II*. New York: Wiley.

Millon, T. (1983). *Millon Clinical Multiaxial Inventory manual* (3rd ed.). Minneapolis: National Computer Systems.

Millon, T. (1996). *Disorders of personalit* (2nd ed.). New York: Wiley.

Millon, T. (1997). *Millon clinical multiaxial inventory—III* (2nd ed.). Minneapolis: NCS.

Millon, T., & Everly, G. S., Jr. (1985). *Personality and its disorders*. New York: Wiley.

Millon, T., & Everly, G., Jr. (1985). *Personality and its disorders*. New York: Wiley.

Millon, T., Crossman, S., Meagher, S., Millon, C., & Everly, G. S., Jr. (1999). *Personality-guided therapy*. New York: Wiley.

Millon, T., Green, C. J., & Meagher, R. B. (1982). *Millon Behavioral Health Inventory manual* (3rd ed.). Minneapolis: National Computer Systems.

Millon, T., Grossman, S., Meagher, S., Millon, C., & Everly, G. S., Jr. (1999). *Personality-guided therapy*. New York: Wiley.

Mirowsky, J. (1995). Age and the sense of control. *Social Psychology Quarterly, 58*(1), 31–43.

Mitchell, C. M., & Drossman, D. (1987). The irritable bowel syndrome. *Annals of Behavioral Medicine, 9*, 13–18.

Mitchell, J. T. (1983). When disaster strikes ... the Critical Incident Stress Debriefing process. *Journal of Emergency Medical Services, 8*, 36–39.

Mitchell, J. T. (1983). When disaster strikes ... The Critical Incident Stress Debriefing process. *Journal of Emergency Medical Services, 8*(1), 36–39.

Mitchell, J. T., & Everly, G. S. (2000). The CISD and CISM: Evolution, effects and outcomes. In B. Raphael & J. Wilson (Eds.), *Psychological debriefing* (pp. 71–90). Cambridge: Cambridge University Press.

Mitchell, J. T., & Everly, G. S. (1997). Scientific evidence for CISM. *Journal of Emergency Medical Services, 22,* 87–93.

Mitchell, J. T., & Everly, G. S., Jr. (2001). *Critical Incident Stress Debriefing: An operational guide to group crisis intervention.* Ellicott City, MD: Chevron.

Mitchell, J. T., Schiller, G., Eyler, V., & Everly, G. S., Jr. (1999). Community crisis intervention: The Coldenham tragedy revisited. *International Journal of Emergency Mental Health, 1,* 227–236.

Mittelman, B., & Wolff, H. G. (1942). Emotions and gastroduodenal function. *Psychosomatic Medicine, 4,* 5–19.

Mittleman, M. A., Maclure, M., Sherwood, J. B., Mulry, R. P., Tofler, G. H., Jacobs, S. C., Friedman, R., Benson, H., & Muller, J. E. (1995). Triggering of acute myocardial infarction onset by episodes of anger. Determinants of myocardial infarction onset study investigators. *Circulation, 92*(7), 1720–1725.

Monroe, R. (1970). *Episodic behavioral disorders.* Cambridge, MA: Harvard University Press.

Monroe, R. (1982). Limbic ictus and atypical psychosis. *Journal of Nervous and Mental Disease, 170,* 711–716.

Monroe, S. (1983). Major and minor life events as predictors of psychological distress. *Journal of Behavioral Medicine, 6,* 189–206.

Moore, J. I. (1992). *Pharmacology.* New York: Springer-Verlag.

Moore, N. (1965). Behavior therapy in bronchial asthma: A controlled study. *Journal of Psychosomatic Research, 1,* 257–276.

Moos, R., & Engel, B. (1962). Psychophysiological reactions in hypertensive and arthritic patients. *Journal of Psychosomatic Research, 6,* 222–241.

Moran, M. G. (1995). Pulmonary and rheumatologic diseases. In A. Stoudemire (Ed.), *Psychological factors affecting medical conditions* (pp. 141–158). Washington, DC: American Psychiatric Press.

Morris, M. C., Beckett, L. A., Scherr, P. A., Hebert, L. E., Bennett, D. A., Field, T. S., & Evans, D. A. (1998). Vitamin E and vitamin C supplement use and risk of incident Alzheimer disease. *Alzheimer Disease and Associated Disorders, 12,* 121–126.

Moser, D. K., Dracup, K., Woo, M. A., & Stevenson, L. W. (1997). Voluntary control of vascular tone by using skin-temperature biofeedback-relaxation in patients with advanced heart failure. *Alternative Therapies in Health and Medicine, 3*(1), 51–59.

Mossey, J. M., & Shapiro, E. (1982). Self-rated health: A predictor of mortality among the elderly. *American Journal of Public Health, 72*(8), 800–808.

Moynihan, J. A., Brenner, G. J., Cocke, R., Karp, J. D., Breneman, S. M., Dopp, J. M., Ader, R., Cohen, N., Grota, L. J., & Felten, S. Y. (1994). Stress-induced modulation of immune function in mice. In R. Glaser & J. K. Kiecolt-Glaser (Eds.), *Handbook of human stress and immunity* (pp. 1–22). New York: Academic Press.

Mullen, B. (1989). *Advanced BASIC meta-analysis.* Hillsdale, NJ: Erlbaum.

Mullen, B. (1989). *BASIC Meta-analysis.* Hillsdale, NJ: Erlbaum.

Muller, N., & Ackenheil, M. (1995). The immune system and schizophrenia. In B. Leonard & K. Miller (Eds.), *Stress, the immune system and psychiatry* (pp. 137–164). Chichester, UK: Wiley.

Murphy, M., & Donovan, S. (1984). *Contemporary meditation research.* San Francisco: Esalen Institute.

Murphy, M., & Donovan, S. (1988). *The physical and psychological effects of meditation* (2nd ed.). San Rafael, CA: Esalen Institute Study of Exceptional Functioning.

Murray, C. J. L., & Lopez, A. D. (Eds.). (1996) *The global burden of disease.* Cambridge, MA: Harvard School of Public Health.

Musaph, H. (1977). Itching and other dermatoses. In E. Wittower & H. Wames (Eds.), *Psychosomatic medicine* (pp. 307–316). New York: Harper & Row.

Myers, D. (2001). Weapons of mass destruction and terrorism: Mental health consequences and implications for planning and services. In *American Red Cross* (Ed.), *The ripple Effects from Ground Zero: Coping with mental health needs in times of tragedy and terror.* Washington, DC: ARC.

Nance, D. M., Rayson, D., & Carr, R. I. (1987). The effects of lesions in the lateral septal and hippocampal areas on the humoral immune response of adult female rats. *Brain, Behavior, and Immunity, 1,* 292–305.

Naranjo, C., & Ornstein, R. (1971). *On the psychology of meditation.* New York: Viking.

Nauta, W. (1979). Expanding borders of the limbic system concept. In T. Rasmussen & R. Marino (Eds.), *Functional neurosurgery* (pp. 7–23). New York: Raven Press.

Nauta, W., & Domesick, V. (1982). Neural associations of the limbic system. In A. Beckman (Ed.), *Neural substrates of behavior* (pp. 3–29). New York: Spectrum.

Newman, E. C. (2000). Group crisis intervention in a school setting following an attempted suicide. *International Journal of Emergency Mental Health, 2,* 97–100.

Niaura, R., & Goldstein, M. G. (1995). Cardiovascular disease, Part II: Coronary artery disease and sudden death and hypertension. In A. Stoudemire (Ed.), *Psychological factors affecting medical conditions* (pp. 39–56). Washington, DC: American Psychiatric Press.

North, T. C., McCullagh, P., & Tran, Z. V. (1990). Effects of exercise on depression. *Exercise and Sport Sciences Reviews, 18,* 379–415.

O'Halloran, J. P., Jevning, R., Wilson, A. F., Skowsky, R., Alexander, C., & Walsh, R. N. (1985). Hormonal control in a state of decreased activation: Potentiation of arginine vasopressin secretion. *Physiology and Behavioral, 35,* 591–595.

Occupational Safety and Health Administration. (1996). *Guidelines for preventing workplace violence for health care and social service workers—OSHA 3148-1996.* Washington, DC: Author.

Occupational Safety and Health Administration. (1998). *Recommendations for workplace violence prevention programs in late-night retail establishments—OSHA 3153-1998.* Washington, DC: Author.

Ogden, E., & Shock, N. (1939). Voluntary hypercirculation. *American Journal of the Medical Sciences, 98,* 329–342.

Omer, H., & Everly, G. S., Jr. (1988). Psychological influences on pre-term labor. *American Journal of Psychiatry, 145*(12), 1507–1513.

Orme-Johnson, D., & Farrow, J. (1978). *Scientific research on the transcendental meditation program* [Collected paper]. New York: Maharishi International University Press.

Ornish, D. (1990). *Dr. Dean Ornish's program for reversing heart disease.* New York: Ballantine.

Ornish, D., Schwerwitz, L. W., Billings, J. H., Gould, L., Merritt, T. A., Sparler, S., Armstrong, W. T., Ports, T. A., Kirkeeide, R. L., Hogeboom, C., & Brand, R. J. (1998). Intensive lifestyle changes for reversal of coronary heart disease. *Journal of the American Medical Association, 280,* 2001–2007.

Ornstein, R. (1972). *The psychology of consciousness.* San Francisco: Freeman.

Overmier, J. B., & Seligman, M. E. P. (1967). Effects of inescapable shock upon subsequent escape and avoidance learning. *Journal of Comparative and Physiological Psychology, 63,* 28–33.

Oxman, T. E., Freeman, D. H., & Manheimer, E. D. (1995). Lack of social participation or religious strength and comfort as risk factors for death after cardiac surgery in the elderly. *Psychosomatic Medicine, 57,* 5–15.

Packard, R. C., & Ham, L. P. (1996). EEG biofeedback in the treatment of Lyme disease: A case study. *Journal of Neurotherapy, 1*(3), 22–31.

Paffenbarger, R. S., Hyde, R., & Wing, A. (1986). Physical activity, all-cause mortality, and longevity of college alumni. *New England Journal of Medicine, 314,* 605–613.

Pagano, R. (1981). Recent research in the physiology of meditation. In G. Adam, I. Meszaros, & E. Banyai (Eds.), *Brain and behavior: Advances in physiological sciences* (Vol. 17, pp. 443–451). Budapest: Pergamon Press.

Palan, B., & Chandwani, S. (1989). Coping with examination stress through hypnosis: An experimental study. *American Journal of Clinical Hypnosis, 31*, 173–180.

Papez, J. (1937). A proposed mechanism of emotion. *Archives of Neurology and Psychiatry, 38*, 725–743.

Parad, L., & Parad, H. (1968). A study of crisis oriented planned short-term treatment: Part II. *Social Casework, 49*, 418–426.

Pargament, K. I. (1990). God help me: Toward a theoretical framework of coping for the psychology of religion. *Research in the Social Scientific Study of Religion, 2*, 195–224.

Pargament, K. I., Echemendia, R. J., Johnson, S., Cook, P., McGath, C., Myers, J., & Brannick, M. (1987). The conservative church: Psychological advantages and disadvantages. *American Journal of Community Psychology, 15*, 269–286.

Parkinson, B., & Manstead, A. S. R. (1992). Appraisal as a cause of emotion. In M. Clark (Ed.), *Emotion* (pp. 122–149). Newbury Park, CA: Sage.

Parslow, T. G. (1994). Lymphocytes and lymphoid tissues. In D. Stites, A. I. Terr, & T. G. Parslow (Eds.), *Basic and clinical immunology* (8th ed., pp. 22–39). Norwalk, CT: Appleton & Lange.

Partridge, C., & Johnston, M. (1989). Perceived control of recovery from physical disability: Measurement and prediction. *British Journal of Clinical Psychology, 28*, 53–60.

Pate, R. R., Pratt, M., Blair, S. N., Haskell, W. L., Macera, C. A., Bouchard, C., Buchner, D., Ettinger, W., Heath, G. W., King, A. C., Kriska, A., Leon, A. S., Marcus, B. H., Morris, J., Paffenbarger, R. S., Partrick, K., Pollock, M. L., Rippe, J. M., Sallis, J., & Wilmore, J. H. (1995). Physical activity and public health: A recommendation from the centers for disease control and prevention and the American College of Sports Medicine. *Journal of the American Medical Association, 273*, 402–407.

Patel, C. (1993). Yoga-based therapy. In P. M. Lehrer & R. L. Woolfolk (Eds.), *Principles and practice of stress management* (2nd ed., pp. 89–137). New York: Guilford.

Patel, C., & Marmot, M. (1988). Can general practitioners use training in relaxation and management of stress to reduce mild hypertension? *British Medical Journal, 296*, 21–24.

Paul, G. (1967). Strategy of outcome research in psychotherapy. *Journal of Consulting and Clinical Psychology, 31*, 109–118.

Paykel, E., Myers, J., Dienelt, M., Klerman, G., Lindenthal, J., & Pepper, J. (1969). Life events and depression: A controlled study. *Archives of General Psychiatry, 21*, 753–760.

Peek, C. J. (1995). A primer of biofeedback instrumentation. In M. S. Schwartz & associates (Eds.), *Biofeedback: A practioner's guide* (pp. 45–95). New York: Guilford.

Peeters, M. C. W., Buunk, B. P., & Schaufeli, W. B. (1995). The role of attributions in the cognitive appraisal of work-related stressful events: An event-recording approach. *Work and Stress, 9*, 463–474.

Pekala, R. J., & Forbes, E. J. (1988). Hypnoidal effects associated with several stress management techniques. *Australian Journal of Clinical and Experimental Hypnosis, 16*, 121–132.

Pekala, R. J., & Forbes, E. J. (1990). Subjective effects of several stress management strategies: With reference to attention. *Behavioral Medicine, 16*, 39–43.

Pekala, R. J., Forbes, E. J., & Contrisciani, P. A. (1988). Assessing the phenomenological effects of several stress management strategies. *Imagination, Cognition and Personality, 8*, 265–281.

Penfield, W. (1975). *The mystery of the mind*. Princeton, NJ: Princeton University Press.

Peniston, E. G., & Kulkosky, P. J. (1999). Neurofeedback in the treatment of addictive disorders. In J. R. Evans (Ed.), *Introduction to quantitative EEG and neurofeedback* (pp. 157–179). San Diego: Academic Press.

Pennebaker, J. (1999). Effects of traumatic disclosure on physical and mental health. *International Journal of Emergency Mental Health, 1*, 9–18.

Pennebaker, J. W. (1999). The effects of traumatic exposure on physical and mental health: The values of writing and talking about upsetting events. *International Journal of Emergency Mental Health, 1*, 9–18.

Pennebaker, J. W., & Beall, S. K. (1986). Confronting a traumatic event: Toward an understanding of inhibition and disease. *Journal of Abnormal Psychology, 95*, 274–281.

Pennebaker, J. W., Kiecolt-Glaser, J. K., & Glaser, R. (1988). Disclosure of traumas and immune function: Health implications for psychotherapy. *Journal of Consulting and Clinical Psychology, 56*(2), 239–245.

Péronnet, F., & Szabo, A. (1993). Sympathetic response to acute psychosocial stressors in humans: Linkage to physical exercise and training. In P. Seraganian (Ed.), *Exercise psychology: The influence of physical exercise on psychological processes*. New York: Wiley.

Perry, S., Fishman, B., Jacobsberg, L., & Frances, A. (1992). Relationships over 1 year between lymphocyte subsets and psychosocial variables among adults with infection by human immunodeficiency virus. *Archives of General Psychiatry, 49*, 396–401.

Peterson, C., & Seligman, M. E. P. (1984). Causal explanations as a risk factor for depression: Theory and evidence. *Psychological Review, 91*(3), 347–374.

Pitts, F., & McClure, J. (1967). Lactate metabolism in anxiety neurosis. *New England Journal of Medicine, 277*, 1329–1336.

Platman, S. R. (1999). Psychopharmacology and posttraumatic stress disorder. *International Journal of Emergency Mental Health, 3*, 195–199.

Polivy, J., & Herman, C. P. (1999). Distress and eating: Why do dieters overeat? *International Journal of Stress Management, 5*(1), 57–75.

Post, R. (1985). Stress sensitization, kindling, and conditioning. *Behavioral and Brain Sciences, 8*, 372–373.

Post, R. (1986). Does limbic system dysfunction play a role in affective illness? In B. Doane & K. Livingston (Eds.), *The limbic system* (pp. 229–249). New York: Raven Press.

Post, R. M., Weiss, S., & Smith, M. (1995). Sensitization and kindling. In M. J. Friedmean, D. Charney, & A. Deutch (Eds.), *Neurobiological, and clinical consequences of stress* (pp. 203–224). Philadelphia: Lippincott-Raven.

Post, R., & Ballenger, J. (1981). Kindling models for the progressive development of psychopathology. In H. van Pragg (Ed.), *Handbook of biological psychiatry* (pp. 609–651). New York: Marcel Dekker.

Post, R., Rubinow, D., & Ballenger, J. (1986). Conditioning and sensitisation in the longitudinal course of affective illness. *British Journal of Psychiatry, 149*, 191–201.

Post, R., Uhde, T., Putnam, F., Ballenger, J., & Berrettini, W. (1982). Kindling and carbamazepine in affective illness. *Journal of Nervous and Mental Disease, 170*, 717–731.

Powell, L. (1984). Type A behavior pattern: An update on conceptual assessment and intervention research. *Behavioral Medicine Update, 6*, 7–10.

Praeger-Decker, I., & Decker, W. (1980). Efficacy of muscle relaxation in combating stress. *Health Education, 11*, 39–42.

Pratico, D., Tangirala, R. K., Rader, D. J., Rokach, J., & Fitzgerald, G. A. (1998). Vitamin E suppresses isoprostane generation *in vivo* and reduces atherosclerosis in ApoE-deficient mice. *National Medicine, 4*(10), 1189–1192.

Pronnet, F., & Szabo, A. (1993). Sympathetic response to acute psychosocial stressors in humans: Linkage to physical exercise and training. In P. Seraganian (Ed.), *Exercise psychology: The influence of physical exercise on psychological processes* (pp. 172–217). New York: Wiley.

Propst, L. R., Ostrom, R., Watkins, P., Dean, T., & Mashburn, D. (1992). Comparative efficacy of religious and nonreligious cognitive-behavioral therapy for the treatment of clinical depression in religious individuals. *Journal of Consulting and Clinical Psychology, 60*, 94–103.

Pryor, W. A. (2000). Vitamin E and heart disease: Basic science to clinical intervention trials. *Free Radical Biology and Medicine, 28*, 141–164.

Puchalski, C. M., & Larson, D. B. (1998). Developing curricula in spirituality and medicine. *Academic Medicine, 73*, 970–974.

Rabkin, J. G. (1982). Stress and psychiatric disorders. In L. Goldberger & S. Brenitz (Eds.), *Handbook of stress* (pp. 566–584). New York: Free Press.

Rachman, S. (1968). The effect of muscular relaxation or desensitization therapy. *Behavior Therapy and Research, 6*, 159–166.

Racine, R., Tuff, L., & Zaide, J. (1976). Kindling unit discharge patterns and neural plasticity. In J. Wada & R. Ross (Eds.), *Kindling* (pp. 19–39). New York: Raven Press.

Rakowski, W., & Cryan, C. D. (1990). Associations among health perceptions and health status within three age groups. *Journal of Aging and Health, 2*(1), 58–80.

Raphael, B., Meldrum, L., & McFarlane, A. (1995). Does debriefing after psychological trauma work? *British Medical Journal, 310*, 1479–1480.

Raphael, B., Wilson, J., Meldrum, L., & McFarlane, A. (1996). Acute preventive interventions. In B. van der Kolk, et al. (Eds.), *Traumatic stress* (pp. 463–479). New York: Guilford.

Raskin, M., Bali, L. R., & Peeke, H. V. (1980). Muscle biofeedback and transcendental meditation. *Archives of General Psychiatry, 37*, 93–97.

Raskin, N. (1985). Migraine. In W. Dorfinan & L. Cristofar (Eds.), *Psychosomatic illness review* (pp. 11–22). New York: Macmillan.

Ravindran, A. V., Griffiths, J., Merali, Z., & Anisman, H. (1995). Lymphocyte subsets associated with major depression and dysthymia: Modification by antidepressant treatment. *Psychosomatic Medicine, 57*, 555–563.

Ray, C., Lindop, J., & Gibson, S. (1982). The concept of coping. *Psychological Medicine, 12*, 385–395.

Redmond, D. E. (1979). New and old evidence for the involvement of a brain norepinephrine system in anxiety. In W. Fann, I. Karacan, A. Pikomey, & R. Williams (Eds.), *Phenomenology and treatment of anxiety* (pp. 153–204). New York: Spectrum.

Redmond, D. E., & Huang, Y. (1979). New evidence for a locus ceruleus–norepinephrine connection with anxiety. *Life Sciences, 25*, 2149–2162.

Reed, G. M. (1989). *Stress, coping, and psychological adaptation in a sample of gay and bisexual men with AIDS.* Unpublished doctoral dissertation, University of California, Los Angeles.

Reed, G. M., Taylor, S. E., & Kemeny, M. E. (1993). Perceived control and psychological adjustment in gay men with AIDS. *Journal of Applied Social Psychology, 23*(10), 791–824.

Reid, G. J., & McGrath, P. J. (1996). Psychological treatments for migraine. *Biomedical Pharmacotherapy, 50*(2), 58–63.

Reiman, E., Raichle, M. E., Robins, E., Butler, F. K., Herscovitch, P., Fox, P., & Perlmutter, J. (1986). The application of positron emission tomography to the study of panic disorder. *American Journal of Psychiatry, 143*, 469–477.

Rejeski, W. J., & Thompson, A. (1993). Historical and conceptual roots of exercise psychology. In P. Seraganian (Ed.), *Exercise psychology: The influence of physical exercise on psychological processes* (pp. 3–35). New York: Wiley.

Reynolds, G. P. (1992). The amygdala and the neurochemistry of schizophrenia. In J. P. Aggleton (Ed.), *The amygdala* (pp. 561–574). New York: Wiley-Liss.

Ribisl, P. (1984). Developing an exercise prescription for health. In N. Miller, J. D. Matarazzo, S. W. Weiss, A. J. Herd, & S. M. Weiss (Eds.), *Behavioral health* (pp. 448–466). New York: Wiley.

Richards, D. (1999, April). *A field study of CISD vs. CISM.* Paper presented at the 5th World Congress on Stress, Trauma, and Coping, Baltimore, MD.

Richards, L., & Pohl, P. (1999). Therapeutic interventions to improve upper extremity recovery and function. *Clinical Geriatric Medicine, 15*(4), 819–832.

Richards, P. S., & Bergin, A. E. (1997). *A spiritual strategy for counseling and psychotherapy.* Washington, DC: American Psychological Association.

Robinson, H., Sigman, M. & Wilson, J. (1997). Duty-related stressors and PTSD symptoms in suburban police officers. *Psychological Reports, 81*, 835–845.

Robinson, R., & Mitchell, J. (1995). Getting some balance back into the debriefing debate. *Bulletin of the Australian Psychological Society, 17,* 5–10.

Rochefort, G. J., Rosenberger, J., & Saffran, M. (1959). Depletion of pituitary corticotropin by various stresses and by neurohypophyseal preparations. *Journal of Physiology, 146,* 105–116.

Rodin, J., & Langer, E. J. (1977). Long-term effects of a control-relevant intervention with the institutionalized aged. *Journal of Personality and Social Psychology, 35*(12), 897–902.

Rodin, J., & Timko, C. (1992). Sense of control, aging, and health. In M. G. Ory, R. P. Abeles, & P. D. Lipman (Eds.), *Aging, health, and behavior* (pp. 174–206). Newbury Park, CA: Sage.

Roessler, R., & Greenfield, M. (Eds.). (1962). *Physiological correlates of psychological disorders.* Madison: University of Wisconsin Press.

Rokicki, L. A., Holroyd, K. A., France, C. R., Lipchik, G. L., France, J. L., & Kvaal, S. A. (1997). Change mechanisms associated with combined relaxation/EMG biofeedback training for chronic tension headache. *Applied Psychophysiology and Biofeedback, 22*(1), 21–41.

Roldan, E., Alvarez-Pelaez, P., & de Molina, F. (1974). Electrographic study of the amygdaloid defense response. *Physiology and Behavior, 13,* 779–787.

Romano, J. (1982). Biofeedback training and therapeutic gains. *Personnel and Guidance Journal, 60,* 473–475.

Rosch, P. (1986). Foreword. In J. Humphrey (Ed.), *Human stress* (pp. ix–xi). New York: American Management Systems Press.

Rosch, P. J. (1995). Future directions in psychoneuroimmunology: Psychoelectroneuro-immunology? In B. Leonard & K. Miller (Eds.), *Stress, the immune system and psychiatry* (pp. 206–231). Chichester, UK: Wiley.

Rose, S., & Bisson, J. (1998). Brief early psychological interventions following trauma: A systematic review of literature. *Journal of Traumatic Stress, 11,* 697–710.

Roseman, L. (1984). Cognitive determinants of emotion. In P. Shaver (Ed.), *Review of personality and social psychology* (pp. 11–36). Beverly Hills, CA: Sage.

Rosen, G. M. (1999). Treatment fidelity and research on eye movement desensitization and reprocessing (EMDR). *Journal of Anxiety Disorders, 13*(1–2), 173–184.

Rosenbaum, M. (1985). Ulcerative colitis. In W. Dorfman & L. Cristofar (Eds.), *Psychosomatic illness review* (pp. 61–75). New York: Macmillan.

Rosenberg, S., Hayes, J., & Peterson, R. (1987). Revising the Seriousness of Illness Rating Scale. *International Journal of Psychiatry in Medicine, 17,* 85–92.

Rosenman, R., & Friedman, M. (1974). *Type A behavior and your heart.* New York: Knopf.

Rosenzweig, M., & Leiman, A. (1982). *Physiological psychology.* Lexington, MA: Heath.

Rossi, E. R. (1986). *The psychobiology of mind–body healing.* New York: Norton.

Rossier, J., Bloom, F., & Guillemin, R. (1980). In H. Selye (Ed.), *Selye's guide to stress research* (pp. 187–207). New York: Van Nostrand Reinhold.

Rostad, F. G., & Long, B. C. (1996). Exercise as a coping strategy for stress: A review. *International Journal of Sport Psychology, 27,* 197–222.

Rothbaum, B. O. (1997). A controlled study of eye movement desensitization and reprocessing in the treatment of posttraumatic stress disordered sexual assault victims. *Bulletin of the Menninger Clinic, 61,* 317–334.

Rotter, J. B. (1954). *Social learning theory and clinical psychology.* Englewood Cliffs, NJ: Prentice-Hall.

Rotter, J. B. (1966). Generalized expectancies for internal versus external control of reinforcement. *Psychological Monographs, 80* (1, Whole No. 609).

Rowe, J. W., & Kahn, R. L. (1987). Human aging: Usual and successful. *Science, 237,* 143–149.

Rubin, L. R. (1977). *Reanimation of the paralyzed face.* St. Louis, MD: Mosby.

Rubin, L. R. (1977). *Reanimation of the paralyzed face.* St. Louis: Mosby.

Ryan, A. (1974). A history of sports medicine. In A. Ryan & F. Allman (Eds.), *Sports medicine* (pp. 1–3). New York: Academic Press.

Sabbioni, M. E., Bovbjerg, D. H., Jacobsen, P. D., Manne, S. L., & Redd, W. H. (1992). Treatment related psychological distress during adjuvant chemotherapy as a conditioned response. *Annals of Oncology, 3,* 393–398.

Sahs, J. A., Goetz, R., Reddy, M., Rabkin, J. G., Williams, J. B. W., Kertzner, R., & Gorman, J. M. (1994). Psychological distress and natural killer cells in gay men with and without HIV infection. *American Journal of Psychiatry, 151*(10), 1479–1484.

Salk, J. (1973). *The survival of the wisest.* New York: Harper & Row.

Sanderson, W. C., Rapee, R. M., & Barlow, D. H. (1989). The influence of an illusion of control on panic attacks induced via inhalation of 5.5% carbon dioxide-enriched air. *Archives of General Psychiatry, 46,* 157–162.

Sano, M., Ernesto, C., Thomas, R. G., Klauber, M. R., Schafer, K., Grundman, M., Woodbury, P., Growdon, J., Cotman, C. W., Pfeiffer, E., Schneider, L. S., & Thal, L. J. (1997). A controlled trial of seleqiline, alpha-ocopherol, or both as treatment for Alzheimer's disease: The Alzheimer's Disease Cooperative Study. *New England Journal of Medicine, 336*(17), 1216–1222.

Sapp, M. (1992). Relaxation and hypnosis in reducing anxiety and stress. *Australian Journal of Clinical Hypnotherapy and Hypnosis, 13,* 39–55.

Sarafino, E. P. (1998). *Health psychology: Biopsychosocial interactions* (3rd ed.). New York: Wiley.

Sarason, I. G. (1957). Effect of anxiety and two kinds of motivating instructions on verbal learning. *Journal of Abnormal and Social Psychology, 54,* 166–171.

Sarason, I., Johnson, J., & Siegel, J. (1978). Assessing the impact of life changes. *Journal of Consulting and Clinical Psychology, 46,* 932–946.

Sarnoff, D. (1982). Biofeedback: New uses in counseling. *Personnel and Guidance Journal, 60,* 357–360.

Saunders, J. T., Cox, D. J., Teates, C. D., & Pohl, S. L. (1994). Thermal biofeedback in the treatement of intermittent claudication in diabetes: A case study. *Biofeedback and Self-Regulation, 19*(4), 337–345.

Scheck, M., Schaeffer, J., & Gillette, C. (1998). Brief psychological intervention with traumatized young women: The efficacy of eye movement desensitization and reprocessing. *Journal of Traumatic Stress, 11,* 25–44.

Schleifer, S. J., Keller, S. E., Camerino, M., Thornton, J. C., & Stein, M. (1983). Suppression of lymphocyte stimulation following bereavement. *Journal of the American Medical Association, 250,* 374–377.

Schmale, A., & Iker, H. (1966). The psychological setting of uterine cervical cancer. *Annals of the New York Academy of Sciences, 125,* 807–813.

Schmidt, N. B., Trakowski, J. H., & Staab, J. P. (1997). Extinction of panicogenic effects of a 35% CO_2 challenge in patients with panic disorder. *Journal of Abnormal Psychology, 106*(4), 630–638.

Schneider, C. J. (1989). A brief history of biofeedback. *Biofeedback, 17*(1), 4–7.

Schnore, M. M. (1959). Individual patterns of physiological activity as a function of task differences and degree of arousal. *Journal of Experimental Psychology, 58,* 117–128.

Schulz, R., & Hanusa, B. H. (1978). Long-term effects of control and predictability enhancing interventions: Findings and ethical issues. *Journal of Personality and Social Psychology, 36,* 1194–1201.

Schulze, G. E., Benson, R. W., Paule, M. G., & Roberts, D. W. (1988). Behaviorally conditioned suppression of murine T-cell dependent but not T-cell independent antibody responses. *Pharmacology, Biochemistry and Behavior, 30,* 859–865.

Schwartz, G. (1977). Psychosomatic disorders and biofeedback: A psychobiological model of disregulation. In J. Maser & M. Seligman (Eds.), *Psychopathology: Experimental models* (pp. 270–307). San Francisco: Freeman.

Schwartz, G. (1979). The brain as a health care system. In C. Stone, F. Cohen, & N. Adler (Eds.), *Health psychology* (pp. 549–573). San Francisco: Jossey-Bass.

Schwartz, G., Fair, P., Mandel, M., Salt, P., Mieske, M., & Klerman, G. (1978). Facial electromyography in the assessment of improvement in depression. *Psychosomatic Medicine, 40,* 355–360.

Schwartz, M. S. (1987). *Biofeedback.* New York: Guilford.

Schwartz, M. S. (1995). *Biofeedback: A practioner's guide* (2nd ed.). New York: Guilford.

Schwartz, M. S., & Kelly, M. F. (1995). Raynaud's disease: Selected issues and considerations in using biofeedback therapies. In M. Schwartz and Associates (Eds.), *Biofeedback: A practioner's guide* (2nd ed., pp. 429–444). New York: Guilford.

Scotton, B., Chinen, A., & Battista, J. (1996). *Textbook of transpersonal psychiatry and psychology.* New York: Basic Books.

Sedaleck, K., & Taub, E. (1996). Biofeedback treatment of Raynaud's disease. *Professional Psychology: Research and Practice, 27*(6), 548–553.

Seif, B. B. (1982). Hypnosis in a man with fear of voiding in public facilities. *America Journal of Clinical Hypnosis, 24,* 288–289.

Seifert, A. R., & Lubar, J. F. (1975). Reduction of epileptic seizures through EEG biofeedback training. *Biological Psychology, 3,* 157–184.

Seifert, W. (Ed.). (1983). *Neurobiology of the hippocampus.* New York: Academic Press.

Seligman, M. E. P. (1975). *Helplessness: On depression, development and death.* San Francisco: Freeman.

Seligman, M. E. P. (1995). The effectiveness of psychotherapy. *American Psychologist, 50,* 993–994.

Seligman, M. E. P. (1996). Science as an ally of practice. *American Psychologist, 51,* 1072–1079.

Seligman, M. E. P., & Csikszentmihalyi, M. (2000). Positive psychology: An introduction. *American Psychologist, 55*(1), 5–14.

Seligman, M. E. P., & Maier, S. F. (1967). Failure to escape traumatic shock. *Journal of Experimental Psychology, 74,* 1–9.

Selye, H. (1936). A syndrome produced by diverse noxious agents. *Nature, 138,* 32–33.

Selye, H. (1951). The General Adaptation Syndrome and the gastrointestinal diseases of adaptation. *American Journal of Proctology, 2,* 167–184.

Selye, H. (1956). *The stress of life.* New York: McGraw-Hill.

Selye, H. (1974). *Stress without distress.* Philadelphia: Lippincott.

Selye, H. (1976). *Stress in health and disease.* Boston: Butterworth.

Seraganian, P. (1993). *Exercise psychology: The influence of physical exercise on psychological processes.* New York: Wiley.

Serban, G. (1975). Stress in schizophrenics and normals. *British Journal of Psychiatry, 126,* 397–407.

Sethi, A. S. (1989). *Meditation as an intervention in stress reactivity.* New York: American Management Services Press.

Shader, R. (1984). Epidemiologic and family studies. *Psychosomatics, 25*(Suppl.), 10–15.

Shagass, C., & Malmo, R. (1954). Psychodynamic themes and localized muscular tension during psychotherapy. *Psychosomatic Medicine, 16,* 295–313.

Shalev, A., Peri, T., Canetti, L., & Schreiber, S. (1996). Predictors of PTSD in injured survivors of trauma: A prospective study. *American Journal of Psychiatry, 153,* 219–225.

Shapiro, D. H. (1978). *Precision nirvana.* Englewood Cliffs, NJ: Prentice-Hall.

Shapiro, D. H. (1985). Clinical use of meditation as a self-regulation strategy. *American Psychologist, 40,* 719–722.

Shapiro, D. H., & Giber, D. (1978). Meditation and psychotherapeutic effects. *Archives of General Psychiatry, 35,* 294–302.

Shapiro, D. H., & Walsh, R. N. (Eds.). (1984). *Meditation: Classic and contemporary perspectives.* New York: Aldine.

Shapiro, D. H., Jr., & Astin, J. (1998). *Control Therapy: An integrated approach to psychotherapy, health, and healing.* New York: Wiley.

Shapiro, D. H., Jr., & Astin, J. A. (1998). *Control therapy: An integrated approach to psychotherapy, health, and healing.* New York: Wiley.

Shapiro, F. (1989). Efficacy of the eye movement desensitization procedure in the treatment of traumatic memories. *Journal of Traumatic Stress, 2,* 199–223.

Shapiro, F. (1995). *Eye movement desensitization and reprocessing: Basic principles, protocols, and procedures.* New York: Guilford.

Shapiro, F. (1999). Eye movement desensitization and reprocessing (EMDR) and the anxiety disorders: Clinical and research implications of an integrated psychotherapy treatment. *Journal of Anxiety Disorders, 13*(1–2), 35–67.

Shapiro, F., & Solomon, R. (1995). Eye movement desensitization and reprocessing: Neuro-cognitive information processing. In G. S. Everly, Jr. (Ed.), *Innovations in disaster and trauma psychology: Vol. 1. Applications in emergency services and disaster response* (pp. 217–237). Ellicott City, MD: Chevron.

Shapiro, S. L., Schwartz, G. E., & Bonner, G. (1998). Effects of mindfulness-based stress reduction on medical and premedical students. *Journal of Behavioral Medicine, 21*(6), 581–599.

Sharkey, B. J. (1990). *Physiology of fitness* (3rd. ed). Champaign, IL: Human Kinetics.

Sharpley, C. F., & Rogers, H. (1984). A meta-analysis of frontal EMG levels with biofeedback and alternative procedures. *Biofeedback and Self-Regulation, 9,* 385–393.

Shealy, C. N., Smith, T., Liss, S., & Borgmeyer, V. (2000, November). *EEG alterations during absent "healing."* Paper presented at the meeting of the American Institute of Stress, Kohala Coast, Hawaii.

Shearn, D. W. (1962). Operant conditioning of heart rate. *Science, 137,* 530–531.

Sheehan, P. (1972). *The function and nature of imagery.* New York: Academic Press.

Shellenberger, R., & Green, J. (1986). From the ghost in the box to successful biofeedback training. Greeley, CO: Health Psychology.

Shellenberger, R., & Green, J. (1987). Specific effects of biofeedback versus biofeedback-assisted self-regulation training. *Biofeedback and Self-Regulation, 12*(3), 185–209.

Shepherd, J., & Weiss, S. (Eds.). (1987). Behavioral medicine and cardiovascular disease. *Circulation, 76* (entire Monograph 6).

Shoemaker, J., & Tasto, D. (1975). Effects of muscle relaxation on blood pressure of essential hypertensives. *Behaviour Research and Therapy, 13,* 29–43.

Shouse, M. N., & Lubar, J. F. (1978). Physiological bases of hyperkinesis treated with methylphenidate. *Pediatrics, 62,* 343–351.

Sicher, F., Targ, E., Moore, D., & Smith, H. (1998). A randomized double-blind study of the effect of distant healing in an advanced AIDS population. *Western Journal of Medicine, 169,* 356–363.

Silverman, J. (1986). PTSD. *Advances in Psychosomatic Medicine, 16,* 115–140.

Sime, W. (1984). Psychological benefits of exercise training in the healthy individual. In J. Matarazzo, S. Weiss, J. Heid, N. Miller, & S. Weiss (Eds.), *Behavioral health* (pp. 488–508). New York: Wiley.

Simon, H. B., & Levisohn, S. R. (1987). *The athlete within: A personal guide to total fitness.* Boston: Little, Brown.

Simonton, C., Matthews-Simonton, S., & Sparks, T. (1980). Psychological intervention in the treatment of cancer. *Psychosomatics, 21,* 226–233.

Sklar, L. S., & Anisman, H. (1979). Stress and coping factors influence tumor growth. *Science, 205,* 513–515.

Small, R., Lumley, J., Donohue, L., Potter, A., & Waldenstrom, U. (2000). Randomised controlled trial of midwife led debriefing to reduce maternal depression after operative childbirth. *British Medical Journal, 321,* 1043–1047.

Smith, K. J., Everly, G. S., & Johns, T. (1992, December). A structural modeling analysis of the mediating role of cognitive-affective arousal in the relationship between job stressors and illness among accountants. Paper presented to the Second APA/NIOSH Conference on Occupational Stress, Washington, DC.

Smith, K. J., Everly, G. S., & Johns, T. (1993). The role of stress arousal in the dynamics of the stressor-to-illness process among accountants. *Contemporary Accounting Research, 9*, 432–449.

Smith, M. L., Glass, G. V., & Miller, T. I. (1980). *The benefits of psychotherapy.* Baltimore: Johns Hopkins University Press.

Smith, W. P., Compton, W. C., & West, W. B. (1995). Meditation as an adjunct to a happiness enhancement program. *Journal of Clinical Psychology, 51*(2), 269–273.

Solomon, G. F., & Moos, R. H. (1964). Emotions, immunity and disease: A speculative theoretical integration. *Archives of General Psychiatry, 11*, 657–674.

Solomon, G. F., Segerstrom, S. C., Grohr, P., Kemeny, M., & Fahey, J. (1997). Shaking up immunity: Psychological and immunologic changes after a natural disaster. *Psychosomatic Medicine, 59*, 114–127.

Solomon, Z., & Benbenishty, R. (1986). The role of proximity, immediacy, and expectancy in frontline treatment of combat stress reaction among Israelis in the Lebanon War. *American Journal of Psychiatry, 143*, 613–617.

Sonstroem, R. J. (1997). Physical activity and self-esteem. In W. Morgan (Ed.), *Physical activity and mental health* (pp. 127–144). Washington, DC: Taylor & Francis.

Sorg, B. A., & Kalivas, P. (1995). Stress and neuronal sensitization. In M. J. Friedman, D. Charney, & A. Deutch (Eds.), *Neurobiological, and clinical consequences of stress* (pp. 83–102). Philadelphia: Lippincott-Raven.

Soskis, D. A., Orne, E. C., Orne, M. T., & Dinges, D. F. (1989). Self-hypnosis and meditation for stress management: A brief communication. *International Journal of Clinical and Experimental Hypnosis, 37*, 285–289.

Sothers, K., & Anchor, K. (1989). Prevention and treatment of essential hypertension with meditation-related methods. *Medical Psychotherapy: An International Journal, 2*, 137–156.

Speilberger, C. D. (1983). *State–Trait Anxiety Inventory.* Palo Alto, CA: Consulting Psychologists Press.

Spiegel, D. A., Wiegel, M., Baker, S. L., Greene, K. A. I. (2000). Pharmacological management of anxiety disorders. In D. I. Mostofsky & D. H. Barlow (Eds.), *The management of stress and anxiety in medical disorders* (pp. 36–65). Needham Heights, MA: Allyn & Bacon.

Spielberger, C. D., Gorsuch, R., & Luchene, R. (1970). *The STAI manual.* Palo Alto, CA: Consulting Psychologists Press.

Spilka, B., Shaver, P., & Kirkpatrick, L. A. (1985). A general attribution theory for the psychology of religion. *Journal for the Scientific Study of Religion, 24*, 1–20.

Stahl, S. M. (2000). *Essential psychopharmacology* (2nd ed.). New York: Cambridge University Press.

Stamm, B. H. (1996). *Measurement of stress, trauma, and adaptation.* Luthereville, MD: Sidran Press.

Stanton, H. E. (1989). Hypnosis and rational-emotive therapy—a de-stressing combination: A brief communication. *International Journal of Clinical and Experimental Hypnosis, 37*, 95–99.

Steif, B. B. (1982). Hypnosis in a man with fear of voiding in public facilities. *American Journal of Clinical Hypnosis, 24*, 288–289.

Stephenson, P. (1977). Physiologic and psychotropic effects of caffeine on man. *Journal of the American Dietetic Association, 71*, 240–247.

Steplewski, Z., & Vogel, W. H. (1986). Total leukocytes, T cell subpopulation, and natural killer (NK) cell activity in rats exposed to resistant stress. *Life Science, 38*, 2419–2427.

Steptoe, A. (1981). *Psychological factors in cardiovascular disorders.* New York: Academic Press.

Sterman, M. B. (1973). Neurophysiological and clinical studies in an epileptic following sensorimotor EEG biofeedback training: Some effects on epilepsy. In L. Birk (Ed.), *Biofeedback: Behavioral medicine.* New York: Grune & Stratton.

Sterman, M. B., & Friar, L. (1972). Suppression of seizures in an epileptic following sensorimotor EEG feedback training. *Electroencephalography and Clinical Neurophysiology, 33*, 89–95.

Stern, R., Ray, W., & Davis, C. (1980). *Psychophysiological recording*. New York: Oxford University Press.

Sternbach, R. (1966). *Principles of psychophysiology*. New York: Academic Press.

Stone, J. (1986). Presentations of doctor and office to facilitate hypnosis. In B. Zilbergard, M. G. Edelstein, & D. Araoz (Eds.), *Hypnosis questions and answers* (pp. 69–75). New York: Norton.

Stoudemire, A. (Ed.). (1995). *Psychological factors affecting medical conditions*. Washington, DC: American Psychiatric Press.

Stoyva, J. M. (1976). Self-regulation and stress-related disorders: A perspective on biofeedback. In D. I. Mostofsky (Ed.), *Behavior control and modification of physiological activity*. Englewood Cliffs, NJ: Prentice-Hall.

Stoyva, J. M. (1979). Musculoskeletal and stress-related disorders. In O. Pomerleau & J. Brady (Eds.), *Behavioral medicine* (pp. 155–176). Baltimore: Williams & Wilkins.

Stoyva, J. M. (1983). Guidelines in the training of general relaxation. In J. Basmajian (Ed.), *Biofeedback principles and practices for clinicians* (2nd ed., pp. 92–111). Baltimore: Williams & Wilkins.

Stoyva, J. M., & Anderson, C. (1982). A coping-rest model of relaxation and stress management. In L. Goldberger & S. Breznitz (Eds.), *Handbook of Stress* (pp. 745–763). New York: Free Press.

Stoyva, J. M., & Budzynski, T. H. (1974). Cultivated low-arousal: An anti-stress response? In L. DiCara (Ed.), *Recent advances in limbic and autonomic nervous systems research* (pp. 369–394). New York: Plenum Press.

Stoyva, J. M., & Budzynski, T. H. (1993). Biofeedback methods in the treatment of anxiety and stress disorders. In P. Lehrer & R. Woolfolk (Eds.), *Principles and practice of stress management* (2nd ed., pp. 263–300). New York: Guilford.

Strecher, V. J., Becker, M. H., Kirscht, J. P., Eraker, S. A., & Graham-Tomasi, R. P. (1985). Psychosocial aspects of changes in cigarette-smoking behavior. *Patient Education and Counseling, 7,* 249–262.

Strelau, J., Farley, F., & Gale, A. (1985). *The biological basis of personality and behavior*. New York: McGraw-Hill.

Stroebel, C. F. (1979, November). *Non-specific effects and psychodynamic issues in self-regulatory techniques*. Paper presented at the Johns Hopkins Conference in Clinical Biofeedback, Baltimore, MD.

Strupp, H. H. (1970). Specific vs. nonspecific factors in psychotherapy and the problem of control. *Archives of General Psychiatry, 23,* 393–401.

Strupp, H. H. (1980). Success and failure in time-limited psychotherapy. *Archives of General Psychiatry, 37,* 947–954.

Suler, J. R. (1985). Meditation and somatic arousal reduction: A comment on Holme's review. *American Psychologist, 40,* 717.

Suter, S. (1986). *Health psychophysiology*. Hillsdale, NJ: Erlbaum.

Swanson, W. C., & Carbon, J. B. (1989). Crisis intervention: Theory and technique. In Task Force report of the American Psychiatric Association, *Treatments of psychiatric disorders* (pp. 2520–2531). Washington, DC: American Psychiatric Press.

Swanson, W. C., & Carbon, J. B. (1989). Crisis intervention: Theory and technique. In Task Force Report of the American Psychiatric Association, *Treatments of psychiatric disorders* (pp. 2520–2531). Washington, DC: American Psychological Association Press.

Swingle, P. G. (1998). Neurofeedback treatment of pseudoseizure disorder. *Biological Psychiatry, 44*(11), 1196–1199.

Tart, C. (1975). *States of consciousness*. New York: Dutton.

Taub, E., & Stroebel, C. (1978). Biofeedback in the treatment of vasonconstrictive syndromes. *Biofeedback and Self-Regulation, 3,* 363–374.

Taylor, A., Jacques, P. F., & Epstein, E. M. (1995). Relations among aging, antioxidant status, and cataracts. *American Journal of Nutrition, 62,* 14395–14475.

Taylor, C. B. (1978). Relaxation training and related techniques. In W. S. Agras (Ed.), *Behavioral modification* (pp. 30–52). Boston: Little, Brown.

Taylor, J. (1953). A scale for manifest anxiety. *Journal of Abnormal and Social Psychology, 48,* 285–290.

Taylor, M., & Abrams, R. (1975). Acute mania. *Archives of General Psychiatry, 32,* 863–865.

Taylor, R. E. (1985). Imagery for the treatment of obsessional behavior: A case study. *American Journal of Clinical Hypnosis, 27,* 175–179.

Taylor, S. E., Lichtman, R. R., & Wood, J. V. (1984). Attributions, beliefs about control, and adjustment to breast cancer. *Journal of Personality and Social Psychology, 46,* 489–502.

Terry, D. J., Tonge, L., & Callan, V. J. (1995). Employee adjustment to stress: The role of coping resources, situational factors, and coping resources. *Anxiety, Stress, and Coping, 8,* 1–24.

Thankachan, M. V., & Mishra, H. (1996). Behavioural management with peptic ulcer cases. *Indian Journal of Clinical Psychology, 23*(2), 135–141.

Thibodeau, G. A., & Patton, K. T. (1993). *Anatomy and physiology* (2nd ed.). St. Louis: Mosby.

Thomas, C., & McCabe, L. (1980). Precursors of premature disease and death: Habits of nervous tension. *Johns Hopkins Medical Journal, 147,* 137–145.

Thompson, B., Geller, N. L., Hunsberger, S., Frederick, M., Hill, R., Jacob, R. G., Smith E. A., Kaufmann, P., Freedman, R. R., Wigley, F. M., & Bielory, L. (1999). Behavioral and pharmacologic interventions: The Raynaud's Treatment Study. *Control Clinical Trials, 20*(1), 52–63.

Thompson, S. C. (1981). Will it hurt less if I can control it? A complex answer to a simple question. *Psychological Bulletin, 90*(1), 89–101.

Thompson, S. C., Armstrong, W., & Thomas, C. (1998). Illusions of control, underestimations, and accuracy: A control heuristic explanation. *Psychological Bulletin, 123*(2), 143–161.

Tkachuk, G. A., & Martin, G. L. (1999). Exercise therapy for patients with psychiatric disorders: Research and clinical implications. *Professional Psychology: Research and Practice, 30*(3), 275–282.

Tomita, T. (1975). Action of catecholamines on skeletal muscles. In S. Geigor (Ed.), *Handbook of physiology,* (Vol. 6, pp. 537–552). Washington, DC: American Physiological Society.

Tortora, G. J. (1990). *Principles of anatomy and physiology* (6th ed.). New York: Harper & Row.

Tortora, G. J. (2000). *Principles of anatomy and physiology* (9th ed.). New York: Wiley.

Tosi, D. J. (1974). *Youth toward personal growth: A rational-emotive approach.* Columbus, OH: Charles Merrill.

Tosi, D., Howard, L., & Gwynne, P. H. (1982). The treatment of anxiety neurosis through rational stage directed hypnotherapy: A cognitive–experiential perspective. *Psychotherapy: Theory, Research and Practice, 191,* 95–101.

Tower, J. F. (1984). *A meta-analysis of the relationships among stress, social supports, and illness and their implications for health professions education.* Unpublished doctoral dissertation, University of Pennsylvania, Philadelphia.

Tracey, T. J. (1991). The structure of control and influence in counseling and psychotherapy: A comparison of several definitions and measures. *Journal of Counseling Psychology, 38*(3), 265–278.

Tucker, L. A., & Bagwell, M. (1991). The relation between aerobic fitness and serum cholesterol levels in a large employed population. *American Journal of Health Promotion, 6*(1), 17–23.

Turnbull, G., Busuttil, W., & Pittman, S. (1997). Psychological debriefing for victims of acute burn trauma. *British Journal of Psychiatry, 171,* 582.

Tuson, K. M., & Sinyor, D. (1993). On the affective benefits of acute exercise: Taking stock after twenty years of research. In P. Seraganian (Ed.), *Exercise psychology: The influence of physical exercise on psychological processes* (pp. 80–121). New York: Wiley.

Tyc, V. L., Mulhern, R. K., Barclay, D. R., Smith, B. F., & Bieberich, A. A. (1997). Variables associated with anticipatory nausea and vomiting in pediatric cancer patients receiving ondansetron antiemetic therapy. *Journal of Pediatric Psychology, 22*(1), 45–58.

Tyrey, L., & Nalbandov, A. V. (1972). Influence of anterior hypothalamic lesions or circulating antibody titers in the rat. *American Journal of Physiology, 222,* 179–185.

U.S. Department of Defense. (2001, October). Consensus workshop on mass violence and early intervention. Warrenton, Virginia.

U.S. Department of Health and Human Services. (1999). *Mental health: Report of the surgeon general.* Rockville, MD: Author.

U.S. Public Health Service. (1979). *Healthy people.* Washington, DC: U.S. Government Printing Office.

Usdin, E., Kretnansky, R., & Kopin, L. (1976). *Catecholamines and stress.* Oxford, UK: Pergamon Press.

van der Kolk, B. A. (1987). *Psychological trauma.* Washington, DC: American Psychiatric Press.

van der Kolk, B. A., Greenberg, M., Boyd, H., & Krystal, J. (1985). Inescapable shock, neurotransmitters, and addition to trauma. *Biological Psychiatry, 20,* 314–325.

van Dixhoorn, J. (1998). Cardiorespiratory effects of breathing and relaxation instruction in myocardial infarction patients. *Biological Psychology, 49*(1–2), 123–135.

Van Etten, M., & Taylor, S. (1998). Comparative efficacy of treatments for posttraumatic stress disorder: A meta-analysis. *Clinical Psychology and Psychotherapy, 5,* 126–144.

Van Hoesen, G. W. (1982). The para-hippocampal gyrus. *Trends in Neuroscience, 5,* 345–350.

Van Peski-Oosterbaan, A. S., Spinhoven, P., van Rood, Y., Van der Does, W. A. J., & Bruschke, A. J. V. (1997). Cognitive behavioural therapy for unexplained noncardiac chest pain: A pilot study. *Behavioural and Cognitive Psychotherapy, 25*(4), 339–350.

Vanderhoof, L. (1980). *The effects of a simple relaxation technique on stress during pelvic examinations.* Unpublished master's thesis, University of Maryland School of Nursing, Baltimore.

Verrier, R., & Lown, B. (1984). Behavioral stress and cardiac arrhythmias. *Annual Review of Physiology, 46,* 155–176.

Vessey, S. H. (1964). Effects of grouping on levels of circulating antibodies in mice. *Proceedings of Social and Experimental Biological Medicine, 115,* 252–255.

Violanti, J. M. (1996). Police suicide: Risks and relationships. *Frontline Counselor, 4,* 6.

Wagner, G., Rabkin, J., & Rabkin, R. (1998). Exercise as a mediator of psychological and nutritional effects of terstosterone therapy in HIV+ men. *Medicine and Science in Sports and Exercise, 30*(6), 811–817.

Wallace, R. K., Benson, H., & Wilson, A. F. (1971). A wakeful hypometabolic physiologic state. *American Journal of Physiology, 22*(3), 795–799.

Walsh, R. (1996). Meditation research: The state of the art. In B. Scotton, A. Chinen, & J. Battista (Eds.), *Textbook of transpersonal psychiatry and psychology* (pp. 167–175). New York: Basic Books.

Watts, R. (1994). The efficacy of critical incident stress debriefing for personnel. *Bulletin of the Australian Psychological Society, 16,* 6–7.

Wearden, A. J., Morriss, R. K., Mullis, R., Strickland, P. L., Pearson, D. J., David, J., Appleby, L., Campbell, I. T., & Morris, J. A. (1998). Randomised, double-blind, placebo-controlled treatment trial of fluoxetine and graded exercise for chronic fatigue syndrome. *British Journal of Psychiatry, 172*(6), 485–490.

Wee, D. F., Mills, D. M., & Koelher, G. (1999). The effects of Critical Incident Stress Debriefing on emergency medical services personnel following the Los Angeles civil disturbance. *International Journal of Emergency Mental Health, 1,* 33–38.

Wei, X., Ghosh, S. K., Taylor, M. E., Johnson, V. A., Emini, E. A., Deutsch, P., Lifson, J. D., Bonhoeffer, S., Nowak, M. A., Hahn, B. H., Saag, M. S., & Shaw, G. M. (1995). Viral dynamics in human immunodeficiency virus type 1 infection. *Nature, 373,* 117–122.

Weil, J. (1974). *A neurophysiological model of emotional and intentional behavior.* Springfield, IL: Charles C. Thomas.

Weiner, H. (1977). *Psychobiology and human disease.* New York: Elsevier.

Weiner, H., Thaler, M., Reiser, M., & Mfirsky, L. (1957). Etiology of duodenal ulcer. *Psychosomatic Medicine, 19,* 1–10.

Weinstock, L., & Cluse, R. (1987). A focused overview of gastrointestinal physiology. *Annals of Behavioral Medicine, 9,* 3–6.

Weiss, D. S., Marmar, C., Metzler, T., & Ronfeldt, H. (1995). Predicting symptomatic distress in emergency services personnel. *Journal of Consulting and Clinical Psychology, 63,* 361–368.

Weiss, D., & Marmar, C. (October, 1993). The impact of debriefings on emergency services personnel workers: Effects of site and service. International Society for Traumatic Stress Studies Annual Meeting. San Antonio, Texas.

Weiss, J. M. (1968). Effects of coping responses on stress. *Journal of Comparative Physiological Psychology, 65,* 251–260.

Weiss, R. S. (1975). *Marital separation.* New York: Basic Books.

Weller, D., & Everly, G. S., Jr. (1985). Occupational health through physical fitness programming. In G. S. Everly & R. Feldman (Eds.), *Occupational health promotion* (pp. 127–146). New York: Macmillan.

Weller, D., & Everly, G. S., Jr. (1985). Occupational health through physical fitness programming. In G. S. Everly, Jr. and R. Feldman (Eds.), *Occupational health promotion* (pp. 127–146). New York: Macmillian.

Wenger, M. A., Clemens, T., Darsie, M. L., Engel, B. T., Estess, F. M., & Sonnenschien, R. R. (1960). Autonomic response patterns during intravenous infusion of epinephrine and norepinephrine. *Psychosomatic Medicine, 22,* 294–307.

Wessley, S., Rose, S., & Bisson, J. (1998). A systematic review of brief psychological interventions (debriefing) for the treatment of immediate trauma related symptoms and the prevention of post traumatic stress disorder (Cochrane Review). Cochrane Library, Issue 3, Oxford, UK: Update Software.

Western Management Consultants. (1996). *The Medical Services Branch CISM evaluation report.* Vancouver, BC: Author.

Weyerer, S., & Kupfer, B. (1994). Physical exercise and psychological health. *Sports Medicine, 17,* 108–116.

Whitehead, W. E. (1992). Biofeedback treatment of gastrointestinal disorders. *Biofeedback and Self Regulation, 17*(1), 59–76.

Whitehouse, W. G., Dinges, D. F., Orne, E. C., Keller, S. E., Bates, B. L., Bauer, N. K., Morahan, P., Haupt, B. A., Carlin, M. M., Bloom, P. B., Zaugg, L., & Orne, M. T. (1996). Psychosocial and immune effects of self-hypnosis training for stress management throughout the first semester of medical school. *Psychosomatic Medicine, 58,* 249–263.

Whiteside, R. G. (1998). *The art of using and losing control: Adjusting the therapeutic stance.* Bristol, PA: Brunner/Mazel.

Whitney, E. N., Cataldo, C. B., & Rolfes, S. R. (1998). *Understanding nutrition* (8th ed.). Belmont, CA: West Wadsworth.

Whitney, E. N., Hamilton, E. M., & Rolfes, S. R. (1990). *Understanding nutrition* (5th ed.). St. Paul, MN: West.

Widiger, T., & Frances, A. (1985). Axis II personality disorders. *Hospital and Community Psychiatry, 36,* 619–627.

Wiklund, I., & Sanne, A. (1984). Emotional reaction, health preoccupation and sexual activity two months after a myocardial infarction. *Scandinavian Journal of Rehabilitation Medicine, 46,* 47–56.

Wilder, J. (1950). The law of initial values. *Psychosomatic Medicine, 12,* 392–401.

Williams, M. H. (1999). *Nutrition for health, fitness, and sport* (5th ed.). Boston: McGraw-Hill.

Williams, R. B. (1984). Type A behavior and coronary artery disease. *Behavioral Medicine Update, 6,* 29–33.

Williams, R. B. (1986). Patterns of reactivity and stress. In K. Matthews, R. R. Williams, S. B. Manuck, B. Faulkner, T. Dembroski, T. Detre, & S. M. Weiss (Eds.), *Handbook of stress, reactivity, and cardiovascular disease* (pp. 109–125). New York: Wiley.

Williams, R. B. (1995). Somatic consequences of stress. In M. J. Friedman, D. Charney, & A. Deutch (Eds.), *Neurobiological, and clinical consequences of stress* (pp. 381–402). Philadelphia: Lippincott-Raven.

Williams, R. B., Haney, T., Lee, K., Kong, Y., Blumenthal, J., & Whalen, R. (1980). Type A behavior, hostility, and artherosclerosis. *Psychosomatic Medicine, 42*, 539–549.

Wilson, J., Friedman, M., & Lindy, J. (Eds). (2001). *Treating psychological trauma & PTSD* New York: Guilford.

Wilson, S. A., Becker, L. A., & Tinker, R. H. (1995). Eye movement desensitization and reprocessing: Effectiveness and autonomic correlates. *Journal of Behavior Therapy and Experimental Psychiatry, 27*, 219–229.

Wilson, S. A., Becker, L. A., & Tinker, R. H. (1997). Fifteen-month follow-up of eye movement desensitization and reprocessing (EMDR) treatment for PTSD and psychological trauma. *Journal of Consulting and Clinical Psychology, 63*, 1047–1056.

Wolf, S. (1985). Peptic ulcer. In W. Dorfman & L. Cristofar (Eds.), *Psychosomatic illness review* (pp. 52–60). New York: Macmillan.

Wolf, S., & Glass, G. B. (1950). Correlation of conscious and unconscious conflicts with changes in gastric function and structure. In H. G. Wolff & S. Wolf (Eds.), *Life stress and bodily disease* (pp. 17–35). Baltimore: Williams & Wilkins.

Wolfe, J., & Kimerling, R. (1998). Assessment of PTSD and gender. In J. Wilson & T. M. Keene (Eds.), *Assessing psychological trauma and PTSD*. New York: Plenum.

Wolff, H. G. (1963). *Headache and other head pain*. New York: Oxford University Press.

Wolpe, J. (1958). *Psychotherapy by reciprocal inhibition*. Stanford, CA: Stanford University Press.

Wolpe, J., & Lazarus, A. A. (1966). *Behavior therapy techniques*. Elmsford, NY: Pergamon Press.

Wooten, P. (1996). Humor: An antidote for stress. *Holistic Nursing Practice, 10*(2), 49–56.

Worthington, E. L., Kurusu, T. A., McCullough, M. E., & Sandage, S. J. (1996). Empirical research on religion and psychotherapeutic processes and outcomes: A 10-year review and research prospectus. *Psychological Bulletin, 119*, 448–487.

Wright, P., Takei, N., Rifkin, L., & Murray, R. M. (1995). Maternal influenza, obstetric complications, and schizophrenia. *American Journal of Psychiatry, 152*(12), 1714–1720.

Wurtman, J., & Suffes, S. (1997). *The serotonin solution: To achieve permanent weight control*. New York: Ballentine Books.

Wyler, R. A., Masuda, M., & Holmes, T. H. (1968). Seriousness of illness rating scale. *Journal of Psychosomatic Research, 11*, 363–374.

Yalom, I. (1970). *Group psychotherapy*. New York: Basic Books.

Yamada, S., DePasquale, M., Patlak, S., & Cserr, H. F. (1991). Albumin outflow into deep cervical lymph from different regions of rabbit brain. *American Journal of Physiology, 261*(4, Pt. 2), H1197–H1204.

Yehuda, R., Giller, E., Levengood, R., Southwick, S., & Siever, L. (1995). Hypothalamic–pituitary–adrenal-functioning in post-traumatic stress disorder. In M. J. Friedman, D. Charney, & A. Deutch (Eds.), *Neurobiological, and clinical consequences of stress*, (pp. 351–366). Philadelphia: Lippincott-Raven.

Young, L., Richter, J., Bradley, L., & Anderson, K. (1987). Disorders of the upper gastrointestinal system. *Annals of Behavioral Medicine, 9*, 7–12.

Youngstedt, S. D., O'Conner, P. J., Crabbe, J. B., & Dishman, R. K. (1998). Acute exercise reduces caffeine-induced anxiogenesis. *Medicine and Science in Sports and Exercise, 30*(5), 740–745.

Yuwiler, A. (1976). Stress, anxiety and endocrine function. In R. Grenell & S. Gabay (Eds.), *Biological foundations of psychiatry* (pp. 889–943). New York: Raven Press.

Zajonc, R. B. (1984). On the primacy of affect. *American Psychologist, 39*(2), 117–123.

Zalcman, S., Kerr, L., & Anisman, H. (1991). Immunosuppression elicited by stressors and stressor-related odors. *Brain Behavior and Immunity, 5,* 262–273.

Zalcman, S., Richter, M., & Anisman, H. (1989). Alterations of immune functioning following exposure to stressor-related cues. *Brain, Behavior and Immunity, 3,* 99–109.

Zamarra, J. W., Schneider, R. H., Besseghini, I., Robinson, D. K., & Salerno, J. W. (1996). Usefulness of the transcendental meditation program in the treatment of patients with coronary artery disease. *American Journal of Cardiology, 77*(10), 867–870.

Zeller, J. M., McCain, N. L., McCann, J. J., Swanson, B., & Colletti, M. A. (1996). Methodological issues in psychoneuroimmunology research. *Nursing Research, 45*(5), 314–318.

Zhang, J., Harper, R., & Ni, H. (1986). Cryogenic blockade of the central nucleus of the amygdala attenuates aversively conditioned blood pressure and respiratory responses. *Brain Research, 386,* 136–145.

Ziegler, R. G., Mayne, S. T., & Swanson, C. A. (1996). Nutrition and lung cancer. *Cancer Causes and Control, 7*(1), 157–177.

Zuckerman, M. (1960). The development of an affect adjective checklist for the measurement of anxiety. *Journal of Consulting Psychology, 24,* 457–462.

Zuckerman, M., & Lubin, B. (1965). *Manual for the Multiple Affect Adjective Checklist.* San Diego: Educational and Industrial Testing Service.

About the Authors

George S. Everly, Jr., Ph.D. is Chairman of the Board Emeritus of the International Critical Incident Stress Foundation, a United Nations—affiliated organization providing consultation and training in emergency mental health and disaster response. Dr. Everly also serves on the adjunct faculties of Loyola College in Maryland and Johns Hopkins University. Formerly Chief Psychologist and Director of Behavioral Medicine at the Johns Hopkins Homwood Hospital Center, Dr. Everly has also held appointments at Harvard University and Harvard Medical School. He has authored or edited 12 other texts, including *Psychotraumatology: Key Papers and Core Concepts in Posttraumatic Stress* (with J. Lating), *Critical Incident Stress Management* (with J. Mitchell), and *Personality and Its Disorders* (with T. Millon). Dr. Everly has given invited lectures in 22 countries on six continents.

Jeffrey M. Lating, Ph.D. is Director of Clinical Training at Loyola College in Maryland's Doctor of Psychology Program. He was formerly the Chief Psychologist and Director of Clinical Training at the Union Memorial Hospital in Baltimore. He earned his B.A. in psychology at Swarthmore College and his Ph.D. in clinical psychology at the University of Georgia. He also completed a postdoctoral fellowship in medical psychology at the Johns Hopkins Hospital. He is coeditor of the text *Psychotraumatology: Key Papers and Core Concepts in Posttraumatic Stress* (with G. Everly) and the Managing Editor of the *International Journal of Emergency Mental Health*.

Index